Pediatric Sleep Medicine Update

Guest Editors

JUDITH A. OWENS, MD, MPH
JODI A. MINDELL, PhD

PEDIATRIC CLINICS
OF NORTH AMERICA

www.pediatric.theclinics.com

June 2011 • Volume 58 • Number 3

SAUNDERS an imprint of ELSEVIER, Inc.

W.B. SAUNDERS COMPANY
A Division of Elsevier Inc.

1600 John F. Kennedy Boulevard • Suite 1800 • Philadelphia, Pennsylvania 19103-2899

http://www.theclinics.com

THE PEDIATRIC CLINICS OF NORTH AMERICA Volume 58, Number 3
June 2011 ISSN 0031-3955, ISBN-13: 978-1-4557-0483-5

Editor: Kerry Holland
Developmental Editor: Donald Mumford

The Pediatric Clinics of North America (ISSN 0031-3955) is published bimonthly by Elsevier Inc., 360 Park Avenue South, New York, NY 10010-1710. Months of issue are February, April, June, August, October, and December. Periodicals postage paid at New York, NY and additional mailing offices. Subscription prices are $179.00 per year (US individuals), $423.00 per year (US institutions), $243.00 per year (Canadian individuals), $563.00 per year (Canadian institutions), $289.00 per year (international individuals), $563.00 per year (international institutions), $87.00 per year (US students and residents), and $149.00 per year (international and Canadian residents and students). To receive students/resident rare, orders must be accompanied by name of affiliated institution, date of term, and the signature of program/residency coordinator on institution letterhead. Orders will be billed at individual rate until proof of status is received. Foreign air speed delivery is included in all *Clinics* subscription prices. All prices are subject to change without notice. **POSTMASTER:** Send address changes to *The Pediatric Clinics of North America*, Elsevier Health Sciences Division, Subscription Customer Service, 3251 Riverport Lane, Maryland Heights, MO 63043. **Customer Service: 1-800-654-2452 (US and Canada). From outside of the US and Canada: 1-314-447-8871. Fax: 1-314-447-8029. For print support, E-mail: JournalsCustomerService-usa@elsevier.com. For online support, E-mail: JournalsOnlineSupport-usa@elsevier.com.**

Reprints. For copies of 100 or more, of articles in this publication, please contact the Commercial Reprints Department, Elsevier Inc., 360 Park Avenue South, New York, NY 10010-1710. Tel.: 212-633-3812; Fax: 212-462-1935; E-mail: reprints@elsevier.com.

The Pediatric Clinics of North America is also published in Spanish by McGraw-Hill Inter-americana Editores S.A., Mexico City, Mexico; in Portuguese by Riechmann and Affonso Editores, Rua Comandante Coelho 1085, CEP 21250, Rio de Janeiro, Brazil; and in Greek by Althayia SA, Athens, Greece.

The Pediatric Clinics of North America is covered in *MEDLINE/PubMed (Index Medicus), Excerpta Medica, Current Contents, Current Contents/Clinical Medicine, Science Citation Index, ASCA, ISI/BIOMED*, and *BIOSIS*.

Printed and bound by CPI Group (UK) Ltd, Croydon, CR0 4YY

Transferred to Digital Print 2011

GOAL STATEMENT
The goal of the *Pediatric Clinics of North America* is to keep practicing physicians and residents up to date with current clinical practice in pediatrics by providing timely articles reviewing the state-of-the-art in patient care.

ACCREDITATION
The *Pediatric Clinics of North America* is planned and implemented in accordance with the Essential Areas and Policies of the Accreditation Council for Continuing Medical Education (ACCME) through the joint sponsorship of the University Of Virginia School Of Medicine and Elsevier. The University Of Virginia School of Medicine is accredited by the ACCME to provide continuing medical education for physicians.

The University of Virginia School of Medicine designates this educational activity for a maximum of 15 *AMA PRA Category 1 Credits*™ for each issue, 90 credits per year. Physicians should only claim credit commensurate with the extent of their participation in the activity.

The American Medical Association has determined that physicians not licensed in the US who participate in this CME activity are eligible for a maximum of 15 *AMA PRA Category 1 Credits*™ for each issue, 90 credits per year.

Credit can be earned by reading the text material, taking the CME examination online at http://www.theclinics.com/home/cme, and completing the evaluation. After taking the test, you will be required to review any and all incorrect answers. Following completion of the test and evaluation, your credit will be awarded and you may print your certificate.

FACULTY DISCLOSURE/CONFLICT OF INTEREST
The University of Virginia School of Medicine, as an ACCME accredited provider, endorses and strives to comply with the Accreditation Council for Continuing Medical Education (ACCME) Standards of Commercial Support, Commonwealth of Virginia statutes, University of Virginia policies and procedures, and associated federal and private regulations and guidelines on the need for disclosure and monitoring of proprietary and financial interests that may affect the scientific integrity and balance of content delivered in continuing medical education activities under our auspices.

The University of Virginia School of Medicine requires that all CME activities accredited through this institution be developed independently and be scientifically rigorous, balanced and objective in the presentation/discussion of its content, theories and practices.

All authors/editors participating in an accredited CME activity are expected to disclose to the readers relevant financial relationships with commercial entities occurring within the past 12 months (such as grants or research support, employee, consultant, stock holder, member of speakers bureau, etc.). The University of Virginia School of Medicine will employ appropriate mechanisms to resolve potential conflicts of interest to maintain the standards of fair and balanced education to the reader. Questions about specific strategies can be directed to the Office of Continuing Medical Education, University of Virginia School of Medicine, Charlottesville, Virginia.

The faculty and staff of the University of Virginia Office of Continuing Medical Education have no financial affiliations to disclose.

The authors/editors listed below have identified no financial or professional relationships for themselves or their spouse/partner:
Debra A. Babcock, MD; Dean W. Beebe, PhD; Alyssa Cairns, PhD; Mary A. Carskadon, PhD; Jamie Cassoff, BSc; Penny Corkum, PhD; Fiona Davidson, BSc; Reut Gruber, PhD; Chantelle N. Hart, PhD; Carla Holloway, (Acquisitions Editor); Ellissa Jelalian, PhD; Oskar G. Jenni, MD; Barbel Knauper, PhD; Amy S. Lewandowski, PhD; Marilyn MacPherson, MD, FRCPC; Beth A. Malow, MD, MS; Lisa J. Meltzer, PhD; Hawley E. Montgomery-Downs, PhD; Tonya M. Palermo, PhD; Ghazala H. Quraishi, MD; Karen Rheuban, MD (Test Author); Ann M. Reynolds, MD; Teresa M. Ward, RN, PhD; Helene Werner, PhD; Manisha Witmans, MD, FRCPC, FAAP, FAASM; and Rochelle Young, RN, BA, BSN.

The authors/editors listed below identified the following professional or financial affiliations for themselves or their spouse/partner:
Jeffrey S. Durmer, MD, PhD is a consultant for UCB Pharma, Inc.
Jodi A. Mindell, PhD (Guest Editor) is a consultant for Johnson's Baby, Merck, and GlaxoSmithKline; and is on the Speakers' Bureau and Advisory Committee/Board for Johnson's Baby.
Judith A. Owens, MD, MPH (Guest Editor) receives grant support from Shire, Boehringer-Ingleheim, and Rhodes; is a consultant for Cephalon, Takeda, Rhodes, Shionogi Pharma, NeuroPro, and Transcept; is on the Speakers' Bureau for Eli Lilly; and is on the Advisory Board for Eli Lilly, Shire, and Isis Biopolymer.
James K. Wyatt, PhD, FAASM, D.ABSM is an industry funded research/investigator for the Respironics Sleep and Respiratory Research Foundation.

Disclosure of Discussion of Non-FDA Approved Uses for Pharmaceutical Products and/or Medical Devices
The University of Virginia School of Medicine, as an ACCME provider, requires that all faculty presenters identify and disclose any off-label uses for pharmaceutical and medical device products. The University of Virginia School of Medicine recommends that each physician fully review all the available data on new products or procedures prior to clinical use.

TO ENROLL
To enroll in the Pediatric Clinics of North America Continuing Medical Education program, call customer service at 1-800-654-2452 or visit us online at www.theclinics.com/home/cme. The CME program is available to subscribers for an additional fee of $223.00.

Contributors

GUEST EDITORS

JUDITH A. OWENS, MD, MPH
Director of Sleep Medicine, Division of Pulmonary and Sleep Medicine, Children's
National Medical Center, Washington, DC

JODI A. MINDELL, PhD
Professor, Department of Psychology, Saint Joseph's University; Associate Director,
Sleep Center, Children's Hospital of Philadelphia, Philadelphia, Pennsylvania

AUTHORS

DEBRA A. BABCOCK, MD
Altos Pediatric Associates, Los Altos, California

DEAN W. BEEBE, PhD
Associate Professor of Pediatrics, Program Director, Neuropsychology Program, Division
of Behavioral Medicine and Clinical Psychology, Cincinnati Children's Hospital Medical
Center, University of Cincinnati College of Medicine, Cincinnati, Ohio

ALYSSA CAIRNS, PhD
Postdoctoral Research Fellow, Department of Psychiatry and Human Behavior,
The Warren Alpert Medical School of Brown University; Weight Control and Diabetes
Research Center, The Miriam Hospital, Providence, Rhode Island

MARY A. CARSKADON, PhD
Professor, Psychiatry and Human Behavior, Warren Alpert Medical School of Brown
University; Director of Chronobiology and Sleep Research, Bradley Hospital Sleep Lab,
E.P. Bradley Hospital, Providence, Rhode Island

JAMIE CASSOFF, BSc
Attention, Behavior and Sleep Lab, Douglas Mental Health University Institute;
Department of Psychology, McGill University, Montreal, Quebec, Canada

PENNY CORKUM, PhD
Associate Professor, Department of Psychology, Dalhousie University, Halifax, Nova
Scotia, Canada

FIONA DAVIDSON, BSc
Graduate Student, Department of Psychology, Dalhousie University, Halifax, Nova Scotia,
Canada

JEFFREY S. DURMER, MD, PhD
Chief Medical Officer, Fusion Sleep Medicine Program; Adjunct Professor, School
of Health Professions, Department of Respiratory Therapy, College of Health and
Human Sciences, Georgia State University, Atlanta, Georgia

REUT GRUBER, PhD
Attention, Behavior and Sleep Lab; Department of Psychiatry, McGill University, Douglas Mental Health University Institute, Verdun, Quebec, Canada

CHANTELLE N. HART, PhD
Assistant Professor (Research), Department of Psychiatry and Human Behavior, The Warren Alpert Medical School of Brown University; Staff Psychologist, Weight Control and Diabetes Research Center, The Miriam Hospital, Providence, Rhode Island

ELISSA JELALIAN, PhD
Associate Professor, Department of Psychiatry and Human Behavior, The Warren Alpert Medical School of Brown University; Staff Psychologist, Weight Control and Diabetes Research Center, The Miriam Hospital, Providence, Rhode Island

OSKAR G. JENNI, MD
Director, Child Development Center, University Children's Hospital Zurich, Zurich, Switzerland

BÄRBEL KNÄUPER, PhD
Associate Professor, Department of Psychology, McGill University, Montreal, Quebec, Canada

AMY S. LEWANDOWSKI, PhD
Acting Assistant Professor, Department of Anesthesiology and Pain Medicine, Seattle Children's Hospital Research Institute, University of Washington School of Medicine, Seattle, Washington

MARILYN MACPHERSON, MD, FRCPC
Pediatrician, Colchester East Hants Health Authority, Truro, Nova Scotia, Canada

BETH A. MALOW, MD, MS
Professor of Neurology and Pediatrics and Kennedy Center Investigator, Vanderbilt University School of Medicine, Nashville, Tennessee

LISA J. MELTZER, PhD
Assistant Professor of Pediatrics, Department of Pediatrics, National Jewish Health, Denver, Colorado

JODI A. MINDELL, PhD
Professor, Department of Psychology, Saint Joseph's University; Associate Director, Sleep Center, Children's Hospital of Philadelphia, Philadelphia, Pennsylvania

HAWLEY E. MONTGOMERY-DOWNS, PhD
Assistant Professor of Psychology, Department of Psychology, West Virginia University, Morgantown, West Virginia

JUDITH A. OWENS, MD, MPH
Director of Sleep Medicine, Division of Pulmonary and Sleep Medicine, Children's National Medical Center, Washington, DC

TONYA M. PALERMO, PhD
Professor, Departments of Anesthesiology and Pediatrics, University of Washington School of Medicine, Seattle, Washington

GHAZALA H. QURAISHI, MD
Clinical Faculty, Fusion Sleep Medicine Program, Atlanta, Georgia

ANN M. REYNOLDS, MD
Associate Professor of Pediatrics, Department of Pediatrics, The Children's Hospital, University of Colorado Denver School of Medicine, Aurora, Colorado

TERESA M. WARD, RN, PhD
Assistant Professor, Department of Family and Child Nursing, University of Washington School of Nursing, Seattle, Washington

HELENE WERNER, PhD
Postdoctoral Research Fellow, Child Development Center, University Children's Hospital Zurich, Zurich, Switzerland

MANISHA WITMANS, MD, FRCPC, FAAP, FAASM
Assistant Professor, Division of Pediatric Respiratory Medicine, University of Alberta; Director, Northern Alberta Pediatric Sleep Centre, Stollery Children's Hospital, Edmonton, Alberta, Canada

JAMES K. WYATT, PhD, FAASM
Diplomate, American Board of Sleep Medicine; Director, Sleep Disorders Service and Research Center, Rush University Medical Center; Associate Professor of Behavioral Sciences, Rush Medical College, Chicago, Illinois

ROCHELLE YOUNG, RN, BA, BSN
Sleep Program Coordinator, Stollery Children's Hospital, Alberta, Canada

Contents

1600s. Clinicians must consider potential mimics, comorbid, and associated conditions when evaluating children with RLS symptoms. The traditional differentiation of RLS from periodic limb movement disorder (PLMD) is noted in children as well as adults. Because current pediatric RLS research is sparse, this article provides the most up-to-date evidence-based as well as consensus opinion-based information on the subject of childhood RLS and PLMD. Prevalence, pathophysiology, diagnosis, treatment, and clinical associations are discussed.

This article begins with a review of the major central nervous system functional systems that allow for optimal alertness during the waking day, and the rapid initiation and good maintenance of sleep at night. Subsequent sections discuss each of the 6 primary circadian rhythm sleep disorders. Attention is paid to known or suspected pathophysiology, diagnostic criteria and assessment methodology, and treatment options. The article concludes with a discussion of challenges that must be met to improve the recognition and treatment of these quite impactful sleep disorders.

A reduction in sleep amount from late childhood through the second decade has long been known; however, the weight of current evidence holds that sleep need does not decline across this span. This article will describe how the loss of sleep through adolescence is not driven by lower need for sleep but arises from a convergence of biologic, psychological, and socio-cultural influences.

This article summarizes correlational, case-control, quasi-experimental, and experimental studies that have examined whether sleep during childhood and adolescence is related to daytime functioning. Published findings suggest that inadequate sleep quality and/or quantity can cause sleepiness, inattention and, very likely, other cognitive and behavioral deficits that significantly impact children and adolescents in functional settings. This article then integrates findings from longitudinal studies within a developmental psychopathology model. Important questions remain, but evidence supports the integration of sleep screening and interventions into routine clinical care and also supports advocacy for public policy changes to improve the sleep of children and adolescents.

Children with attention-deficit/hyperactivity disorder (ADHD) have high rates of sleep problems and sleep disorders. It is critical that pediatricians assess for sleep problems during the course of ADHD assessment and when treating children with stimulant medication. Sleep must be considered in the differential diagnosis and in terms of comorbidity with ADHD. The most common sleep problem in children with ADHD is insomnia, and the first line of treatment should be the implementation of behavioral interventions rather than medication. More research is needed to determine if children with ADHD respond to behavioral interventions in a similar manner as typically developing children.

Sleep disorders are common in children with autism spectrum disorders and have a significant effect on daytime function and parental stress. The cornerstone of treatment is to establish the cause of the sleep concern, which is often multifactorial. Identifying and treating sleep disorders may result not only in more consolidated sleep, more rapid time to fall asleep, and avoidance of night waking but also favorably affect daytime behavior and parental stress. Targeting effective treatment strategies is dependent on understanding the underlying causes of sleep problems in children with Autism spectrum disorders, therefore further research is paramount.

Untreated sleep disturbances and sleep disorders pose significant adverse daytime consequences and place children at considerable risk for poor health outcomes. Sleep disturbances occur at a greater frequency in children with acute and chronic medical conditions compared with otherwise healthy peers. Sleep disturbances in medically ill children can be associated with sleep disorders, comorbid with acute and chronic conditions, or secondary to underlying disease-related mechanisms, treatment regimens, or hospitalization. Clinical management should include a multidisciplinary approach with particular emphasis on routine, regular sleep assessments and prevention of daytime consequences, and promotion of healthy sleep habits and health outcomes.

The purpose of this review is to provide a comprehensive update of epidemiologic studies that have assessed the association between sleep and obesity risk. Data suggest that short sleep is associated with an increased risk for being or becoming overweight/obese or having increased body fat. Late bedtimes are also a risk factor for overweight/obesity. Findings also suggest that changes in eating pathways may lead to increased body fat. Future experimental studies are needed to enhance our understanding of the underlying mechanisms through which sleep may play a role in the development and maintenance of childhood obesity.

THE CLINICS ARE NOW AVAILABLE ONLINE!

Access your subscription at:
www.theclinics.com

Preface

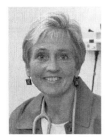 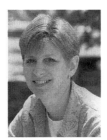

Judith A. Owens, MD, MPH   Jodi A. Mindell, PhD
Guest Editors

There are a number of seminal events to which we might attribute the "birth" of pediatric sleep medicine: the creation of the first manual on scoring of infant sleep by Anders, Emde, and Parmelee in 1971, the Guilleminault and coworkers' 1976 article on sleep apnea in children in the journal *Pediatrics*, and the publication of the first edition of Richard Ferber's book *Solve Your Child's Sleep Problems* in 1985. What matters most is that all of these developments introduced a number of novel key concepts: that sleep in children is fundamentally similar to but at the same time distinctly different from sleep in adults, that sleep disorders in the pediatric population are both common and clinically important, and that disturbances in sleep in children often have profound acute and chronic effects on mood, behavior, cognition, performance, and quality of life. The importance of this paradigm shift from a prevailing sense that children "simply don't have trouble sleeping" to the recognition of the vital importance of sleep to all aspects of children's physical and mental health cannot be overstated.

In this volume, the wide range of topics covered, the wealth of information included, and the quality of research encompassed provide not only compelling evidence for how far we have come, but also offer a template for future clinical and research directions. The updates on the pathophysiology, diagnosis, and treatment of key sleep disorders of childhood (eg, sleep disordered breathing, insomnia, restless legs syndrome), as well as strategies for addressing sleep problems in the primary care setting, provide the clinician with a state-of-the-art approach to evaluation and management. Fundamental aspects of the ontogeny of sleep and the role of sleep in cognitive development are also covered in detail. The relatively recent focus on sleep in special pediatric populations is given particular attention in articles on sleep in children with chronic medical disorders, attention deficit hyperactivity disorder, and autism spectrum disorders. Furthermore, important psychosocial aspects of sleep in children are discussed within the context of family and cultural considerations that impact sleep practices, attitudes, and beliefs about sleep, and ultimately on clinical issues such as how families define a sleep "problem" and what are acceptable intervention strategies. Finally, educational and public health aspects of sleep are highlighted in articles on teaching about healthy sleep in the primary care practice setting and on the important link between insufficient sleep and obesity in children.

Pediatr Clin N Am 58 (2011) xv–xvi
doi:10.1016/j.pcl.2011.04.001
0031-3955/11/$ – see front matter © 2011 Elsevier Inc. All rights reserved.

pediatric.theclinics.com

It is our hope that the information provided will be of real-world practical use to the clinicians who are encountering sleep problems in their patients on a daily basis, and also to health care practitioners who may be interested in learning more about developments in the field of pediatric sleep medicine. At the end of the day, it is our patients and their families who will benefit most from an increased awareness of and emphasis on the vital role that sleep plays in children's lives.

Judith A. Owens, MD, MPH
Division of Pulmonary and Sleep Medicine
Children's National Medical Center
111 Michigan Avenue NW
Washington, DC 20010, USA

Jodi A. Mindell, PhD
Department of Psychology
Saint Joseph's University
5600 City Avenue
Philadelphia, PA 19131, USA

E-mail addresses:
owensleep@gmail.com (J.A. Owens)
jodi.mindell@gmail.com (J.A. Mindell)

Evaluating Sleep and Sleep Disorders in the Pediatric Primary Care Setting

Debra A. Babcock, MD

KEYWORDS

• Sleep • Sleep disorders • Pediatrics • Primary care • Children

Every physician faces the same challenges every day. Why has the patient come to the office? Is there a problem that can be managed by the physician? At what point should a referral be made? Sleep is no different. Almost all childhood issues, from normal development to disease, have a sleep component: separation fears, colic, fever, otitis media, gastroenteritis, and school anxiety, just to name a few. When the child does not sleep well, the parents do not either. But according to the 2004 Sleep in America Poll from the National Sleep Foundation, 52% of physicians do not ask about a child's sleep habits. When parents were asked in that same poll about their children's sleep, 69% said their children experience one or more sleep problems at least a few nights a week.[1] Clearly, there is a disconnect here that must be addressed.

Sleep is so basic a function that for a long time it seemed almost unworthy of much attention. In the last 60 years or so, however, sleep has been shown to be so much more. Research in the field has exploded, and now there are subspecialties within medicine to address the new knowledge.

This article highlights the day-to-day experiences of the general pediatrician as an educator and a guidance counselor, not the sleep specialist, in evaluating the sleep of children. There is much pediatricians can do to help families through these hard times. As pediatricians educate themselves about sleep, they can pass that knowledge on to families and help them anticipate the next developmental change, understand sleep disruption in the presence of illness or psychological stress, and provide tools to help everyone in the family sleep better. Pediatricians, almost by definition, are educators. The mission of pediatricians has always been to help parents navigate the changes inherent in their children as they grow, to educate them and to provide guidance for what to expect with each developmental stage. Being awake and alert is key to being able to function at a peak level. Evaluating sleep and educating patients and parents about good sleep habits are the first steps to reaching that goal (**Table 1**).

The author has nothing to disclose.
Altos Pediatric Associates, 842 Altos Oaks Drive, Los Altos, CA 94024, USA
E-mail address: deb@rosekind.com

Pediatr Clin N Am 58 (2011) 543–554
doi:10.1016/j.pcl.2011.03.001   pediatric.theclinics.com

Table 1 Normal sleep amounts		
Age	Total Sleep	Average Total Sleep (h)
Newborn (0–2 mo)	10–19 h	13.0–14.5
Infants (2–12 mo)	9–10 h at night + 3–4 h of nap	12–13
Toddlers (1–3 y)	9.5–10.5 h at night + 2–3 h of nap	11–13
Preschool (3–5 y)	9–10 h	9–10
School age (6–12 y)	9–10 h	9–10
Adolescents (13–18 y)	9–9.5 h needed (most get 7.0–7.5 h)	9.25 needed

Data from Mindell JA, Owens J. Sleep in infancy, childhood, and adolescence. In: A clinical guide to pediatric sleep: diagnosis and management of sleep problems, 2nd edition. Philadelphia: Lippincott Williams & Wilkins; 2009. p. 12–29.

EVALUATING INFANTS

Changes in sleep patterns are virtually characteristic of infant developmental stages. The newborn wakes every 2 to 4 hours, whereas a 1-year-old child generally sleeps a consolidated night of 10 hours plus takes two 1- to 2-hour naps.[2] Therefore, in evaluating the sleep of infants, the age and developmental stage are key.

Parents of newborns often do not know what to expect, and they themselves are often so sleep deprived that they do not remember one day to the next. These parents usually know that the baby needs to feed every 2 to 4 hours and wakes to do so. But these parents are often concerned that the baby seems to sleep during the day and be awake at night, just the opposite of the parents' daily rhythm.[3] It is as though as the pregnant mother moves through the day the fetus is calm; at night when the mother is quiet, the fetus is more active. This pattern does not change immediately at the time of birth; newborn sleep patterns take 2 to 3 weeks to change. Waking the baby at 2- to 3-hour intervals during the day helps, as well as exposure to light during the daytime and quiet darkness at night.[3]

Asking about the sleeping arrangement for infants is important. It is now well accepted that infants should be placed on their backs for sleep to reduce the risk of sudden infant death syndrome.[4] Once babies are able to roll from back to front, at about 5 to 6 months of age, their nighttime position is less crucial. Many newborns sleep in the same room as their parents and sometime in the same bed. This arrangement makes nighttime nursing easier for parents during the first few months when babies wake to feed. However, once the baby is able to consolidate sleep for 6 to 8 hours, cosleeping becomes more of a choice than a necessity. Many families choose cosleeping for cultural or sentimental reasons. There is evidence that cosleeping increases the number of arousals for both the parents and the child,[5] so this is an important issue to discuss if parents come in with concerns about frequent nighttime awakenings. Once parents are educated about the physiologic processes of sleep, they can make an informed decision about wanting to continue.

Other issues related to the evaluation of infant sleep are often brought up by parents, such as questions of normal versus abnormal sleep behavior. Most of these problems are easily identified as normal after a discussion of normal infant sleep. The twitching and eye rolling seen in newborn infants is typical of active sleep and is easily distinguished from seizure activity. The inability at times to wake young infants is likely related to the depth of sleep they experience in quiet sleep. Of course, further questioning to rule out serious illness must be done, that is, if there is fever, vomiting, general lethargy, or other system involvement.

One of the symptoms of the condition known as colic is sleep disruption. The other main symptoms are fussiness and crying. Colic is a poorly understood phenomenon even today. Whether the origin is feeding intolerance and abdominal pain, immaturity of the nervous system, or irritability, the lack of sleep experienced by the family unit as a result of a colicky baby is perhaps the most significant issue. In this case, evaluation of the sleep of the parents is as important as the sleep of the infant. Interventions to help the parents, such as trading off baby care, enlisting a grandparent or other adult, or other options, give them some respite. Sleep-deprived parents may make poor decisions and exhibit labile emotions toward the baby and each other. In fact, in about 10% of families with infants, the baby's sleep habits cause significant stress on family relationships.[1]

Older infants, ages 6 to 12 months, have sleep issues related to their emerging brain development. These infants begin to see patterns in their experiences and come to expect a particular outcome after a particular behavior. At this time, sleep associations begin to become important. Parents may ask about the frequent nighttime awakenings of their baby. Certainly medical illness must be ruled out, for example, pain from otitis media or gastroesophageal reflux, upper airway congestion, and itching from eczema. Once it is clear that there is no medical reason for the wakening, the possibility of a trained nighttime feeder, who expects to be fed whenever awake, or a baby with separation fears may become more evident.

At this stage of development, the older infant, it is often helpful to discuss good sleep habits with parents. Sleep habits are learned behaviors; a baby who is successful at calling a parent to the bedside may become a signaler, whereas the baby that can comfort itself may become a self-soother.[2]

Sleep problems in infancy typically do not require referral to a sleep specialist. Some cases of sleep disruption in the young infant are caused by medical concerns, and treating the underlying illness improves sleep. Those babies with specific medical problems may need referral to a medical specialist. As the infant gets a bit older, behavioral issues and parenting style are often the cause of poor sleep. At this point, discussions between the pediatrician and the parents are often all that is needed. Parents who are overwhelmed by taking care of an infant, or a mother with postpartum depression, may themselves require referrals to counselors, but the main intervention at this time is education of the parents about normal sleep processes, guidance about what to expect with each developmental phase, and ways to develop good sleep habits (eg, set bedtimes, establishment of a bedtime routine).

EVALUATING TODDLERS

The toddler years, ages 1 to 4 years, are a time of explosive development. The brain has enlarged almost 40%, and the child transitions from a preverbal, barely independently walking infant to a verbal, willful, socially interactive individual. Along with these major changes in physical and emotional development, the sleep/wake cycle matures as well. At this time, toddlers generally sleep 10 to 11 hours at night and move from 2 naps a day at age 1 year to none at age 4 years.[2] Evaluating sleep in children of this age group means looking at behavior. Significant chronic medical problems have likely been identified by now and their effect on sleep reduced or at least understood.

Most appointments to the pediatrician at this time are not made because of a sleep complaint. Usually, sleep problems are secondary to an acute illness, resulting from pain, fever, illness, or stimulating medications, such as albuterol. When the medical issue has been resolved, sleep returns to normal, unless behavioral issues have intervened and the child has realized a secondary gain from waking at night.

Asking about sleep should be a part of every routine physical examination. This opportunity allows parents to bring up and discuss issues that they might otherwise think are normal, are embarrassed to talk about, or have just given up on solving. Questions to explore include

- When does the child go to bed?
- Is there a bedtime routine? What is it?
- Who puts the child to bed?
- Where does the child sleep, alone or with a sibling or parent?
- What happens when the parent leaves?
- Does the child wake during the night? What happens then?
- What time does the child wake in the morning?
- Does the child take a nap?
- What is the child's daytime functioning like?
- How much sleep does the parent get? How is the parent functioning during the day?

Ideally, children blissfully go to bed in their own crib or bed after a short bedtime routine, say night-night, fall asleep quickly, and wake 11 hours later. However, there are sometimes bumps in this scenario. If a child cannot fall asleep without the aid of a parent, in an environment other than his/her own bed, or wakes frequently, the issue may be that the child simply has not yet learned good sleep behaviors. Once parents understand what they need to teach the child, hopefully they can implement change. The use of a transitional object, such as a blanket or a doll, may be helpful. Bedtime is often the first real parenting challenge parents face. Do they do what is right for the child's health and development, or do they give in to the child and do what is easy for them and makes the child happy? The pediatrician can gain much insight into family dynamics and parenting style when evaluating this problem. Passive parents are more likely to give in, whereas assertive parents are more likely to insist on the child following the prescribed program and are more willing to stick with it. The child has no motivation to change, that is, the child likes being with parents at night. It is the parents who must impose the change on the child, preferably in a gentle way using positive reinforcement, and they must be willing to deal with some push back.

Parents who themselves are not sleeping well may have less patience dealing with the tantrums and typical behavioral issues of toddlers. About 70% of parents report that their toddler wakes them up at night.[1] Evaluating daytime functioning of the parents, then, is important for overall family dynamics.

It is unusual to make a referral to a sleep specialist during the toddler years. More likely, outside help from counselors and behavior specialists may be warranted, although there are sleep specialists who focus on behavioral issues. Occasionally, a toddler might exhibit enough snoring or apnea to warrant a sleep study or an otolaryngology referral, but most of the problems in children of this age group are behavioral. Some sleep problems, as defined for older children and adults, are actually normal for toddlers, for example, daytime sleepiness and enuresis (toddlers normally take naps and cannot control their urine during the night).

The other caveat for needing a sleep specialist in this age group is for children with disabilities. Developmental disabilities typically become more apparent between the ages of 1 and 4 years. Conditions such as autism, pervasive developmental disorder, and developmental delay can affect a child's daily rhythm and sleep (see the articles by Dean Beebe; and Reynolds and Marlow elsewhere in this issue for further exploration of this topic). These children are often seen by many specialists who may be able to design treatment plans that also help sleep. However, a pediatric sleep specialist can often give particularly helpful guidance.

The toddler years are a time to develop good sleep habits, proper sleep associations, and a positive attitude toward sleep for everyone in the family. Educating parents about normal sleep processes and behaviors in the developing toddler is essential. There may be times when enough of an issue exists that a separate visit with the pediatrician may be helpful so that both parents might attend, hear the same information, and come up with a plan together for dealing with the sleep of a difficult toddler (**Box 1**).

EVALUATING CHILDREN

By the time a child is 5- to 12-years old, sleep habits have typically become ingrained. Toddlers with sleep refusal often become children with poor sleep habits. Although some sleep problems are elicited at well-child visits on routine questioning about sleep, parents of school-age children are more likely than parents of toddlers to make a specific appointment to address a sleep disturbance.

During the well-child examination, pediatricians have always asked about eating habits and, in the past 30 years or so, are more concerned about exercise habits as ways to emphasize a healthy lifestyle. It is just as important to ask about sleep habits, especially as children enter school age. Evaluating children's sleep and teaching them the importance of sleep will go a long way in ensuring optimum health and mental alertness, both crucial for school success. Questions should include

- What time do they go to bed?
- What time do they get up?
- Do they snore?
- How do they feel during the day?
- If it is difficult to wake them in the morning, it may be because they are not going to bed early enough. Why not?
- Do they have sleep refusal, separation anxiety, fear of the dark, or of a stranger coming into the house?

This is the classic age of fears of monsters under the bed or in the closet. Children at this age are reading stories and seeing videos that can frighten them. Some children are more aware of loss, whether it be the death of a relative or a pet, or a friend's relative or pet, or the perceived potential for the loss of a parent. For these children, separation at bedtime leads to the fear that they may never see their loved ones again. Some children have experienced a home break-in or fear this possibility. These children need to check every door and window and strive to remain vigilant, and awake, all night long. It is understandable, then, how these fears can affect a child's ability to fall asleep. Falling asleep means losing control over the environment. If the child can be reassured that someone is looking out for him/her or can be given a tool to help send away the monsters, the child may be able to relax and give in to sleep.

Often the first time that bedtime and wake time need to be enforced is at school entry. Here again, parents with difficulty in setting limits are bound to have children who fight bedtime. Parents know that children need a good night's sleep, but they may not realize that this sleep means 10 hours for children in elementary school. Allowing children to have electronics in their bedrooms is a known cause of bedtime delay,[6] which only gets worse as school-age children become teenagers, but in fact 43% of school-age children have a television in their room.[1] This is a good time to begin the rule that all electronics, including televisions, phones, and computers, stay out of the bedroom at bedtime.

Box 1
Screening questions

Infants/babies

What are the sleeping arrangements? Where? Cosleeping?

What is the sleep routine? Is there a schedule?

How do the parents handle nighttime awakenings?

Are there medical problems? (colic, otitis, reflux, congestion, eczema, and so forth)

How are the parents sleeping?

Toddlers

What time does the child go to bed and get up in the morning?

What is the bedtime routine? (who helps, what does it include, where does it happen)

Where does the child sleep? Is he/she alone? With a sibling or a parent?

What happens at separation, when the parent leaves? Is there a transitional object?

Are there nighttime arousals? What happens then?

Does the child nap? When? Where?

How does the child function during the day?

How are the parents sleeping? How are they doing during the day?

Children

What time does the child go to bed and get up in the morning?

What is the bedtime routine?

What is in the sleep environment? Electronics?

Are there nighttime arousals? What happens then?

Does the child snore?

Is there sleep refusal, separation anxiety, fear of the dark, or fear of strangers?

Is the child enuretic?

How does the child function during the day? How does he/she feel?

Teenagers

Is there a regular bedtime? Wake time? When?

Is there a presleep routine?

What is the cause of delay in going to sleep? Homework or socializing?

Does the teenager nap?

Are there electronics in the bedroom?

How does the teenager feel during the day? How is he/she functioning?

Are there after school activities or commitments?

Does the teenager complain of fatigue?

Fatigue

Ask about these issues:

Medical: acute illness, thyroid dysfunction, anemia, Epstein-Barr virus disease, muscle disease, medications, snoring, diabetes, poor nutrition, medications

Psychological: depression, anxiety, school refusal, drug use, stress

Sleep related: phase delay, overscheduling, late bedtime, caffeine use, naps, electronics, cataplexy

After age 5 years, some of the sleep-related behaviors that were considered normal for toddlers are now considered abnormal. Sleepwalking, sleep talking, night terrors, and similar partial arousals are more concerning to parents at this age, although these behaviors are not usually pathologic. In evaluating these behaviors, the frequency, severity, and length of the episode should be determined and the context within the family, discussed. Is there a pattern to the timing of the events? Is the child overtired or stressed in some way? Is there a familial component? These episodes occur in deep sleep so they are typically seen in the first third of the night.[7] Events occurring later may need reevaluation as to the accuracy of the diagnosis. A child who is over-tired from an active day or has a sleep debt incurred by inadequate sleep the night before is more prone to partial arousals by virtue of sleeping more deeply.[7] Typically all that is required for treatment by the pediatrician is to reassure parents of the benign nature of these events and encourage adequate hours of sleep. Keeping a sleep diary can help elucidate a pattern. There may be some intractable cases that do not respond to the usual measures. These children may require a medication to lessen the depth of sleep (benzodiazepines have been shown to be effective[7]) or a referral to a sleep specialist. Evaluation of snoring and symptoms of sleep apnea should also be considered, given their association with partial arousal parasomnias.

Another sleep-related problem, although not a sleep disorder per se, in childhood is enuresis. This issue may not be brought to the attention of the pediatrician out of embarrassment of the child or parent, so it should always be asked about during routine physical examinations. About 90% of children are dry at night by age 6 years (97% by age 12 years).[8] Until that age, bed-wetting is considered normal and children often sleep too deeply to be able to succeed with behavioral treatments. Enuresis is classified as primary, meaning the child has never been completely dry at night, or secondary, meaning that there has been a dry period of about a year or more. Ninety percent of cases are primary. Secondary cases are more likely due to another medical condition, for example, urinary tract infection, spina bifida occulta, diabetes, seizures, or obstructive sleep apnea.[8] Enuresis may run in families, that is, if one parent was enuretic, the chance of the child being a bed wetter is about 45%. If both parents have a positive history, the likelihood of the child being affected is about 75%.[9] Enuresis seems to have a maturational component also. Children who lag behind their peers in motor skill development are more likely to wet at night. On physical examina-tion, the physician should look for abdominal masses, abnormal deep tendon reflexes or sensation, genitourinary anomalies, and skin findings at the sacrum, such as dimpling or excessive hair growth, which might indicate a medical condition.

Most cases of uncomplicated enuresis can be treated by the pediatrician. Encour-agingly, there is a spontaneous cure rate of about 15% each year.[10] Reassurance can be given that many other children of the same age have the same problem, they just do not talk about it. Explaining the anatomy of the urologic system and voluntary control by the brain using pictures is also helpful, so the child can visualize what is supposed to happen. Bed-wetting alarm systems (using a wetness sensor linked to a buzzer) are the most effective treatments, with about a 75% success rate,[11,12] but these systems do require a commitment on the part of both the child and the parent. If the child does not hear the alarm, the parent must go in and wake the child. Typically, success occurs after 4 to 6 weeks of conditioning. Using positive reinforcement, such as a star chart on the calendar for dry nights coupled with a reward, can help. Other skill-based treat-ments, such as retention control training (to increase bladder capacity), stream inter-ruption, visualization, and responsibility training, or having the parent wake the child before the expected time of wetting are perhaps helpful but less effective than the alarm. The advent of the use of desmopressin (DDAVP) for enuresis has saved many a camping trip or overnight stay. DDAVP is an antidiuretic hormone that causes overall increased concentration of the urine. DDAVP can cause hyponatremia, which in turn can cause seizures, but in the doses used for enuresis, this side effect is uncommon.[13] Taken at bedtime, it usually eliminates nighttime wetting. Although the use of DDAVP does not usually result in long-term cure, it can be very effective for short-term use.

Parents often ask if children should be put in cotton underwear or allowed to stay in pull-ups. Although the ideal is to have the child in underwear, realistically, many families cannot deal with the associated nightly linen change. Often a combination of cotton underwear worn under pull-ups keeps sanity in the family.

Pediatricians should always be on the lookout for sleep-disordered breathing (SDB) in children (see the article by Witmans and Young elsewhere in this issue for further exploration of this topic). Whenever children are brought in for an examination, whether it be for a routine physical examination or for an illness, the throat is almost always examined. The observation of enlarged tonsils, which is common in childhood, should prompt the question of snoring at night. How loud? How frequent? Is it related to position? Is there apnea? Parents may not realize that snoring is an abnormal condition even in children, the result of an anatomically or functionally narrowed airway. If loud breathing only occurs during times of upper airway illness and is not severe, watchful waiting may be all that is necessary. In this age of digital electronics, it is fairly easy for a parent to actually bring in a video of their child sleeping, which can greatly aid in the diagnosis of SDB.

Once the issue of SDB has been raised, there should follow a discussion of the best way to proceed. Although it may be more academically correct to obtain an overnight sleep study at an accredited center to quantify the respiratory distress index and lowest oxygen saturation, there are times when that may not be necessary. If a parent observes significant SDB with or without apnea and the physical examination is positive for enlarged tonsils, direct referral to an otolaryngologist is acceptable. If there is any question, however, a sleep study can be very helpful in convincing both the parent and the otolaryngologist that surgical intervention is helpful. Because most children are symptomatic because of airway obstruction from the tonsils and adenoids, both of these should be removed.[14] It is also important to remember that there is a set of lingual tonsils that are not easily seen. These tonsils should also be evaluated and considered for removal.

Sometimes a discussion of SDB in children leads to the question of whether or not a parent snores. It is not unusual to find parents who snore, so this question is always reasonable to ask. There are cases of significant obstructive sleep apnea and drowsy driving that have been discovered after a visit with the pediatrician, an action taken by the parent, and a potentially catastrophic situation averted.

Not all children present with nighttime symptoms, even on questioning during a well-child visit. Some children show fatigue or boredom during the day, poor school performance, or even hyperactivity (see the article by Corkum and colleagues elsewhere in this issue for further exploration of this topic). The pediatrician needs to be alert for these potential symptoms of disordered nighttime sleep and include evaluation of sleep in any workup of altered daytime functioning.

Neuropsychological and neurocognitive conditions become more apparent during the school-age years. These conditions include attention-deficit disorder, attention-deficit/hyperactivity disorder, learning disabilities, and psychological disorders, which are covered more in-depth in articles elsewhere in this issue. Most of these disorders first come to the attention of the pediatrician who must at least be aware of how sleep affects and is affected by these disorders. Sometimes it is difficult to assess which came first, the sleep disruption or the daytime problem. Referral to psychoeducational testing can help clarify the situation as can a sleep study if there is any question that nighttime symptoms exist. Regardless, making sure that the child has the opportunity for good sleep is beneficial. A regular bedtime routine and proper sleep associations certainly help.

EVALUATING ADOLESCENTS

Sleep is often given the lowest priority by this age group because homework, sports, and socializing seem so much more important to them. It is difficult to educate adolescents about the importance of sleep because their adolescent brains recognize concrete, short-term goals much better than somewhat abstract, long-term goals.[15] It is rare in general pediatrics to find a teenager who is not chronically sleep deprived and often suffering the associated consequences of fatigue and psychological dysfunction. Although the amount of sleep needed by teenagers is 9 hours per night,[16] the 2006 Sleep in America Poll found that the average sixth grader gets 8.4 hours of sleep on weeknights and the average eleventh grader only 6.9 hours. More than one-quarter of teenagers reported falling asleep in school at least once a week.[17] In addition, the reasons for staying up later change. A simple survey of about 100 middle- and high-school students done in an independent school in California in 2006 as part of a college outreach project found that 89% of seventh graders stayed up to do homework. In contrast, only 44% of twelfth graders stayed up to do homework, whereas the remainder were watching television and messaging.[18] Sixth graders stay up to do homework, but seniors in high school stay up for socializing.

According to the 2006 Sleep in America Poll, more than half of the teenagers say that they know they are getting less sleep than they should. Then why do they do that? Probably because they do not understand the consequences. When it is brought to their attention that an extra hour (or two) of sleep would help them in so many ways, teenagers often do not believe, even in the face of overwhelming research (see article elsewhere in this issue).

As in every previous age group, teenagers should be questioned about their sleep habits at every routine physical examination; they should be asked about bedtime, wake time, presleep routine, electronics in the bedroom, and even napping. Inevitably, it is found that these teenagers are not sleeping enough, which is a good starting point for a discussion of sleep needs in the adolescent. It is understandable that these children feel so squeezed; most of them have after-school commitments to add to their homework load. Some teenagers have very early school start times, and some sacrifice sleep for their beauty routine. It is practically impossible to educate teenagers and parents about the sleep needs of teenagers at these routine physicals; other important topics need to be covered as well (eg, nutrition, exercise, adolescent risk behaviors). There is a pressing need for handout materials, Web sites, and education geared toward adolescents that can be quickly accessed and distributed.

Unlike in previous age groups, teenagers and their parents come to the pediatrician for the specific complaint of fatigue. The evaluation of this symptom is time consuming, and the time allotted for this visit should reflect that. Sometimes more than one visit is necessary. There should be a thorough investigation of all possible factors: medical, psychological, and sleep related.

Medical

Look for acute or chronic illness, thyroid dysfunction, anemia, Epstein-Barr virus disease, muscle disease, medication reactions, snoring, cardiac or respiratory problems, nutrition or calorie deficiency, and diabetes.

Psychological

Look for depression, anxiety, school refusal, drug use, family or personal stress. An evaluation by a mental health specialist may be in order.

Sleep related

Look for phase delay, overscheduling and late bedtimes, electronic addiction, frequent use of caffeine, napping, and cataplexy.

Sometimes it is helpful to keep a daily log of sleep, daytime activity, meals, and mental status to clarify the complaint. A laboratory workup and possibly a sleep study should be performed. In most cases, teenage fatigue is multifactorial, but there are very few situations in which simply getting more sleep would not help. Accomplishing that, however, is not so easy. Many teenagers would rather be told that they are anemic or have hypothyroidism and that simply taking a pill would make them better. Trying to implement a fairly major behavioral change, to go to bed earlier, is difficult. If teenagers and their families can be made to understand the benefits of appropriate sleep, they may be more motivated to change. In simple cases, information on time management, avoidance of stimulating drugs or medications, and/or relaxation skills might suffice. However, the help of a specialist in sleep or psychology may be required. Most pediatricians simply do not have the time or the expertise to treat families with significant issues.

Fatigue in teenagers has become a cultural phenomenon. It is seen as a badge of honor to claim to have slept for only 4 hours the night before. Indeed, teenagers have more to do now. Our society rewards individuals who excel in sports (lots of practice time), excel in academics (lots of study time), are artists/musicians (lots of practice time), do many hours of community service, and perhaps work part-time as well. Even our educational institutions often give the wrong message. One side of a sign at a local California high school seen in 2002 displayed a demanding finals schedule, on the opposite side was prominently written "Sleep is for Slackers" (Mark Rosekind, PhD, Mountain View, CA, personal communication, 2002). Teenagers feel invincible; they want to do it all, for their own self-esteem and perhaps to ensure acceptance to the college of their choice. Electronics now allow connection to the outside world 24/7, encroaching even more on sleep time. The result is burned-out, phase-delayed, tired teenagers who do not realize that they are jeopardizing the very things they want. Parents are often at a loss to know what to do. Previously passive parents are helpless; assertive parents come up against a suddenly more assertive child who bristles against limits set by his/her parents. Parents have less control over children in this age group than children of any previous age. It is not unusual for parents to stop enforcing bedtime, who actually go to bed earlier than their children. In evaluating fatigue, then, the family dynamics are often as crucial to understand as the evidence for medical or sleep-related symptoms.

Teenage sleep disorders often require more specialty referrals than other ages, except perhaps for the children who are seen by an otolaryngologist for airway management. Teenage sleep problems are more ingrained, sometimes evolving from sleep issues in childhood. If a teenager continues to complain of excessive fatigue or sleepiness despite a normal medical and psychological workup and appropriate nighttime sleep, he/she should be referred to a sleep specialist. Likewise, if the teenager has phase delay that is refractory to simple measures or other symptoms suspicious for a true sleep disorder, such as cataplexy, movements during sleep, and so forth, expert sleep help should be sought. If there are concerns of psychological or true psychiatric symptoms or substance abuse, appropriate referrals to a mental health provider should be made (**Box 2**).

Box 2
Healthy sleep habits

For all ages

    A regular daily schedule

    An environment conducive to sleep: cool, dark, quiet

    Morning light exposure

Infants and toddlers

    Establish a regular sleep schedule, including regularly scheduled naps

    Establish a good bedtime routine; transitional objects help

    Avoid falling asleep and sleeping in an environment other than their own bed (car, couch, parent's bed[a])

    Avoid bright lights in the bedroom and during the night

Children

    Establish a regular consistent bedtime routine

    Reduce stimulating play at bedtime

    Set and enforce a regular bedtime and wake time

    Do not allow electronics in the bedroom

Teenagers

    Set an appropriate bedtime, aim for 9 hours of sleep

    Get up at a reasonable time, even on weekends, to avoid having trouble falling asleep on Sunday night

    Get exposure to morning light

    Eliminate caffeine after noon

    Avoid nicotine and alcohol

    Avoid electronics in the bedroom

    Establish a curfew on messaging

[a] Unless the parents actively choose cosleeping

INCORPORATING SLEEP INTO PEDIATRIC PRACTICE

The evaluation of sleep in children should be as natural and routine for the pediatrician as is the evaluation of nutrition, exercise, and development. Good sleep is vital for a healthy mind and body, every bit as important as eating and breathing. The body cannot exist without food, air, or sleep.

Pediatricians should be comfortable with a basic knowledge of normal sleep and good sleep habits to be able to recognize when things are not right and when a specialist referral should be made. Whether the issue is medical, psychological, related to parenting problems, or a true sleep disorder, recognition must precede treatment and resolution.

Overall, the most important intervention is sleep education. Sleep basics can be outlined by the physician in 10 to 20 minutes as part of a routine physical examination or at a separate appointment. However, there is no way the subject can be given its due in that amount of time. Sleep education needs to be addressed by schools or by the family; online tools, minicourses in the health curriculum, and seminars are all possible if sleep is seen as a valuable subject to teach.

The pediatrician's job as an educator is much easier if children (and their parents) had already been taught the basics about sleep and health, so as to imprint on them the benefits of a good night's sleep and the consequences of not getting enough sleep.

REFERENCES

1. Sleep in America poll. Washington, DC: National Sleep Foundation; 2004.
2. Mindell JA, Owens J. Sleep in infancy, childhood, and adolescence. In: Mindell JA, Owens J, editors. A clinical guide to pediatric sleep: diagnosis and management of sleep problems. 2nd edition. Philadelphia: Lippincott Williams & Wilkins; 2009. p. 12–29.
3. Terman M, Terman JS. Light therapy. In: Kryger MH, Roth T, Dement WC, editors. Principles and practice of sleep medicine. 4th edition. Philadelphia: Elsevier Science; 2005. p. 1424–42.
4. Task Force on Sudden Infant Death Syndrome. Policy statement: the changing concept of sudden infant death syndrome: diagnostic coding shifts, controversies regarding the sleeping environment, and new variables to consider in reducing risk. Pediatrics 2005;116(5):1245–55.
5. McKenna J, Mosko S, Dungy C, et al. Sleep and arousal patterns of co-sleeping human mother/infant pairs: a preliminary study with implication for the study of sudden infant death syndrome (SIDS). Am J Phys Anthropol 1990;83:331.
6. Cain N, Gradisal M. Electronic media use and sleep in school aged children and adolescents: a review. Sleep Med 2010;11(8):735–42.
7. Rosen G, Mahowald M. Disorders of arousal in children. In: Sheldon SH, Ferber R, Kryger M, editors. Principles and practices of pediatric sleep medicine. Philadelphia: Elsevier Saunders; 2005. p. 293–302.
8. Sheldon SH. Sleep-related enuresis. In: Sheldon SH, Ferber R, Kryger M, editors. Principles and practices of pediatric sleep medicine. Philadelphia: Elsevier Saunders; 2005. p. 317–25.
9. Ferber R. Bedwetting. In: Ferber R, editor. Solve your child's sleep problems. New York: Simon and Schuster; 1985. p. 174–89.
10. Forsythe W, Redmond A. Enuresis and spontaneous cure rate study of 1129 enuretics. Arch Dis Child 1974;39:259.
11. Doleys DM. Behavioral treatments for nocturnal enuresis in children: a review of the recent literature. Psychol Bull 1977;84:30.
12. Werry J. The conditioning treatments of enuresis. Am J Psychiatry 1966;123:226.
13. Thompson S, Rey JM. Functional enuresis: is desmopressin the answer? J Am Acad Child Adolesc Psychiatry 1995;34:226–71.
14. Marcus CL. Treatment of obstructive sleep apnea syndrome in children. In: Sheldon SH, Ferber R, Kryger M, editors. Principles and practices of pediatric sleep medicine. Philadelphia: Elsevier Saunders; 2005. p. 235–47.
15. Shafer MB, Irwin CE Jr. The adolescent patient: growth and development. In: Rudolph AM, editor. Rudolph's pediatrics. Norwalk (CT): Appleton and Lange; 1991. p. 39–44.
16. Carskadon MA, Harvey K, Duke P, et al. Pubertal changes in daytime sleepiness. Sleep 1980;2:453–60.
17. Sleep in America poll. Washington, DC: National Sleep Foundation; 2006.
18. Rosekind AA. Menlo sleep survey: project for sleep and dreams class. Stanford University; 2006.

Pediatric Insomnia

Judith A. Owens, MD, MPH[a],*, Jodi A. Mindell, PhD[b,c]

KEYWORDS

• Insomnia • Infants • Children • Adolescents

Similar to many other presenting complaints in the pediatric population, such as headaches or shortness of breath, insomnia in children and adolescents should be viewed as a symptom or constellation of symptoms that result from a wide range of possible causes. The causes of childhood insomnia are varied, and include both primarily medical (eg, medication-related, pain-induced) and behavioral (eg, associated with lack of a regular sleep schedule or negative sleep-onset associations) issues, and are often the result of a combination of these factors. In a general sense, the working definition of insomnia in children may be construed as similar to that in adults, (eg, significant difficulty initiating or maintaining sleep); however, from a clinical standpoint, the most frequent manifestations of childhood insomnia, particularly in younger children, are bedtime refusal or struggles, difficulty falling asleep after "lights out," or frequent or prolonged night wakings requiring parental intervention.

The diagnosis of insomnia in children may be more challenging than in adults for several reasons. First, the patient rarely presents with a complaint of sleeplessness; caregiver concerns and their subjective observations regarding a child's sleep patterns and behaviors often serve to define sleep disturbances in the clinical context. Parents' ability and willingness to recognize and report sleep problems in children also vary across age groups, with parents of infants and toddlers more likely to observe and thus be aware of sleep concerns than parents of school-aged children and adolescents.

In addition, sleep problems in the pediatric population must be viewed against a background of the normal developmental trajectory across childhood and appropriate developmental norms; "normal" bedtime behavior, time to sleep onset, and sleep duration are dramatically different in 6-month-old infants, 6-year-old school-aged children, and 16-year-old adolescents.

Finally, culturally based differences in values and beliefs regarding the meaning, relative importance, and role of sleep in daily life, and sleep practices (eg, sleeping space and the timing of sleep periods, solitary sleep vs bed-sharing, use of transitional

[a] Division of Pulmonary and Sleep Medicine, Children's National Medical Center, 111 Michigan Avenue NW, Washington, DC 20010, USA
[b] Department of Psychology, 5600 City Avenue, Saint Joseph's University, Philadelphia, PA 19131, USA
[c] Sleep Center, Children's Hospital of Philadelphia, 34th Street and Civic Center Boulevard, Philadelphia, PA 19104, USA
* Corresponding author.
E-mail address: owensleep@gmail.com

Pediatr Clin N Am 58 (2011) 555–569
doi:10.1016/j.pcl.2011.03.011
0031-3955/11/$ – see front matter © 2011 Elsevier Inc. All rights reserved.

objects) have a profound effect on not only how a parent defines a sleep "problem" but also the relative acceptability of various treatment strategies. Finally, the consequences of childhood insomnia, in addition to or instead of direct repercussions on the child (eg, daytime sleepiness, behavior problems), may principally involve caregiver stress and sleeplessness. For example, several studies have documented secondary effects of childhood sleep problems on parents (eg, maternal depression) and on family stress and functioning.[1–3] This issue is particularly salient in families of children with chronic medical or neurodevelopmental conditions, for whom the additional caregiver burden of chronic sleeplessness and fatigue may be considerable.

PEDIATRIC INSOMNIAS
Behavioral Insomnia of Childhood

Behavioral insomnia of childhood (BIC) is the most common behavioral sleep disorder experienced by young children, and is characterized by bedtime problems and night wakings, as indicated by parent report. For didactic purposes, the sleep-onset association and limit-setting subtypes of BIC are defined as separate entities. However, in reality, the two often coexist, and many children present with both bedtime delays and night wakings, which is the combined subtype.

BIC, sleep-onset association type
BIC, sleep-onset association type (BIC-SOA) presents with frequent and prolonged night wakings that require caregiver intervention to help the child return to sleep. The diagnostic criteria for this disorder include (1) prolonged sleep onset that requires particular conditions, (2) demanding sleep-onset conditions, (3) significant delay of sleep onset in absence of those conditions, and (4) caregiver intervention is required to return the child to sleep after night wakings.[4] Thus, BIC-SOA involves sleep regulation for a child to both fall asleep at bedtime without parental intervention or assistance and fall back asleep after normally occurring brief arousals during the night. Children with BIC-SOA are unable to self-soothe to sleep at bedtime or during the night, but rather signal the caregiver by crying (or coming into the parents' bedroom if the child is no longer in a crib) until the necessary associations are provided.

The capacity to self-soothe begins to develop in the first 12 weeks of life, and is a reflection of both neurodevelopmental maturation and learning. However, the developmental goal of independent self-soothing in infants at bedtime and after night wakings may not be shared by all families, and voluntary or lifestyle bed- or room-sharing between children and parents is a common and accepted practice in many cultures and ethnic groups. Sleep behavior in infancy, in particular, must also be understood in the context of the relationship and interaction between child and caregiver, which impacts greatly on the quality and quantity of sleep.[5,6] Furthermore, a diagnosis of BIC-SOA before the age of 6 months is not typical.

Both internal and external factors affect the risk for and reinforcement of the presence of prolonged night wakings. For example, parental presence while falling asleep, intentional cosleeping, or feeding a child to sleep increase the likelihood that a child will not have the ability to return to sleep independently.[7,8] Medical conditions (eg, reflux) or periodic illness; scheduling changes or vacations; acquisition of typical developmental milestones; or a difficult temperament can also affect the frequency of arousals and the ability of a child to self-soothe. Insecure maternal–child attachment, parental anxiety, and maternal depression are additional risk factors for prolonged night wakings in young children. Finally, sleep disturbances also reflect complex combined influences of biologic, environmental, and cultural factors, and thus may differ substantially across different cultures and in different contexts.[9]

BIC, limit-setting type

The limit-setting type of BIC (BIC-LST) is characterized by noncompliant behaviors at bedtime, such as refusal to go to bed, verbal protests, and repeated demands at bedtime ("curtain calls"), rather than night wakings. These behaviors result in delayed sleep onset generally without prolonged night wakings, although resistant behaviors may occur during the night. Diagnostic criteria include (1) trouble initiating or maintaining sleep, (2) stalling or refusal to go to sleep at bedtime or after night wakings, and (3) lack of or insufficient limits set by caregiver regarding bedtime and sleep behaviors.[4] BIC-LST is most common in children who are preschool-aged and older. If sleep onset is sufficiently prolonged, the delay may result in inadequate sleep. This sleep problem most commonly develops from a caregiver's inability or unwillingness to set consistent bedtime rules and enforce a regular bedtime, and is often exacerbated by the child's oppositional behavior.

Both developmental and external issues can also contribute to the onset and maintenance of bedtime behaviors associated with BIC-LST. For example, the development of the imagination may result in increased nighttime fears. An increase in separation anxiety, especially during the early toddler years, may lead to bedtime resistance and problematic night wakings. Furthermore, an increased need for autonomy and independence may result in increased bedtime resistance. In some cases, however, the child's resistance at bedtime may be from an underlying problem in falling asleep caused by other factors (such as asthma, medication use, restless legs, or anxiety) or a mismatch between the child's intrinsic circadian preferences ("night owl") and parental expectations. Finally, additional factors specific to the parents (eg, permissive parenting style, conflicting parental discipline styles, unrealistic parental expectations) or child (eg, age, temperament, daytime oppositional behavior) may contribute to the sleep problems.

BIC, combined type

Children with the combined type of BIC (BIC-C) typically present with bedtime resistance (eg, multiple requests, refusal) in conjunction with frequent and problematic night wakings.[4] In these cases, caregivers usually set insufficient or no limits at bedtime and these children ultimately require the presence of a negative sleep association to fall and return to sleep.

Prevalence

In general, behavioral insomnia of childhood is a disorder of young children (0–5 years of age), although it can persist into middle childhood and beyond, especially in those with special needs. Prevalence studies of insomnia in children and adolescents, especially for BIC, are hampered by the lack of standardized research criteria in terms of the frequency, severity, and chronicity of symptoms such as "sleep-onset delay" and "problematic night wakings." In general, study definitions of insomnia in children tend to be based on a priori inclusion criteria that can range from the more general (parental report of "difficulty falling asleep") to the more specific ("takes longer than 30 minutes to fall asleep at least 3 nights per week for at least 3 months"), and clearly vary with age and developmental status, although studies indicate considerable variability in cross-cultural studies. For example, in one study asking parents whether their child had a sleep problems, prevalence rates varied from approximately 10% in Vietnam and Thailand to 25% to 30% in the United States and Australia and as high as 75% in China and Taiwan.[10]

Despite this variation in definition, the identified prevalence of sleep disturbances overall in children is remarkably similar across studies (albeit almost all studies cited are conducted in predominantly Caucasian countries). Overall, an estimated 20% to 30% of children in cross-sectional studies are reported to have some significant bedtime problems or night wakings.[6,11,12] For infants and toddlers, night wakings are one of the most common sleep problems, with 25% to 50% of children older than 6 months of age continuing to awaken during the night. Bedtime resistance is found in 10% to 15% of toddlers. However, because these two sleep complaints frequently coexist, and similar treatments strategies may be used for both, many studies do not approach them as separate concerns, and therefore individual prevalence rates are difficult to estimate.

Difficulties falling asleep and night wakings (15%–30%) are also common in preschoolers.[11,13] Although sleep problems were previously believed to be rare in middle childhood, more recent studies have reported an overall prevalence of any parent-reported sleep problem in 25% to 40% of these children, including 15% who experience bedtime resistance and almost 11% of 4- to 0-year-olds who have sleep-related anxiety.[14,15]

Assessment

Typically, behavioral insomnia of childhood is identified based on parent report of sleep concerns. A comprehensive evaluation should include assessment of current sleep patterns, usual sleep duration, and sleep/wake schedule, which is often best assessed using a sleep diary, in which parents record daily sleep behaviors for an extended period (approximately 2 weeks). A review of sleeping arrangements, bedtime routines, and parental behaviors and responses to the child both at bedtime and after night wakings can help assess for factors contributing to the sleep problem. An evaluation for medical contributions is also warranted, especially pain (eg, ear infections) and reflux.

Treatment

When left untreated, bedtime and sleep problems can be chronic, and children rarely "outgrow" them. However, behavioral treatments can yield effective and durable results. Consistent with the conclusions of two previous reviews,[16,17] a recent review of 52 treatment studies indicates that behavioral therapies produce reliable and durable changes in both bedtime resistance and night wakings in young children.[18] Of the studies, 94% found behavioral interventions to be efficacious, with more than 80% of treated children showing clinically significant improvement maintained for up to 3 to 6 months. No study reported detrimental effects. Several studies also found positive effects of sleep interventions on secondary child-related outcome variables, such as daytime behaviors (eg, crying, irritability, detachment, self-esteem, emotional well-being).[18] Behavioral interventions for sleep problems also led to improvements in parental well-being (eg, effects on mood, stress, marital satisfaction) in several studies.[19–22]

Successful treatment of BIC generally involves a combination of behavioral strategies for eliminating inappropriate sleep-onset associations, reducing undesirable nighttime behaviors, and encouraging parental limit-setting. For all of these behavioral strategies, it is critical for parents to be consistent in applying behavioral programs to avoid inadvertent intermittent reinforcement of night wakings. They should also be forewarned that protest behavior frequently temporarily escalates at the beginning of treatment ("post-extinction burst"). Pediatric practitioners can offer several highly effective treatment recommendations:

- Establish a consistent bedtime routine that does not include stimulating activities, such as television viewing

- Introduce more appropriate sleep associations that will be readily available to the child during the night, such as use of a transitional object (eg, blanket, stuffed animal)
- Encourage development of self-soothing skills, that is having children fall asleep independently at bedtime without parental presence
- Practice bedtime fading, which involves temporarily setting the child's bedtime to the current sleep-onset time and then gradually advancing bedtime
- Decrease parental attention for problematic bedtime behaviors, such as stalling and additional requests
- Provide positive reinforcement for appropriate behaviors, such as stickers for remaining in bed
- Teach self-relaxation techniques and cognitive-behavioral strategies, which can also be beneficial in older children.

Psychophysiologic Insomnia

The term *insomnia* that is often used by patients and caregivers typically refers to sleep-onset or sleep-maintenance difficulties. The form of sleep-onset or sleep-maintenance insomnia that is defined in adults as psychophysiologic insomnia occurs primarily in older children and adolescents, rather than young children. This type of insomnia is characterized by a combination of learned sleep-preventing associations and heightened physiologic arousal, resulting in a complaint of sleeplessness.[4] A hallmark of this type of insomnia is excessive worry about sleep and an exaggerated concern regarding the potential daytime consequences. This type of insomnia is frequently the result of predisposing factors (eg, genetic vulnerability, underlying medical or psychiatric conditions) combined with precipitating factors (eg, acute stress) and perpetuating factors (eg, poor sleep habits, caffeine use, maladaptive cognitions about sleep).

Prevalence

A recent study found that the lifetime prevalence of insomnia in 13- to 16-year-old adolescents approaches 11%.[23] In addition, up to 35% of adolescents experience insomnia at least several times a month. Similar to adults, insomnia has an increased prevalence in girls postpuberty. Furthermore, lower socioeconomic status is associated with increased insomnia. In contrast, primary insomnia seems to be uncommon in prepubertal children.

Assessment

As with all sleep disorders, a thorough assessment is critical before the development of a treatment plan.[24] First, a thorough evaluation of other possible causes of sleep-onset and sleep-maintenance difficulties should be conducted, including:

- Negatively contributing sleep habits (eg, erratic sleep schedules, caffeine use) and lifestyle issues (eg, staying up late to socialize, electronics use)
- Presence of other sleep disorders, especially delayed sleep-phase disorder, obstructive sleep apnea, and restless legs syndrome
- Acute and chronic medical disorders (especially pain conditions)
- Psychiatric disorders, especially attention deficit hyperactivity disorder (ADHD), anxiety, and depression
- Concurrent medications, especially psychostimulants
- Smoking and alcohol and drug use.

A sleep diary, typically kept for 2 weeks, can be highly informational. Use of additional diagnostic tools such as polysomnographic evaluation are seldom warranted for routine evaluation of insomnia, but may be appropriate if an underlying sleep disruptor, such as obstructive sleep apnea or periodic limb movements, is suspected.

Treatment

Most studies on the treatment of psychophysiologic or primary insomnia have been conducted with adults, with clear evidence-based support for psychological and behavioral treatments. In a recent review of the literature, five treatments met criteria for empirically supported treatments, including stimulus control therapy, sleep restriction, relaxation, paradoxic intention, and cognitive–behavioral therapy.[25] Very few studies on the nonpharmacologic treatment of psychophysiologic insomnia have been conducted in adolescents, however, and almost none have been conducted in children. Studies evaluating the efficacy of pharmacologic treatment of psychophysiologic insomnia in children and adolescents are even more limited (see section on pharmacologic treatment).

In the pediatric practice, simple changes can often result in significant improvements in insomnia. **Box 1** provides a practice handout on the "Seven Rules for Beating Insomnia."[24] Overall, recommendations by the pediatric practitioner may include:

- Educating the child or adolescent about principles of sleep hygiene, including a developmentally appropriate bedtime, a consistent sleep schedule on weekdays and weekends (both bedtimes and wake times), avoidance of naps,

---

Box 1
Seven rules for beating insomnia

1. Choose a set wake-up time. Wake up at the same time every day, no matter how much sleep you got the night before.

2. Choose a bedtime. Choose the earliest possible bedtime that enables you to get the sleep you need. However, too much time in bed will lead to lighter, more interrupted sleep, so an appropriate bedtime is one that enables you to get the sleep that you need but doesn't let you be in bed too long. You only want to spend the amount of time in bed that you actually need for sleep.

3. Go to bed when you are sleepy, but not before your chosen bedtime. Don't go to bed until you are sleepy. So if you are still wide-awake at your chosen bedtime, wait a while longer until you are sleepy enough to fall asleep quickly.

4. Get out of bed when you can't sleep. If you are lying in bed and can't sleep, get out of bed and do something relaxing out of the bedroom. Read a book, watch television, or do something else relaxing; then go back to bed when you feel sleepy enough to fall asleep quickly. Again, if you do not fall asleep quickly, get up. Keep repeating this cycle until you fall asleep. You need to get out of bed when you can't sleep both at bedtime and in the middle of the night.

5. Don't worry or plan in bed. When lying in bed at night, don't spend the time worrying or planning for the next day. Set aside another time of the day to do these things. If you automatically start thinking and worrying when you get in bed, get up and don't head back to bed until your thoughts won't interfere with falling asleep. Thinking in bed is a habit, and one that you can break.

6. Only use your bed for sleep. Don't do anything but sleep in your bed. That is, don't do other activities, such as eat, watch television, or [do homework].

7. Avoid naps. Naps will interfere with your ability to fall asleep at bedtime, so no naps.

From Mindell JA, Owens JA. Clinical guide to pediatric sleep: diagnosis and management of sleep problems, 2nd edition. Philadelphia: Lippincott Williams & Wilkins; 2009; with permission.

avoidance of caffeine, a sleep-conducive environment, and removal of electronics from the bedroom.

- Recommending behavioral interventions, including instructing the patient to use the bed for sleep only and to get out of bed if unable to fall asleep (stimulus control); restricting time-in-bed to the actual time asleep (sleep restriction); and teaching relaxation techniques to reduce anxiety.
- Teaching the patient to counter inappropriate thoughts using cognitive restructuring, which includes (1) identifying the inappropriate sleep cognition, (2) challenging the validity of each sleep cognition, and (3) replacing the thought with a more productive one.

INSOMNIA IN SPECIAL PEDIATRIC POPULATIONS

Because the evaluation and treatment of insomnia in specific populations, such as children with autism spectrum disorders and chronic medical conditions, are discussed in detail elsewhere in this issue, the following section presents only a brief discussion of some of the factors contributing to the high prevalence of sleep problems in these groups. The concept of "primary" versus "secondary" (ie, resulting from an underlying medical or mental health condition) insomnia has largely been supplanted in favor of describing the insomnia as being "comorbid" or "coexisting" with these conditions, because the latter characterization avoids implying directionality or causality. Furthermore, insomnia in these populations is often different from that in typically developing healthy children in terms of severity, frequency, and chronicity, rather than in the "type" of insomnia; thus, many of the principles of evaluation and management of insomnia in children discussed earlier are applicable.

Children With Neurodevelopmental Disorders

Overall, the prevalence rates of sleep problems in children with a wide variety of neurodevelopmental disorders are very high, ranging from 13% to 85%.[24] For example, that significant sleep problems are estimated to occur in 30% to 80% of children with severe mental retardation and in at least half of children with less-severe cognitive impairment. The types of sleep disorders that occur in these children are generally not unique to these populations, but rather are more frequent and more severe than in the general population, and typically reflect the child's developmental level/IQ rather than chronologic age. Significant problems with settling at bedtime in children with unusual or prolonged bedtime routines, frequent night wakings, shortened sleep duration, irregular sleeping patterns, partial arousal parasomnias, and early morning waking, for example, have been reported in a variety of different neurodevelopmental disorders, including Asperger, Angelman, Rett, Smith-Magenis, and Williams syndromes. Sleep problems, especially in children with special needs, are often chronic in nature and unlikely to resolve without aggressive treatment. In addition, sleep disturbances in these children often have a profound effect on the quality of life of the entire family.

Sleep issues in these children may be related to any number of factors, including intrinsic abnormalities in sleep regulation and circadian rhythms, increased or decreased sensitivity to environmental factors, comorbid medical conditions such as seizures, and medications used to treat these associated conditions.[26,27] Common behavioral contributing factors include maladaptive learned sleep practices, parental reluctance to set appropriate limits, and caregiver stress. Psychiatric disorders such as depression and anxiety in children and adolescents with developmental delays and autistic spectrum disorders, and medications used to treat these disorders (eg, atypical antipsychotics) may further contribute to sleep problems.

Children With Psychiatric Disorders

Sleep disturbances are extremely common in child mental health clinical settings[28] and often have a significant impact on symptom severity and the management of psychiatric disorders in children and adolescents.[9,29,30] Psychiatric disorders can be associated with a range of sleep problems, including hypersomnia and fatigue, irregular sleep–wake patterns, disturbing dreams and nightmares, early morning awakenings, and impairments in sleep initiation and maintenance.[31] Studies of children with major depressive disorder, for example, have reported a prevalence of up to 75% for insomnia and 30% for severe insomnia, and sleep-onset delay in a third of depressed adolescents. Sleep complaints, especially difficulty falling asleep, refusal to sleep alone, increased nighttime fears, and nightmares, are also common in anxious children and children who have experienced severely traumatic events (including physical and sexual abuse). Use of psychotropic medications, which may have significant negative effects on sleep, often complicates the issue. Conversely, growing evidence suggests that insomnia in childhood is a risk factor for developing psychiatric conditions, particularly depressive and anxiety disorders, in adolescence and adulthood.[32]

Clinicians who evaluate and treat children with ADHD frequently report sleep disturbances, especially difficulty initiating sleep and restless and disturbed sleep.[33] Surveys of parents and children with ADHD consistently report an increased prevalence of sleep problems, including delayed sleep onset, poor sleep quality, restless sleep, frequent night wakings, and shortened sleep duration. However, more objective methods of examining sleep and sleep architecture (eg, polysomnography, actigraphy) have overall disclosed minimal or inconsistent differences between children with ADHD and controls, except for increased movements during sleep and more night-to-night variability in sleep patterns.[34,35]

Sleep problems in children with ADHD may have a variety of causes, and potential causes range from bedtime resistance related to a comorbid anxiety or oppositional defiant disorder in some children to psychostimulant-mediated delayed sleep onset in others. In still other children, settling difficulties at bedtime may be related to a resurgence of or even an increase in ADHD behaviors (ie, "rebound") in the evening after the effects of daytime medication are no longer present, or deficits in sensory integration associated with ADHD, whereas an intrinsic circadian phase delay may be the primary cause of bedtime resistance in a percentage of children. From a clinical standpoint, then, an important part of managing the individual child with ADHD should be evaluation of any comorbid sleep problems, followed by an appropriate diagnostically driven behavioral or pharmacologic intervention.

Children With Chronic Medical Disorders

Relatively little data currently exist regarding the impact of sleep problems on both acute and chronic health conditions, such as asthma, diabetes, sickle cell disease, cancer, and juvenile rheumatoid arthritis in children.[36–38] However, the interaction between insufficient or poor quality sleep, particularly in children with chronic pain conditions, is likely to significantly impact on quality of life and clinical management. For example, a recent study found that 3% of children hospitalized for medical issues were treated with sleep medications, suggesting that prescribing medication for sleep in hospitalized children is a fairly common practice.[39]

Several patient, caregiver, and environmental factors, such as the impact of underlying disease processes, repeated hospitalization, caregiver stress, comorbid mood and anxiety disorders, and concurrent medications, are clearly important to consider in assessing the bidirectional relationship of insomnia and chronic illness in children. Specific medical conditions that may also have an increased risk of sleep problems include allergies; atopic dermatitis; asthma[1]; migraine headaches; seizure disorders; juvenile rheumatoid arthritis; other rheumatologic conditions, such as chronic fatigue syndrome and fibromyalgia; and chronic gastrointestinal disorders, such as inflammatory bowel disease. Over-the-counter and prescription medications used to treat medical conditions may significantly affect sleep and should be evaluated within the context of sleep issues.

PHARMACOLOGIC AGENTS IN PEDIATRIC INSOMNIA

Studies have suggested that the use of medications to treat insomnia in children is widespread and that a broad variety of medications are being recommended by both pediatric and child mental health practitioners in community and academic settings for sleep disturbances in children.[40,41] Because no medications, except chloral hydrate, are currently labeled by the U.S. Food and Drug Administration (FDA) for the treatment of insomnia in children, the use of these medications in practice settings seems to be based largely on clinical experience, empirical data derived from adults, or small case series of hypnotics in the pediatric population.

Although pharmacologic interventions as an adjunct to behavioral strategies for the treatment of childhood insomnia may be appropriate in selected clinical situations and in specific populations (eg, children with ADHD or autism spectrum disorders), most sleep disturbances in children can be successfully managed with a combination of behavior therapy and modification of sleep practices alone.

If medication is believed to be potentially therapeutically beneficial in a given clinical situation (ie, appropriately implemented behavioral interventions are not fully effective), the following guidelines should be kept in mind. First, the choice of medication as an option for any given child with insomnia should be diagnostically driven; in other words, the specific cause or causes (eg, medication, pain, anxiety, primary sleep disorders such as obstructive sleep apnea) should first be determined and appropriate treatment, in the case of a primary sleep disorder, should be instituted before hypnotic medication is considered. Medication use should also be viewed in the context of the child's medical history and developmental age, and the risks and benefits weighed in the context of the clinical situation.

Clinicians should determine treatment goals that are both realistic and mutually acceptable to the child, caregivers, and family, and should establish measurable treatment outcomes (eg, reduction in sleep latency or number of night wakings). Finally, contraindications for pharmacotherapy in children include insomnia caused by a self-limited condition that often leads to night wakings such as teething; when the potential exists for drug interactions with concurrent medications (eg, opiates); in the presence of alcohol or illicit substance use; when limitations exist to adequate follow-up and monitoring of side effects (eg, parent frequently misses appointments); when insomnia occurs in the context of a primary sleep disorder (eg, obstructive sleep apnea); and when insomnia is determined to be caused by a developmentally based normal sleep behavior (ie, from inappropriate parent or practitioner expectations regarding child's sleep behaviors).

The pharmacokinetic properties of agents (eg, half-life, onset of action) should be considered in targeting specific sleep symptoms such as delayed sleep onset or night wakings. All medications prescribed for sleep problems should be closely monitored for the emergence of side effects. In addition, patients should be screened for concurrent use of nonprescription sleep aids and other herbal supplements, which may intensify the effect of or interact with hypnotic drugs.

A summary of pharmacologic and clinical properties of medications that are currently most commonly used in the treatment of pediatric insomnia are described in the following sections (to avoid any implied rank order in preference, medication classes are listed in alphabetical order).

Alpha Agonists

Clonidine and guanfacine are noradrenergic α_2-agonists that are widely used in pediatric and psychiatric practice, particularly in children with sleep-onset delay and ADHD. Despite a paucity of data regarding efficacy and safety in children, clonidine is often prescribed to shorten sleep latency in children with ADHD.[42] A case series has also reported that clonidine seems to be beneficial and fairly well tolerated in intractable sleep problems in children and young adults with neurodevelopmental disorders.[43] Guanfacine seems to be less sedating and is associated with fewer anticholinergic and cardiovascular side effects than clonidine because of its more selective α-receptor binding.[44] Clonidine is rapidly absorbed with onset of action in 1 hour and peak effects at 2 to 4 hours; the half-life is 6 to 24 hours. Guanfacine has a greater volume of distribution and longer half-life. Potential side effects include anticholinergic effects, irritability, and dysphoria, and rebound hypertension on abrupt discontinuation. Clonidine has a narrow therapeutic index and has been associated with significant cardiotoxicity and death with overdoses.

Antidepressants

Sedating atypical antidepressants (mirtazapine, nefazodone, and trazodone), selective serotonin reuptake inhibitors, and tricyclic antidepressants are used in clinical practice to treat insomnia in adult and pediatric populations. Antidepressants are believed to mediate sleep promotion through influencing activity of non–γ-aminobutyric acid neurotransmitters that regulate sleep and wakefulness (eg, histamine, acetylcholine, serotonin). Most antidepressants, especially those with anticholinergic effects, suppress rapid eye movement (REM), and increase latency to REM sleep; thus, abrupt withdrawal may lead to increased nightmares (REM rebound). Although frequently used in clinical practice, overall little methodologically rigorous research supports the use of any of the antidepressants for insomnia in adults or children. Thus, the use of antidepressants for insomnia should generally be limited to clinical situations in which concurrent mood issues are present, because treating the underlying mood disorder will often result in improved sleep.

Antihistamines

Parental and provider familiarity tend to make antihistamines an acceptable choice for many families. Over-the-counter sleep aids typically contain diphenhydramine or doxylamine, both of which have shown modest efficacy in reducing sleep latency. A double-blind placebo-controlled study of diphenhydramine in school-aged children showed significant subjective improvement in sleep latency and night waking.[45] However, a more recent study of 44 children aged 6 to 15 months found that diphenhydramine was no better than placebo in reducing night waking.[46] Potential adverse effects include anticholinergic effects (eg, dry mouth, blurred vision, urinary retention), morning "hangover" with daytime drowsiness, and paradoxic excitation. Tolerance to antihistamines may develop, necessitating increasing doses.

Benzodiazepines and Nonbenzodiazepine Gabaminergic Receptor Agonists

GABA is the major inhibitory neurotransmitter in the brain; thus, the hypnotic effect of the benzodiazepines is mediated by their action at GABA type A receptors (GABA A). These medications shorten sleep latency, increase total sleep time, and improve sleep maintenance. The benzodiazepines also have muscle relaxant, anxiolytic, and anticonvulsant properties. Use of longer-acting benzodiazepines may lead to morning "hangover," daytime sleepiness, and compromised daytime functioning. Anterograde amnesia and disinhibition may also occur. Finally, these medications are also associated with a risk of habituation or addiction and with withdrawal phenomena. In general, this class of medication should only be used for short-term or transient insomnia, or in clinical situations in which their other properties (eg, anxiolytic) are advantageous.

The nonbenzodiazepine receptor agonists (NBzRAs) bind more selectively to GABA A receptor complexes. Two short-acting NBzRAs are approved for use in adults (zaleplon and zolpidem). Two NBzdRAs with longer half-lives are also approved for sleep maintenance and sleep-initiation insomnia (zolpidem-CR and eszopiclone). A single published clinical trial of zolpidem in children failed to show efficacy. Potential side effects include dizziness, anterograde amnesia, confusion, hallucinations, and headache.

Melatonin

Melatonin is a hormone secreted by the pineal gland that binds to receptors in the suprachiasmatic nucleus in the hypothalamus. Depending on the dose and timing of administration, exogenous synthetic melatonin has both chronobiotic (ie, shifts the circadian sleep–wake cycle) and mild hypnotic (ie, sedating) effects. For example, studies of melatonin in adults with delayed sleep-phase disorder have reported that smaller doses (eg, 0.5 mg) taken 5 to 7 hours before sleep onset may be more effective in treating sleep-onset delay in the context of a circadian rhythm disorder. Alternatively, because plasma levels of exogenous melatonin peak within 1 hour after administration, it may be most helpful in reducing sleep-onset insomnia not related to a delay in circadian timing when taken in larger doses (eg, 3–5 mg) closer to bedtime.

Several studies have shown efficacy in reducing sleep latency in children with ADHD, based on the premise that some of these children have a circadian-mediated phase delay (ie, delayed sleep onset and offset compared with developmental norms).[47] Additional clinical uses for melatonin include treatment of circadian rhythm disturbances (eg, delayed sleep-phase syndrome) and of children with special needs or neurodevelopmental disorders (eg, blindness, Rett syndrome, autism). Although generally regarded as safe, potential adverse effects of melatonin include suppression of the hypothalamic-gonadal axis (potentially triggering precocious puberty on abrupt discontinuation)[48] and increased reactivity of the immune system in children with immune disorders or who are taking immunosuppressants.

Melatonin Receptor Agonists

Synthetic melatonin receptor agonists act selectively at the MT1 and MT2 receptors, and have been reported to be potentially useful in the pediatric population.[49] Ramelteon is the only drug in this class that is FDA approved for the treatment of insomnia, and is also the only schedule VI approved hypnotic. The sleep-promoting effect of ramelteon is postulated to be related to reduction of alerting output of the suprachiasmatic nucleus. It has shown moderate efficacy in clinical trials in adults in reducing sleep latency.

Other Pharmacologic Agents

Finally, other classes of medications that are not indicated for insomnia but that have been reportedly used in pediatric clinical practice include anticonvulsants (carbamazepine, valproic acid, topiramate, gabapentin), atypical antipsychotics (risperidone, olanzapine, quetiapine), and chloral hydrate. In most instances, these medications are being prescribed for alternative indications (eg, bipolar disorder, aggression), and the side effect of daytime sedation that occurs with these medications is used to promote nighttime sleep.

Although these medications may have sedative effects, they should be used with caution, if at all, for insomnia in children. Data are lacking or limited on safety and tolerability for this indication in either adults or children. Furthermore, the sedating effects may interfere with daytime functioning and learning. These medications can also have negative effects on sleep parameters. For example, many of the newer atypical antipsychotics have weight gain as a significant side effect, and thus can worsen obstructive sleep apnea. Finally, the American Academy of Pediatrics recommends against the use of chloral hydrate in children, except for short-term sedation because of the risk of hepatotoxicity.

FUTURE DIRECTIONS

Further elucidation of fundamental questions regarding the cause and impact of insomnia in children is likely to contribute significantly to the understanding. Key areas for future research include the interactions among genetic susceptibility, environmental factors, developmental stage, and learned behaviors in the genesis of childhood insomnia; elucidation of the scope, magnitude, natural history, and impact of insomnia in children and adolescents in general, and on children with medical, mental health, and developmental disorders; risk and protective factors (eg, race/ethnicity, temperament, parenting styles, poverty) influencing the development of childhood insomnia; the relative efficacy of treatments, including behavioral interventions and pharmacotherapy; and the impact of treatment on the natural history of insomnia into adulthood, including the role of sleep problems in predicting the eventual emergence of psychiatric comorbid conditions (depression, anxiety, bipolar disorder).

The diagnostic features of insomnia in children both common to and distinct from adult insomnia need to be further refined, and the characteristics that differentiate normal developmental variation or self-limited sleep problems from "pathology" across the age spectrum need to be clarified. Evidence-based clinical screening and evaluation tools for insomnia in children that may be easily adapted to primary care must be developed and systematically evaluated. Educational interventions targeted toward health care providers and caregivers to raise awareness of the significance of pediatric insomnia are fundamental to primary and secondary prevention efforts. Finally, the potential substantial impact of childhood insomnia on patients and their families clearly deserves further study.

REFERENCES

1. Adams LA, Rickert VI. Reducing bedtime tantrums: comparison between positive routines and graduated extinction. Pediatrics 1989;84:756–61.
2. Hiscock H, Wake M. Randomised controlled trial of behavioural infant sleep intervention to improve infant sleep and maternal mood. BMJ 2002;324:1062–5.
3. Leeson R, Barbour J, Romaniuk D, et al. Management of infant sleep problems in a residential unit. Child Care Health Dev 1994;20:89–100.

4. American Academy of Sleep Medicine. International classification of sleep disorders. Diagnostic and coding manual. 2nd edition. Westchester (IL): American Academy of Sleep Medicine; 2005.

5. Owens LJ, France KG, Wiggs L. Review article: behavioural and cognitive-behavioural interventions for sleep disorders in infants and children: a review. Sleep Med Rev 1999;3:281–302.

6. Goodlin-Jones BL, Burnham MM, Gaylor EE, et al. Night waking, sleep-wake organization, and self-soothing in the first year of life. J Dev Behav Pediatr 2001;22:226–33.

7. Mindell JA, Sadeh A, Kohyama J, et al. Parental behaviors and sleep outcomes in infants and toddlers: a cross-cultural comparison. Sleep Med 2010;11:393–9.

8. Sadeh A, Mindell JA, Luedtke K, et al. Sleep and sleep ecology in the first 3 years: a web-based study. J Sleep Res 2009;18:60–73.

9. Sadeh A, McGuire JP, Sachs H, et al. Sleep and psychological characteristics of children on a psychiatric inpatient unit. J Am Acad Child Adolesc Psychiatry 1995;34:813–9.

10. Mindell JA, Sadeh A, Wiegand B, et al. Cross-cultural differences in infant and toddler sleep. Sleep Med 2010;11:274–80.

11. Mindell JA, Meltzer LJ, Carskadon MA, et al. Developmental aspects of sleep hygiene: findings from the 2004 National Sleep Foundation Sleep in America Poll. Sleep Med 2009;10:771–9.

12. Burnham MM, Goodlin-Jones BL, Gaylor EE, et al. Nighttime sleep-wake patterns and self-soothing from birth to one year of age: a longitudinal intervention study. J Child Psychol Psychiatry 2002;43:713–25.

13. Kerr S, Jowett S. Sleep problems in pre-school children: a review of the literature. Child Care Health Dev 1994;20:379–91.

14. Blader JC, Koplewicz HS, Abikoff H, et al. Sleep problems of elementary school children. A community survey. Arch Pediatr Adolesc Med 1997;151:473–80.

15. Owens JA, Spirito A, McGuinn M, et al. Sleep habits and sleep disturbance in elementary school-aged children. J Dev Behav Pediatr 2000;21:27–36.

16. Mindell JA. Empirically supported treatments in pediatric psychology: bedtime refusal and night wakings in young children. J Pediatr Psychol 1999;24: 465–81.

17. Kuhn BR, Elliott AJ. Treatment efficacy in behavioral pediatric sleep medicine. J Psychosom Res 2003;54:587–97.

18. Mindell JA, Kuhn B, Lewin DS, et al. Behavioral treatment of bedtime problems and night wakings in infants and young children. Sleep 2006;29:1263–76.

19. Mindell JA, Durand VM. Treatment of childhood sleep disorders: generalization across disorders and effects on family members. J Pediatr Psychol 1993;18: 731–50.

20. Wolfson A, Lacks P, Futterman A. Effects of parent training on infant sleeping patterns, parents' stress, and perceived parental competence. J Consult Clin Psychol 1992;60:41–8.

21. Hiscock H, Bayer J, Gold L, et al. Improving infant sleep and maternal mental health: a cluster randomised trial. Arch Dis Child 2007;92:952–8.

22. Hiscock H, Bayer JK, Hampton A, et al. Long-term mother and child mental health effects of a population-based infant sleep intervention: cluster-randomized, controlled trial. Pediatrics 2008;122:e621–7.

23. Johnson EO, Roth T, Schultz L, et al. Epidemiology of DSM-IV insomnia in adolescence: lifetime prevalence, chronicity, and an emergent gender difference. Pediatrics 2006;117:e247–56.

24. Mindell JA, Owens JA. A clinical guide to pediatric sleep: diagnosis and management of sleep problems. 2nd edition. Philadelphia: Lippincott Williams & Wilkins; 2009.

25. Morin CM, Bootzin RR, Buysse DJ, et al. Psychological and behavioral treatment of insomnia: update of the recent evidence (1998–2004). Sleep 2006;29:1398–414.

26. Wiggs L. Sleep problems in children with developmental disorders. J R Soc Med 2001;94:177–9.

27. Johnson C. Sleep problems in children with mental retardation and autism. Child Adolesc Psychiatr Clin N Am 1996;5:673–81.

28. Owens JA, Rosen C, Mindell JA, et al. Use of pharmacotherapy for insomnia in children and adolescents: a national survey of child psychiatrists. Sleep Med 2010;11:692–700.

29. Sachs H, McGuire J, Sadeh A, et al. Cognitive and behavioural correlates of mother reported sleep problems in psychiatrically hospitalized children. Sleep Research 1994;23:207–13.

30. Dahl RE, Ryan ND, Matty MK, et al. Sleep onset abnormalities in depressed adolescents. Biol Psychiatry 1996;39:400–10.

31. Johnson EO, Chilcoat HD, Breslau N. Trouble sleeping and anxiety/depression in childhood. Psychiatry Res 2000;94:93–102.

32. Curt GA, Breitbart W, Cella D, et al. Impact of cancer-related fatigue on the lives of patients: new findings from the fatigue coalition. Oncologist 2000;5:353–60.

33. Owens JA. The ADHD and sleep conundrum: a review. J Dev Behav Pediatr 2005;26:312–22.

34. Sadeh A, Pergamin L, Bar-Haim Y. Sleep in children with attention-deficit hyperactivity disorder: a meta-analysis of polysomnographic studies. Sleep Med Rev 2006;10:381–98.

35. Cortese S, Lecendreux M, Mouren MC, et al. ADHD and insomnia. J Am Acad Child Adolesc Psychiatry 2006;45:384–5.

36. Lewin DS, Dahl RE. Importance of sleep in the management of pediatric pain. J Dev Behav Pediatr 1999;20:244–52.

37. Bloom BJ, Owens JA, McGuinn M, et al. Sleep and its relationship to pain, dysfunction, and disease activity in juvenile rheumatoid arthritis. J Rheumatol 2002;29:169–73.

38. Sadeh A, Horowitz I, Wolach-Benodis L, et al. Sleep and pulmonary function in children with well-controlled, stable asthma. Sleep 1998;21:379–84.

39. Meltzer LJ, Johnson C, Crosette J, et al. Prevalence of diagnosed sleep disorders in pediatric primary care practices. Pediatrics 2010;125:e1410–8.

40. Owens JA, Rosen CL, Mindell JA. Medication use in the treatment of pediatric insomnia: results of a survey of community-based pediatricians. Pediatrics 2003;111:e628–35.

41. Owens JA, Rosen CL, Mindell JA, et al. Use of pharmacotherapy for insomnia in child psychiatry practice: a national survey. Sleep Med 2010;11:692–700.

42. Prince JB, Wilens TE, Biederman J, et al. Clonidine for sleep disturbances associated with attention-deficit hyperactivity disorder: a systematic chart review of 62 cases. J Am Acad Child Adolesc Psychiatry 1996;35:599–605.

43. Ingrassia A, Turk J. The use of clonidine for severe and intractable sleep problems in children with neurodevelopmental disorders–a case series. Eur Child Adolesc Psychiatry 2005;14:34–40.

44. Arnsten AF, Scahill L, Findling RL. alpha2-Adrenergic receptor agonists for the treatment of attention-deficit/hyperactivity disorder: emerging concepts from new data. J Child Adolesc Psychopharmacol 2007;17:393–406.

45. Russo RM, Gururaj VJ, Allen JE. The effectiveness of diphenhydramine HCl in pediatric sleep disorders. J Clin Pharmacol 1976;284–8.
46. Merenstein D, Diener-West M, Halbower AC, et al. The trial of infant response to diphenhydramine: the TIRED study–a randomized, controlled, patient-oriented trial. Arch Pediatr Adolesc Med 2006;160:707–12.
47. Van der Heijden KB, Smits MG, Gunning WB. Sleep hygiene and actigraphically evaluated sleep characteristics in children with ADHD and chronic sleep onset insomnia. J Sleep Res 2006;15:55–62.
48. Luboshitzky R, Tiosano D, Ben-Harush M, et al. Pseudo-precocious puberty in a male patient and the melatonin-testosterone relationship. J Pediatr Endocrinol Metab 1995;8:295–9.
49. Stigler KA, Posey DJ, McDougle CJ. Ramelteon for insomnia in two youths with autistic disorder. J Child Adolesc Psychopharmacol 2006;16:631–6.

Update on Pediatric Sleep-Disordered Breathing

Manisha Witmans, MD, FRCPC[a,b,]*, Rochelle Young, RN, BA, BSN[b]

KEYWORDS

- Pediatric • Children • Sleep-disordered breathing
- Obstructive sleep apnea

The woods are lovely, dark and deep. But [we] have promises to keep, And miles to go before [we] sleep, And miles to go before [we] sleep.

Robert Frost

Despite the many advances in the field of pediatric sleep medicine over the past decade, the science and knowledge of this area (our woods) are largely unexplored and remain unknown, dark and deep. That an understanding of pediatric sleep has only begun to be formed is reflected in the common clinical view of pediatric sleep-disordered breathing (SDB) as a picture of enlarged tonsils and adenoids requiring surgical intervention. Such a limited perspective veils the complexity of SDB in children and requires a significant re-evaluation to improve the outcomes of children and adolescents affected by this burdensome health problem and its wide-ranging consequences. This article provides readers with the most current knowledge and understanding of pediatric SDB, discusses diagnostic issues and management challenges of SDB in children and adolescents, and builds on a previous *Pediatric Clinics of North America* review of this topic.[1,2]

When dealing with a patient presenting with possible SDB, the primary care provider is confronted with the daunting task of effectively diagnosing and treating the child or adolescent. To facilitate understanding of SDB in the pediatric population, this discussion is limited to otherwise healthy children with suspected SDB who are habitual snorers. Those with high risk of SDB related to genetic or craniofacial syndromes or neuromuscular weakness are beyond the scope of this review. In otherwise healthy children, the spectrum of SDB is best conceptualized as a range of conditions. The spectrum ranges from primary snoring (ie, without associated ventilatory abnormalities) to increased upper airway resistance to the most severe form, obstructive sleep apnea

The authors have nothing to disclose.
[a] Division of Pediatric Respiratory Medicine, University of Alberta, Edmonton, AB, Canada
[b] Northern Alberta Pediatric Sleep Centre, Stollery Children's Hospital, Edmonton, AB, Canada
* Corresponding author. 5H2.31 Walter Mackenzie Health Sciences Centre, 8440-112 Street, Edmonton, AB T6R 2J3, Canada.
E-mail address: manisha.witmans@albertahealthservices.ca

(OSA), characterized by repetitive prolonged partial or complete upper airway obstruction leading to fragmented sleep and gas exchange abnormalities. To appropriately identify children suspected of having SDB, the American Academy of Pediatrics published practice guidelines[3,4] almost a decade ago recommending an overnight sleep study or nocturnal polysomnogram (PSG) as the gold standard for diagnosing SDB in otherwise healthy children without comorbidity. This recommendation was put forth by the American Academy of Pediatrics based on studies that failed to find any combination of history and physical findings that reliably identify those children with SDB. Despite the practice guidelines, PSG still are not routinely used in clinical practice. Approximately 10% of children with chronic snoring referred for adenotonsillectomy actually have the PSG to confirm the diagnosis.[5] The huge disparity between the recommendations and what is current practice must be addressed. What are the reasons for the gap between the practice guidelines and the reality of clinical practice? Why does it matter and what should be done to bridge the gaps and advance the field? This review attempts to address these important clinical questions by summarizing what is currently known about SDB in children, including discussions of causes, consequences, and treatment options.

PATHOPHYSIOLOGY OF SDB

Several elegant discussions regarding alterations in the upper airway and subsequent increased airway resistance resulting in SDB are available in the literature.[6–10] In brief, the cause of SDB is likely related to a combination of several factors that results in upper airway dysfunction during sleep. These factors can include any of the following: structural abnormalities anywhere along the entire airway from the nose to the trachea, soft tissue hypertrophy (typically adenotonsillar hypertrophy), craniofacial dysmorphology (posteriorly placed mandible or micrognathia or midfacial hypoplasia), neuromuscular or neuromotor dysfunction,[11] and alterations in sensation of the upper airway.[12] Other important factors that help determine the airway's ability to compensate appropriately in the face of obstruction include neuromotor activation,[13] arousal thresholds, and central nervous system ventilatory control. Inflammation also likely plays a role in the pathophysiology of SDB; the resulting disruption of the homeostasis from sleep fragmentation and hypoxemia may lead to inflammation at the cellular level and the ability of the airway to respond appropriately may be limited in the context of inflammation. There are also be genetic and environmental factors that further influence the imbalance causing upper airway dysfunction and subsequent SDB because the presence of one of these factors alone does not always guarantee the presence of the disorder. Although the exact mechanism involving SDB in children needs to be elucidated further, an increasingly important risk factor in the pediatric population is obesity[7,8,14–21] because parapharyngeal fat deposition associated with obesity may add further load to an already compromised airway by increasing critical airway closing pressure and altering chest wall mechanics.[8] Identifying the underlying factors contributing to SDB in individual children is important because it affects not only the choice of treatment (likelihood that an adenotonsillectomy is warranted) but also the likely efficacy of treatment and outcomes. For example, in children with swallowing dysfunction or altered sensation at the level of the upper airway, in the context of inadequate neuromuscular compensation, addressing only the structural elements of the obstruction by removing the tonsils and adenoids may not cure the SDB but may worsen it. This is challenging in the clinical setting because there are no readily available, specific measures to assess and weigh the significance of these factors and their interaction for each individual patient.

RISK FACTORS THAT CONTRIBUTE TO SDB

Epidemiologic studies, mostly based on parent-report questionnaires, have identified various risk factors for SDB.[22–24] SDB seems more common in boys and African American children.[22,25] Another putative risk factor is recurrent otitis media,[26] which is most likely related to chronic adenotonsillar hypertrophy. Disorders of the upper and lower respiratory system, including asthma and persistent wheezing[21,27–29] and recurrent sinus infections, are also risk factors.[30] Environmental tobacco smoke exposure and maternal smoking during pregnancy not only exacerbate these other respiratory disorders but also have been shown to result in higher rates of snoring and likely SDB.[31] Epidemiologic studies have also suggested that children with a past history of prematurity are at increased risk of SDB.[22,25] One recent study showed that in children with delayed motor milestones, prenatal and perinatal stressors play a role in predisposing children to moderate or severe SDB.[25] All these wide-ranging risk factors together suggest that the mechanisms involved in SDB likely involve gene and environment interactions resulting in morbidity.

Furthermore, many studies, using different methodologies, have identified obesity as a major risk factor for the development, persistence, and recurrence of SDB, conferring up to a 4-fold increase in the risk for SDB.[32] Not all obese children have SDB[8]; therefore, further studies are required to determine which obese children are more vulnerable to developing SDB and how to identify and stratify their risk factors in a clinical setting for optimizing treatment. Preliminary studies of SDB phenotypes in children have suggested that older children with SDB are more likely to be obese and to present with a more adult-like clinical picture, including excessive daytime sleepiness; they may also have a higher risk of end-organ dysfunction.[7,33] The mechanism related to excessive daytime sleepiness and SDB is complex because not all individuals with SDB have excessive daytime sleepiness. Nevertheless, clinicians should maintain a high index of suspicion for SDB in obese children and adolescents, and these individuals should be systematically screened and evaluated for symptoms of SDB.

CONSEQUENCES OF SDB IN CHILDREN

It is difficult to know whether the negative outcomes related to SDB result primarily from the sleep disruption and fragmentation related to frequent arousals, from end-organ effects of related hypoxemia, or from both. Most of the relationships between end-organ dysfunction and SDB are documented using pretreatment and post-treatment studies for SDB in small numbers of patients. Overall, the evidence to date suggests that the end-organ effects of SDB are widespread and that untreated disease may have significant measurable consequences. Although it is not clearly established, there may even be a period of increased vulnerability during specific developmental periods, such that the delay in diagnosis and treatment may have long-term, potentially irreversible sequalae.[25] What is known is that children who have SDB have significantly higher health care use costs and that treatment reduces these expenditures by lowering hospitalization rates, emergency room visits, and medication use.[34,35] What is not known is how individual susceptibility and environmental interactions merge together for individual children, such that there is end-organ dysfunction and morbidity because the severity of the SDB alone may not be enough to determine the type and timing of intervention. Thus, treating children for SDB can result in improvements in various domains but it is not possible to predict which children will benefit and to what extent.[36–44]

NEUROCOGNITIVE DYSFUNCTION

The challenge in trying to distinguish neurocognitive dysfunction resulting from SDB from other factors, such as genetics, environment, and social factors, is a complex one. There are several excellent reviews for interested readers.[36,45,46] Briefly, investigators have attempted to identify whether any specific neurocognitive or psychological tests can identify those at risk for PSG confirmed SDB. Because various studies have used different parameters and criteria to characterize neurocognitive functioning and have also used a variety of PSG-related cutoff values to define SDB, making comparisons across studies is challenging. Several studies in children with primary snoring (defined as apnea-hypopnea index >1/h and <5 events/h) have been shown to have performance deficits compared with controls (apnea-hypopnea index <1 event/h) on measures related to attention, overall cognitive functioning, language, and visuospatial abilities[47,48] and to score higher on measures of anxiety and depression. Even mild SDB may be associated with impairments in behavior and neuropsychological functioning as a result of the perturbations in sleep or gas exchange parameters[37,49] but only one study did not find such an association.[50] The explanation for this discrepancy may be that the children in the latter group are younger and there is more scatter in the findings or that group of patients reflects a different genetic vulnerability to end-organ effects of SDB. Although SDB does contribute to neurocognitive dysfunction, the overall morbidity in a patient with neurocognitive dysfunction reflects the combined influence of genetic, environmental, and sociocultural factors in addition to the independent impact of SDB. Furthermore, translating the epidemiologic evidence to the clinical setting does not reflect potential differences in duration of disease, timing of exposure, and other similarly complex relationships because not all children show impairments in functioning that are linked to the severity of the SDB. Furthermore, there may be mediating neuroprotective factors (cytokines, cerebral oxygenation, and other factors) to explain the variance in neurocognitive deficits among children with SDB.[51] Given the evidence, it is reasonable to conclude that all children with learning or attention problems or poor academic functioning should be evaluated for SDB in the clinical setting.

CARDIOVASCULAR DYSFUNCTION

In adults, the relationship between SDB and related cardiovascular morbidity and mortality is well established. Although the data in children are limited predominantly to studies of small samples of school-aged and older children, the evidence to date is compelling. These studies have established an increased risk of cardiovascular dysfunction in children with SDB, ranging from increases in blood pressure and abnormal echocardiographic findings to more subtle perturbations in autonomic functions and alterations, in inflammatory markers, such as C-reactive protein. For example, there is evidence to suggest that children with SDB have alterations in blood pressure and heart rate during obstructive events similar in magnitude to those described in adults[52] and that there is a strong, dose-dependent relationship between elevated systolic and diastolic blood pressures and severity of SDB.[53–55] This relationship could have tremendous implications for long-term cardiovascular morbidity. In addition, obesity substantially increases the likelihood of having hypertension in the presence of SDB.[56] Echocardiographic evidence of cardiovascular dysfunction, including left ventricular dysfunction, increased pulmonary pressures, and end-diastolic dysfunction, has been reported in children with SDB.[54,55,57–59] Most studies, with one exception,[60] have shown that markers of inflammation, such as C-reactive protein and N-terminal pro–B-type natriuretic peptide, are elevated in children with SDB and decline after therapy.[60–66] Elevated cardiovascular sympathetic activity,[67] in addition to other various inflammatory mediators, which may or may not be directly related to intermittent hypoxemia, could be an important mediator of cardiovascular morbidity. Although children with SDB seem to be at increased risk for cardiovascular dysfunction, the explanation may not be as straightforward because other factors, including disease exposure and genetic permutations, which confer increased vulnerability, may also play a role. In support of that view is recent evidence that shows effects related to cardiovascular dysfunction improve with treatment but may not resolve entirely, particularly if there is a family history of cardiovascular disease.[68–70] These children may continue to be vulnerable after treatment and likely warrant extended follow-up.

METABOLIC DYSFUNCTION

Emerging evidence suggests that metabolic dysfunction is also associated with SDB. The nature of the relationship in the context of obesity and other potential confounding factors needs further study. Metabolic syndrome, defined as a constellation of features, including hypertension, insulin resistance, dyslipidemia, and abdominal obesity, has been increasingly recognized in children. Obesity and SDB are important risk factors for metabolic syndrome. For example, one study found that adolescents with SDB have a 6.5-fold higher risk of metabolic syndrome compared with those without SDB.[71] Other associated features of metabolic dysfunction include fatty liver disease, which has been reported in children with SDB.[72,73] Obese children with SDB seem to have higher levels of insulin resistance but whether this is related to SDB or obesity (or both) requires further study.[74] Some studies have reported post-treatment improvements after adenotonsillectomy in the metabolic profile[44,74,75] but the results are not consistent across studies.

DIAGNOSIS OF SDB

The first step in determining the likelihood of SDB in pediatric patients is to screen for possible symptoms, especially in high-risk groups. In addition to the high-risk groups discussed previously (patients with adenotonsillar hypertrophy, obesity, prematurity, and so forth), children with attention-deficit/hyperactivity disorder are considered high risk because symptoms of SDB are more commonly found in this group. Despite the diagnostic limitations of the history and physical examination (discussed previously), a history of nightly snoring and sleep disruption is an important clue to the possible presence of SDB. An accurate history, however, is largely dependent on the accuracy and quality of a caregiver's observations. It is not clear whether the frequency, severity, and duration of the snoring change the diagnostic yield of SDB. Children with SDB may also primarily exhibit daytime manifestations of poor sleep, such as sleepiness, inattention, or irritability; thus, it is incumbent on primary care clinicians to identify these as potential symptoms of SDB. Although there certainly are challenges to obtaining a valid pediatric patient history, specific and routine questions regarding cardinal symptoms, such as apneic pauses and snoring, should be a part of the assessment. The prevalence of witnessed apneas in children, however, is exceedingly uncommon (<1%); thus, requiring the presence of apneic events as part of the diagnostic criteria may result in underdiagnosis of SDB.[76] Clinicians should ask about other possible symptoms of SDB, such as poor quality or disrupted sleep, evidence of increased work of breathing (nocturnal diaphoresis, paradoxic chest, and abdominal wall movements), or even end-organ dysfunction secondary to SDB, such as hypertension.

In addition to nocturnal symptoms, including restless sleep and secondary enuresis, other aspects of a child's daily functioning that are potentially related to sleep disruption, such as mood, behavior, and daytime sleepiness, should be assessed. Although SDB has been associated with poor academic performance,[36,77–79] other causes of sleep disruption (insufficient sleep, restless legs syndrome, and insomnia) may also contribute to neurobehavioral morbidity.[61] In addition, there is a great deal of overlap between the symptoms that may be attributable to SDB and those associated with other common diagnoses, such as attention-deficit/hyperactivity disorder, which further limits the ability of the clinical history alone to distinguish children who have SDB from those with another disorder.[1,2,80,81] It is imperative for the clinician to maintain a high index of suspicion in such children and regularly evaluate for symptoms of sleep disruption or sleep disorders when children are reported to have a change in level of functioning at school or in the home.

QUESTIONNAIRES

Various questionnaires have been developed to aid in the identification of children who have SDB. In general, they ultimately rely on parent reports when used diagnostically in the clinical setting. For example, the 22-item sleep-related breathing disorder subscale in the Pediatric Sleep Questionnaire, used in screening children ages 2 through 18 for SDB, has reasonable sensitivity (0.85) and specificity (0.87).[82] This questionnaire has been validated in several clinical settings and a score of greater than 0.33 has been shown to predict a 3-fold increased risk of SDB on PSG. Other pediatric SDB questionnaires are limited by the fact that they have undergone limited testing in clinical settings outside the areas of research centers for which they were developed or because they have poor psychometric properties.[83] Although questionnaires can help standardize history-taking inquiry, they may not adequately reflect the entire spectrum of disease presentation and ultimately may not be useful in conclusively determining which individual children require immediate evaluation and treatment in the clinical setting.

PHYSICAL EXAMINATION

Similar to history and questionnaires, physical examination also has limited ability to specifically identify children who will have SDB. There are several reasons for this. First, most physicians and primary care providers are not trained to evaluate aspects of craniofacial morphology, other than adenotonsillar hypertrophy, that may predispose children to SDB, such as malocclusion; position of the palate, maxilla, and mandible; and crowding of the posterior pharynx. Furthermore, end-organ effects from SDB, such as hypertension or altered metabolic parameters, may not be immediately obvious or may occur late in the disease process. The addition of diagnostic radiologic tests may increase the sensitivity of the physical examination. For example, one study reported a sensitivity of 90% using a lateral neck radiograph when combined with findings of upper airway narrowing and enuresis.[84] The constellation of features failed, however, to identify all children with SDB. The bottom line is that children with clinical symptoms, physical findings, and/or risk factors for SDB warrant further evaluation to confirm the diagnosis and help determine both the timing and type of treatment.

IMAGING

Further characterization of the upper airway using sophisticated imaging modalities not only has been shown to distinguish between children with and without SDB but also may help to identify specific airway findings that contribute to the etiology of SDB. Investigators have found differences in the airways of children with SDB using

MRI[85,86] or imaging CT,[87] namely, a smaller cross-sectional area and smaller airway volume. Although these methods may eventually help to predict, triage, and evaluate outcomes of treatment, these testing modalities are not universally available and require sedation, thus are primarily used for research purposes only. Endoscopy of the airway has also been widely used by pediatric otolaryngologists to evaluate the upper airway and identify potential contributory factors (ie, region of collapse, such as laryngomalacia, or obstruction). Visualization under anesthesia may not accurately reflect the appearance of the upper airway during normal sleep, which has been the most significant criticism. Sleep endoscopy, using a standardized technique of evaluating the airway, has been shown to have a positive predictive value of 0.94 and a negative predictive value of 0.8 in children presenting with SDB compared with PSG (Hamdy El-Hakim, MD, unpublished data, University of Alberta, Edmonton, Alberta, 2010). Finally, acoustic pharyngometry accurately predicts associated SDB diagnosed by PSG with high sensitivity (90.9%) and specificity (88.4%) but is also not widely available.[88] In summary, although novel diagnostic methods to evaluate the airway show promise, routine use of imaging tools is not routinely used in primary care practice settings.

PSG AND OTHER TECHNIQUES FOR DIAGNOSING OSA

One important advancement in diagnosing SDB in children is the development of standardized, yet unvalidated, clinical diagnostic criteria for OSA that include symptoms and criteria for PSG.[89] Despite this development, arriving at a diagnosis of SDB does not help clinicians to determine who should be referred for treatment and how urgently treatment is warranted. PSG is considered the diagnostic gold standard for evaluating children and adolescents for SDB.[4] A PSG is a composite of simultaneously recorded physiologic variables, including respiratory variables, heart rate, and sleep stages. Each of the signals has inherent strengths and limitations. Advances in pediatric PSG over the past decade include advances in digital recording techniques, improvements in signal acquisition and processing, improved ability to measure various physiologic parameters, and recognition that a child-friendly atmosphere is necessary when dealing with children.[90] Another significant landmark advancement was the 2007 publication by the Academy of Sleep Medicine of an updated scoring manual for sleep and associated events, which provides explicit rules for scoring various parameters of the PSG in both adults and children[91] and standardizes the process of PSG review, interpretation, and reporting across centers. Although normative reference values have been determined for PSG in some children,[92–95] standardized values are not available for all age groups for PSG. Furthermore, the data generated by PSG does not speak to the various sociocultural or genetic aspects affecting sleep parameters. When diagnostic tests, such as PSG, are used to diagnose OSA in epidemiologic studies, the prevalence rates vary from 1% to 4%.[76] This likely under-represents the actual prevalence of SDB, because the usual basis for initiating PSG testing in clinical settings is the inherent assumption that the presence of habitual snoring (3 or more nights a week) is required.

There are inherent limitations in using the PSG as the sole diagnostic test for SDB. First, PSG is a de facto gold standard, because other methods of making a diagnosis of SDB, including history and physical examination, are inaccurate. PSG is a cumbersome, expensive, resource-intensive, and at times inconvenient, diagnostic procedure. Currently, the lack of sleep laboratories with expertise in studying children limits the accessibility of PSG in many regions, making it a relatively inaccessible test. Furthermore, PSG-derived respiratory parameters, including the apnea-hypopnea index and the number of desaturations and arousals, have not been found to reliably predict the degree of physical or psychological impairment in children with SDB.[42,49,96] More recent research has attempted to examine other specific aspects of sleep (staging, cycle length, and microarchitecture) in an effort to predict outcomes as well as neuro-cognitive dysfunction associated with SDB.[97–101]

The PSG does provide both objective qualitative and quantitative information regarding the key aspects of OSA, including hypoxia indices, hypercapnea, and degree of altered intrathoracic pressures as a measure of upper airway obstruction. It is important for clinicians to keep in mind that children symptomatic for SDB may have normal PSG parameters or, alternatively, that PSG parameters may be abnormal in relatively asymptomatic children. As a result, the American Academy of Sleep Medicine suggests that diagnosis of SDB in children should be based on the integration of the clinical data with the interpretation of the PSG by individuals qualified in the field of pediatric sleep medicine.

Alternatives to in-laboratory PSG are actively being sought, although currently their use is largely limited to research settings. It should be emphasized that each abbreviated testing modality, which uses a fraction or a single aspect of PSG (for example, limited channel monitoring, video, and so forth) or oximetry alone, results in a limited acquisition of information regarding respiratory parameters or sleep disruption or fragmentation, potentially leading to underdiagnosis or detection of only a subset of patients with severe disease.[102–104] The development of more sophisticated techniques evaluating autonomic nervous system tone that enable measurement of arousal and more subtle forms of sleep fragmentation in association with oximetry is worthy of further consideration.[105,106] To date, however, there is insufficient evidence supporting the use in clinical settings of unattended portable monitoring or abbreviated PSG testing in children over the traditional observed in-laboratory monitoring (PSG).

Finally, advances in proteonomics, genomics, and metabolomics have led to attempts to identify biomarkers in the blood or urine that could be used in a primary care setting to either diagnose children at risk for SDB or to identify the end-organ effect consequences of SDB,[49,51,107] such as urine protein metabolites. Preliminary findings suggest a high sensitivity and specificity with a combination of biomarkers and clinical diagnostic criteria.[108] This is still a research tool at present but may be a viable option for diagnosing children in the near future.

TREATMENT OPTIONS
Surgical Treatments

Enlarged tonsils and adenoids constitute just one aspect of the pathophysiologic mechanism of SDB in children, treatment considerations should take into account all possible underlying etiologic factors involved that may contribute to airway dysfunction in the individual child. In contrast to older studies in which adenotonsillectomy was reported as "curative" for OSA, more recent literature using PSG confirmation of outcomes as well as improvement in clinical parameters suggests that treatment failures are increasingly common.[21,109–111] For example, a recent multicenter longitudinal retrospective study of 578 children (mean age 6.9 ± 3.8 y) showed that adenotonsillectomy was curative, as defined by an apnea-hypopnea index less than 1 event per hour of total sleep time, in only 27.2% of children.[21] Treatment failures may be especially prevalent in children with obesity. For example, studies have suggested that predictive factors for failure of adenotonsillectomy include age and body mass index z-score. Not only are obese children at much higher risk of persistent SDB but also data show that the risk of perioperative complications is up to 40-fold higher in obese children with SDB undergoing surgery.[112] Unfortunately, the link between obesity and SDB has not been fully elucidated because some children, even though obese, respond to adenotonsillectomy. This implies a limited role for adenotonsillectomy in obese children much like in adult sleep apnea.

Other predictors of residual SDB across various studies[32,110,111] have included a preoperative apnea-hypopnea index as a marker of severity as well as asthma.[17,113] Asthma and obesity have also both been described as inflammatory states, so that those who are obese may have more asthma-like symptoms and, in turn, children with asthma tend to be more obese.[114] In the same retrospective cohort study,[21] it was found that among non-obese children, asthma also was a predictor of failure. The explanation could be that the underlying inflammation is the putative mechanism that results in an elevated apnea-hypopnea index, or SDB, or asthma. Allergic rhinitis was insignificant as a factor in that study but has previously been reported as a risk factor independent of asthma. The role of asthma and wheezing in association with tonsillar hypertrophy and SDB has been reported by several groups.[22,23,27]

These findings on cure rates in healthy and obese children are based on the assumption that every surgical technique for adenotonsillectomy is equivalent and that for every child, adenotonsillar hypertrophy is the underlying pathophysiologic mechanism for SDB. Current investigations, such as the Randomized Controlled Study of Adenotonsillectomy (CHAT), a multicenter study currently under way with recruitment of more than 200 children, ages 5 to 9, are evaluating the current standard of OSA treatment in affected children. In the CHAT study, an early treatment group will receive adenotonsillectomy within 1 month of enrollment whereas the watchful waiting group will receive treatment within 7 months. Desired outcomes include the determination of which children should be treated and how urgently they should be managed.

There may still be a role for adenotonsillectomy in as the correct first line intervention for a specific phenotype of obstructive sleep apnea in the spectrum of SDB.

Although adenotonsillectomy is beneficial for some children, what is unknown is the magnitude and duration of the benefit of this procedure. The change in growth velocity postsurgery (ie, an increase in height and weight), which used to be a marker for success, has instead been shown consistently across studies to be a predictor of recurrence.[18] One meta-analysis, encompassing 10 studies, evaluated growth and biomarker changes after adenotonsillectomy and found that height, weight, and biomarkers (insulinlike growth factor 1 and insulinlike growth factor binding protein) increased substantially post-treatment, indicating that some evidence of growth failure preoperatively may be related to SDB.[115] Long-term follow-up studies in children up to 3 years postsurgical intervention found improvements in SDB symptoms using validated SDB symptom questionnaires in the short term. Unfortunately, the initial improvements were found to have a tendency to decline.[81] In view of limited resolution or cure after treatment of SDB, it is often recommended that children have PSG preintervention and postintervention. This may not always be practical, however, especially when many children may not even have access to baseline testing. The significance of these shortfalls in diagnostic resources continues to be a challenge for many geographic regions in spite of the substantially increased number of accredited sleep facilities.

Nonpharmacologic Treatments

Positive airway pressure therapy

Those children and adolescents who do not have adenotonsillar hypertrophy, those who are not surgical candidates, or those who have different or additional risk factors for SDB require other treatment considerations. The common endpoint for these patients, irrespective of the underlying cause, is upper airway dysfunction and resulting airway collapse. Continuous positive airway pressure (CPAP) is used widely for treating adult SDB. In some instances, CPAP, even in children and adolescents, may be considered the first line of treatment in children for those who's surgery is considered high risk or contraindicated. The key to establishing successful CPAP use in children involves an approach that engages the child and family that includes an experienced multidisciplinary health care team that is knowledgeable in the management of children or adolescents with SDB.[116–118] Even with the involvement and support of professionals, the data suggest that compliance with treatment is found only in approximately 65% to 70%.[116,119,120] Although few empirical data exist about the efficacy of positive airway pressure therapy in children, the treatment is becomingly more widely used. In contrast to adults, there are few data about the role of positive airway pressure therapy in treating end-organ dysfunction for children, and further research is needed.[121]

Oral appliances

Limited ability to tolerate CPAP has resulted in patients and families seeking out alternative options for treatment of SDB. Oral appliances for treatment of patients with moderate sleep apnea or for those who do not tolerate CPAP have become more widely available for adults. The hesitation for widespread use in children has been the inability to anchor the devices to the primary teeth and potential long-term consequences on myofascial functioning and orthodontia. Oral appliances for treating SDB in children have only been studied in small samples to date, and although improved functional outcomes have been reported in one small study, this was not confirmed by PSG.[122] Rapid maxillary expansion has also been evaluated in a few patients and was reported to result in a significant decrease in the apnea-hypopnea index even up to a year after treatment.[123,124] Although initial results are promising, further research is warranted to determine the utility of such devices in the management of pediatric SDB outside of the research setting.[125]

Pharmacologic Treatments

Previously, nonsurgical treatment, including the use of either intranasal or oral steroids, was used largely as a bridge to surgery. Medications are now are being considered as a viable, routinely used treatment option for those with mild SDB or snoring. The mechanism for the efficacy of steroids has been studied in cell culture from the harvested tonsils of children with PSG-confirmed SDB.[126] A variety of steroids (decreasing in potency from fluticasone to budesonide to dexamethasone) have been shown to reduce proliferation rates of lymphoid tissue in a dose-dependent fashion and to enhance cellular apoptosis.[126] The efficacy of intranasal steroids (budesonide) has also been demonstrated in a rigorous level I trial for mild SDB; the effect persisted after the end of the 8-week medication trial.[127] Although the long-term benefit or the duration of treatment with this method is not known, it is likely beneficial for those children with mild SDB and/or with intermittent, seasonal symptoms, and for those for whom surgery is not indicated.

Tonsillar and adenoidal tissues have also been shown to express an abundance of leukotrienes and their receptors.[128] The leukotriene pathway plays a role in both the inflammatory signaling pathway and the proliferation of adenotonsillar tissue in children with OSA.[129] As a result, leukotriene receptor antagonists may be a useful adjunct in the array of treatments available for children with SDB.[129] A 16-week open-label trial of a leukotriene receptor antagonist in a few children with mild SDB showed an improvement in breathing parameters.[128] One small randomized controlled trial using a combination of intranasal steroids and leukotriene receptor antagonist for 12 weeks showed normalization of sleep parameters in 54% for those with residual SDB post-adenotonsillectomy.[130] What is yet to be determined is which children are most likely to benefit from these pharmacologic treatments either before, in combination with, or in lieu of surgery.

With a better understanding of the mechanisms that cause SDB at the cellular level, development of other novel treatments may be considered. More recently, tonsil proliferating genes are being evaluated. A protein called phosphoserine phosphatase seems to be elevated in those with adenotonsillar hypertrophy. Pharmacologic inhibition of the protein results in reductions in B-cell and T-cell proliferation and apoptosis. Therefore, the development of pharmacologic treatments targeted toward these phosphatases may open up novel forms of nonsurgical treatments for SDB.[131] With novel research such as this, the breadth of interventions for SDB is being expanded beyond the airway to a broader and global focus on prevention and treatment in vulnerable populations of children.

A PROPOSED STRATEGY FOR MANAGEMENT OF CHILDREN WITH SDB

To determine the optimal strategies for treating the SDB epidemic, physicians and allied health professionals must come together. As discussed previously, there are limits inherent to the current treatment paradigm in the ability to accurately diagnose and treat children with SDB using any combination of PSG criteria in association with clinical findings. One approach to treating children with SDB may be tiered access, beginning at the community level, where primary care providers would manage straightforward SDB (such as habitual snoring) with conservative measures and progressing to regionalized centers in which the most severe and complex cases would be managed by an interdisciplinary team. Before the implementation of such a strategy, several key conditions would need to be met. First, an infusion of infrastructure support, through trained personal and equipment, would be needed to manage the large number of existing cases expected in the health regions. Secondly, additional diagnostic methods for defining SDB that are less expensive and more sensitive and specific would need to be developed and validated for pediatric use. Alternatively, a set of criteria for diagnosis of SDB, involving key clinical features and selective laboratory markers of end-organ dysfunction to attempt to characterize severity and subsequent morbidity of SDB, could be developed.[49] This may prove a more feasible and cost-effective means of directing the care of children with SDB.

Irrespective of which particular method is chosen, addressing the management of these children and adolescents will require a concerted effort from sleep medicine professionals to come together to advance the science of pediatric SDB. The increased burden on health care resources, particularly related to obesity and SDB combined, is significant and will become one of the greatest challenges in the management for anyone who is involved in the care of children with sleep disorders.

SUMMARY

Awareness of the deep and dark lack of knowledge regarding the pathogenesis, consequences, and treatment of pediatric SDB has come to the forefront of child health in the past decade, highlighting the growing need for further scientific advances in the field. Although there have been many recent elegant studies that have shown the wide array of negative health effects resulting from end-organ dysfunction related to SDB, the full impact of these findings for affected individuals in the clinical setting has yet to be determined. Despite advances in the diagnosis of SDB, it is not always clear which children must or should be offered treatment and what that treatment should include. Furthermore, the most common current treatment modality for SDB in children, adenotonsillectomy, has come under increasing scrutiny regarding its long-term efficacy in treating SDB in children. Alternate treatment methods need to be investigated and developed because the evidence for current second-line treatments is limited. Development of novel targets that are aimed toward prevention of SDB in high-risk groups must also be explored. It is critical for practitioners caring for children to further bridge research gaps to enable identifying children at risk for SDB and preventing the potentially irreversible long-term sequelae of SDB in children.

REFERENCES

1. D'Andrea LA. Diagnostic studies in the assessment of pediatric sleep-disordered breathing: techniques and indications. Pediatr Clin North Am 2004;51(1):169–86.
2. Rosen CL. Obstructive sleep apnea syndrome in children: controversies in diagnosis and treatment. Pediatr Clin North Am 2004;51(1):153–67, vii.
3. Schechter MS, Section on Pediatric Pulmonology, Subcommittee on Obstructive Sleep Apnea Syndrome. Technical report: diagnosis and management of childhood obstructive sleep apnea syndrome. Pediatrics 2002;109(4):e69.
4. Section on Pediatric Pulmonology, Subcommittee on Obstructive Sleep Apnea Syndrome, American Academy of Pediatrics. Clinical practice guideline: diagnosis and management of childhood obstructive sleep apnea syndrome. Pediatrics 2002;109(4):704–12.
5. Mitchell RB, Pereira KD, Friedman NR. Sleep-disordered breathing in children: survey of current practice. Laryngoscope 2006;116(6):956–8.
6. Katz ES, D'Ambrosio CM. Pathophysiology of pediatric obstructive sleep apnea. Proc Am Thorac Soc 2008;5(2):253–62.
7. Arens R, Muzumdar H. Childhood obesity and obstructive sleep apnea syndrome. J Appl Physiol 2010;108(2):436–44.
8. Arens R, Sin S, Nandalike K, et al. Upper airway structure and body fat composition in obese children with obstructive sleep apnea syndrome. Am J Respir Crit Care Med 2011;183:782–7.
9. Arens R, Sin S, McDonough JM, et al. Changes in upper airway size during tidal breathing in children with obstructive sleep apnea syndrome. Am J Respir Crit Care Med 2005;171(11):1298–304.
10. Arens R, Marcus CL. Pathophysiology of upper airway obstruction: a developmental perspective. Sleep 2004;27(5):997–1019.
11. Huang J, Karamessinis LR, Pepe ME, et al. Upper airway collapsibility during REM sleep in children with the obstructive sleep apnea syndrome. Sleep 2009;32(9):1173–81.
12. Tapia IE, Bandla P, Traylor J, et al. Upper airway sensory function in children with obstructive sleep apnea syndrome. Sleep 2010;33(7):968–72.
13. Marcus CL, Katz ES, Lutz J, et al. Upper airway dynamic responses in children with the obstructive sleep apnea syndrome. Pediatr Res 2005;57(1):99–107.
14. Bhattacharjee R, Kim J, Kheirandish-Gozal L, et al. Obesity and obstructive sleep apnea syndrome in children: a tale of inflammatory cascades. Pediatr Pulmonol 2011;46(4):313–23.
15. Drager LF, Genta PR, Pedrosa RP, et al. Characteristics and predictors of obstructive sleep apnea in patients with systemic hypertension. Am J Cardiol 2010;105(8):1135–9.
16. Goodwin JL, Vasquez MM, Silva GE, et al. Incidence and remission of sleep-disordered breathing and related symptoms in 6- to 17-year old children—the

Tucson children's assessment of sleep apnea study. J Pediatr 2010;157(1): 57–61.

17. Nafiu OO, Green GE, Walton S, et al. Obesity and risk of peri-operative complications in children presenting for adenotonsillectomy. Int J Pediatr Otorhinolaryngol 2009;73(1):89–95.

18. Amin R, Anthony L, Somers V, et al. Growth velocity predicts recurrence of sleep-disordered breathing 1 year after adenotonsillectomy. Am J Respir Crit Care Med 2008;177(6):654–9.

19. Apostolidou MT, Alexopoulos EI, Chaidas K, et al. Obesity and persisting sleep apnea after adenotonsillectomy in greek children. Chest 2008;134(6):1149–55.

20. Kohler MJ, van den Heuvel CJ. Is there a clear link between overweight/obesity and sleep disordered breathing in children? Sleep Med Rev 2008;12(5):347–61 [discussion: 363–4].

21. Bhattacharjee R, Kheirandish-Gozal L, Spruyt K, et al. Adenotonsillectomy outcomes in treatment of obstructive sleep apnea in children: a multicenter retrospective study. Am J Respir Crit Care Med 2010;182(5):676–83.

22. Rosen CL, Larkin EK, Kirchner HL, et al. Prevalence and risk factors for sleep-disordered breathing in 8- to 11-year-old children: association with race and prematurity. J Pediatr 2003;142(4):383–9.

23. Sulit LG, Storfer-Isser A, Rosen CL, et al. Associations of obesity, sleep-disordered breathing, and wheezing in children. Am J Respir Crit Care Med 2005;171(6):659–64.

24. Hibbs AM, Johnson NL, Rosen CL, et al. Prenatal and neonatal risk factors for sleep disordered breathing in school-aged children born preterm. J Pediatr 2008;153(2):176–82.

25. Calhoun SL, Vgontzas AN, Mayes SD, et al. Prenatal and perinatal complications: is it the link between race and SES and childhood sleep disordered breathing? J Clin Sleep Med 2010;6(3):264–9.

26. Gozal D, Kheirandish-Gozal L, Capdevila OS, et al. Prevalence of recurrent otitis media in habitually snoring school-aged children. Sleep Med 2008;9(5):549–54.

27. Kaditis AG, Kalampouka E, Hatzinikolaou S, et al. Associations of tonsillar hypertrophy and snoring with history of wheezing in childhood. Pediatr Pulmonol 2010;45(3):275–80.

28. Peroni DG, Pietrobelli A, Boner AL. Asthma and obesity in childhood: on the road ahead. Int J Obes (Lond) 2010;34(4):599–605.

29. Kuehni CE, Strippoli MP, Chauliac ES, et al. Snoring in preschool children: prevalence, severity and risk factors. Eur Respir J 2008;31(2):326–33.

30. Arens R, Sin S, Willen S, et al. Rhino-sinus involvement in children with obstructive sleep apnea syndrome. Pediatr Pulmonol 2010;45(10):993–8.

31. Ekici M, Ekici A, Keles H, et al. Risk factors and correlates of snoring and observed apnea. Sleep Med 2008;9(3):290–6.

32. Costa DJ, Mitchell R. Adenotonsillectomy for obstructive sleep apnea in obese children: a meta-analysis. Otolaryngol Head Neck Surg 2009;140(4):455–60.

33. Capdevila OS, Kheirandish-Gozal L, Dayyat E, et al. Pediatric obstructive sleep apnea: complications, management, and long-term outcomes. Proc Am Thorac Soc 2008;5(2):274–82.

34. Tarasiuk A, Greenberg-Dotan S, Simon-Tuval T, et al. Elevated morbidity and health care use in children with obstructive sleep apnea syndrome. Am J Respir Crit Care Med 2007;175(1):55–61.

35. Tarasiuk A, Simon T, Tal A, et al. Adenotonsillectomy in children with obstructive sleep apnea syndrome reduces health care utilization. Pediatrics 2004;113(2):351–6.

36. Owens JA. Neurocognitive and behavioral impact of sleep disordered breathing in children. Pediatr Pulmonol 2009;44(5):417–22.
37. Khadra MA, McConnell K, VanDyke R, et al. Determinants of regional cerebral oxygenation in children with sleep-disordered breathing. Am J Respir Crit Care Med 2008;178(8):870–5.
38. Kheirandish L, Gozal D. Neurocognitive dysfunction in children with sleep disorders. Dev Sci 2006;9(4):388–99.
39. Gottlieb DJ, Chase C, Vezina RM, et al. Sleep-disordered breathing symptoms are associated with poorer cognitive function in 5-year-old children. J Pediatr 2004;145(4):458–64.
40. O'Brien LM, Gozal D. Neurocognitive dysfunction and sleep in children: from human to rodent. Pediatr Clin North Am 2004;51(1):187–202.
41. Friedman BC, Hendeles-Amitai A, Kozminsky E, et al. Adenotonsillectomy improves neurocognitive function in children with obstructive sleep apnea syndrome. Sleep 2003;26(8):999–1005.
42. Gozal D, Kheirandish-Gozal L, Bhattacharjee R, et al. Neurocognitive and endothelial dysfunction in children with obstructive sleep apnea. Pediatrics 2010; 126(5):e1161–7.
43. Miano S, Paolino MC, Urbano A, et al. Neurocognitive assessment and sleep analysis in children with sleep-disordered breathing. Clin Neurophysiol 2011; 122(2):311–9.
44. Tsaoussoglou M, Bixler EO, Calhoun S, et al. Sleep-disordered breathing in obese children is associated with prevalent excessive daytime sleepiness, inflammation, and metabolic abnormalities. J Clin Endocrinol Metab 2010; 95(1):143–50.
45. Beebe DW. Neurobehavioral morbidity associated with disordered breathing during sleep in children: a comprehensive review. Sleep 2006;29(9): 1115–34.
46. Bruni O, Ferri R. Neurocognitive deficits in pediatric obstructive sleep apnea: a multifaceted pathogenetic model. Sleep Med 2009;10(2):161–3.
47. O'Brien LM, Holbrook CR, Mervis CB, et al. Sleep and neurobehavioral characteristics of 5- to 7-year-old children with parentally reported symptoms of attention-deficit/hyperactivity disorder. Pediatrics 2003;111(3):554–63.
48. O'Brien LM, Mervis CB, Holbrook CR, et al. Neurobehavioral correlates of sleep-disordered breathing in children. J Sleep Res 2004;13(2):165–72.
49. Gozal D, Kheirandish-Gozal L. New approaches to the diagnosis of sleep-disordered breathing in children. Sleep Med 2010;11(7):708–13.
50. Giordani B, Hodges EK, Guire KE, et al. Neuropsychological and behavioral functioning in children with and without obstructive sleep apnea referred for tonsillectomy. J Int Neuropsychol Soc 2008;14(4):571–81.
51. Gozal D, Sans Capdevila O, McLaughlin Crabtree V, et al. Plasma IGF-1 levels and cognitive dysfunction in children with obstructive sleep apnea. Sleep Med 2009;10(2):167–73.
52. O'Driscoll DM, Foster AM, Ng ML, et al. Acute cardiovascular changes with obstructive events in children with sleep disordered breathing. Sleep 2009; 32(10):1265–71.
53. Li AM, Au CT, Ho C, et al. Blood pressure is elevated in children with primary snoring. J Pediatr 2009;155(3):362.e1–368.e1.
54. Amin RS, Carroll JL, Jeffries JL, et al. Twenty-four-hour ambulatory blood pressure in children with sleep-disordered breathing. Am J Respir Crit Care Med 2004; 169(8):950–6.

55. Amin R, Somers VK, McConnell K, et al. Activity-adjusted 24-hour ambulatory blood pressure and cardiac remodeling in children with sleep disordered breathing. Hypertension 2008;51(1):84–91.
56. Reade EP, Whaley C, Lin JJ, et al. Hypopnea in pediatric patients with obesity hypertension. Pediatr Nephrol 2004;19(9):1014–20.
57. Amin RS, Kimball TR, Bean JA, et al. Left ventricular hypertrophy and abnormal ventricular geometry in children and adolescents with obstructive sleep apnea. Am J Respir Crit Care Med 2002;165(10):1395–9.
58. Amin RS, Kimball TR, Kalra M, et al. Left ventricular function in children with sleep-disordered breathing. Am J Cardiol 2005;95(6):801–4.
59. Kalra M, Kimball TR, Daniels SR, et al. Structural cardiac changes as a predictor of respiratory complications after adenotonsillectomy for obstructive breathing during sleep in children. Sleep Med 2005;6(3):241–5.
60. Apostolidou MT, Alexopoulos EI, Damani E, et al. Absence of blood pressure, metabolic, and inflammatory marker changes after adenotonsillectomy for sleep apnea in greek children. Pediatr Pulmonol 2008;43(6):550–60.
61. Goldbart AD, Levitas A, Greenberg-Dotan S, et al. B-type natriuretic peptide and cardiovascular function in young children with obstructive sleep apnea. Chest 2010;138(3):528–35.
62. Kaditis AG, Alexopoulos EI, Karathanasi A, et al. Adiposity and low-grade systemic inflammation modulate matrix metalloproteinase-9 levels in greek children with sleep apnea. Pediatr Pulmonol 2010;45(7):693–9.
63. Li AM, Chan MH, Yin J, et al. C-reactive protein in children with obstructive sleep apnea and the effects of treatment. Pediatr Pulmonol 2008;43(1):34–40.
64. Gozal D, Crabtree VM, Sans Capdevila O, et al. C-reactive protein, obstructive sleep apnea, and cognitive dysfunction in school-aged children. Am J Respir Crit Care Med 2007;176(2):188–93.
65. Tauman R, O'Brien LM, Gozal D. Hypoxemia and obesity modulate plasma C-reactive protein and interleukin-6 levels in sleep-disordered breathing. Sleep Breath 2007;11(2):77–84.
66. Kheirandish-Gozal L, Capdevila OS, Tauman R, et al. Plasma C-reactive protein in nonobese children with obstructive sleep apnea before and after adenotonsillectomy. J Clin Sleep Med 2006;2(3):301–4.
67. Chaicharn J, Lin Z, Chen ML, et al. Model-based assessment of cardiovascular autonomic control in children with obstructive sleep apnea. Sleep 2009;32(7):927–38.
68. Bhattacharjee R, Gozal D. Cardiovascular disease and sleep disordered breathing: are children vulnerable? Sleep 2009;32(10):1251–2.
69. Bhattacharjee R, Gozal D. Metabolic disease in sleep disordered breathing: puberty! puberty! Sleep 2010;33(9):1133–4.
70. Bhattacharjee R, Kheirandish-Gozal L, Pillar G, et al. Cardiovascular complications of obstructive sleep apnea syndrome: evidence from children. Prog Cardiovasc Dis 2009;51(5):416–33.
71. Redline S, Storfer-Isser A, Rosen CL, et al. Association between metabolic syndrome and sleep-disordered breathing in adolescents. Am J Respir Crit Care Med 2007;176(4):401–8.
72. Verhulst SL, Jacobs S, Aerts L, et al. Sleep-disordered breathing: a new risk factor of suspected fatty liver disease in overweight children and adolescents? Sleep Breath 2009;13(2):207–10.
73. Korner A, Kratzsch J, Gausche R, et al. Metabolic syndrome in children and adolescents–risk for sleep-disordered breathing and obstructive sleep-apnoea syndrome? Arch Physiol Biochem 2008;114(4):237–43.

74. Kelly A, Dougherty S, Cucchiara A, et al. Catecholamines, adiponectin, and insulin resistance as measured by HOMA in children with obstructive sleep apnea. Sleep 2010;33(9):1185–91.

75. Khalyfa A, Bhushan B, Hegazi M, et al. Fatty-acid binding protein 4 gene variants and childhood obesity: potential implications for insulin sensitivity and CRP levels. Lipids Health Dis 2010;9:18.

76. Lumeng JC, Chervin RD. Epidemiology of pediatric obstructive sleep apnea. Proc Am Thorac Soc 2008;5(2):242–52.

77. Honaker SM, Gozal D, Bennett J, et al. Sleep-disordered breathing and verbal skills in school-aged community children. Dev Neuropsychol 2009;34(5):588–600.

78. Ravid S, Afek I, Suraiya S, et al. Sleep disturbances are associated with reduced school achievements in first-grade pupils. Dev Neuropsychol 2009; 34(5):574–87.

79. Perez-Chada D, Perez-Lloret S, Videla AJ, et al. Sleep disordered breathing and daytime sleepiness are associated with poor academic performance in teenagers. A study using the pediatric daytime sleepiness scale (PDSS). Sleep 2007;30(12):1698–703.

80. Cortese S, Faraone SV, Konofal E, et al. Sleep in children with attention-deficit/hyperactivity disorder: meta-analysis of subjective and objective studies. J Am Acad Child Adolesc Psychiatry 2009;48(9):894–908.

81. Weatherly RA, Ruzicka DL, Marriott DJ, et al. Polysomnography in children scheduled for adenotonsillectomy. Otolaryngol Head Neck Surg 2004;131(5):727–31.

82. Chervin RD, Hedger KM, Dillon JE, et al. Pediatric sleep questoinnaire (PSQ): validity and reliability of scales for sleep-disordered breathing, snoring, sleepiness, and behavioral problems. Sleep Med 2000;1:21–32.

83. Spruyt K, Gozal D. Pediatric sleep questionnaires as diagnostic or epidemiological tools: a review of currently available instruments. Sleep Med Rev 2011; 15(1):19–32.

84. Xu Z, Cheuk DK, Lee SL. Clinical evaluation in predicting childhood obstructive sleep apnea. Chest 2006;130(6):1765–71.

85. Arens R, McDonough JM, Costarino AT, et al. Magnetic resonance imaging of the upper airway structure of children with obstructive sleep apnea syndrome. Am J Respir Crit Care Med 2001;164(4):698–703.

86. Arens R, McDonough JM, Corbin AM, et al. Upper airway size analysis by magnetic resonance imaging of children with obstructive sleep apnea syndrome. Am J Respir Crit Care Med 2003;167(1):65–70.

87. Abramson Z, Susarla S, Troulis M, et al. Age-related changes of the upper airway assessed by 3-dimensional computed tomography. J Craniofac Surg 2009;20(Suppl 1):657–63.

88. Gozal D, Burnside MM. Increased upper airway collapsibility in children with obstructive sleep apnea during wakefulness. Am J Respir Crit Care Med 2004;169(2):163–7.

89. American Academy of Sleep Medicine. In: International classification of sleep disorders: diagnostic and coding manual. 2nd edition. Westchester (IL): American Academy of Sleep Medicine; 2005.

90. Beck SE, Marcus CL. Pediatric polysomnography. Sleep Med Clin 2009;4(3):393–406.

91. Iber C, Ancoli-Israel S, Chesson A, et al. The AASM manual for the scoring of sleep and associated events: rules, terminology and technical specifications. 1st edition. Chicago (IL): American Academy of Sleep Medicine; 2007.

92. Tapia IE, Karamessinis L, Bandla P, et al. Polysomnographic values in children undergoing puberty: pediatric vs. adult respiratory rules in adolescents. Sleep 2008;31(12):1737–44.

93. Montgomery-Downs HE, O'Brien LM, Gulliver TE, et al. Polysomnographic characteristics in normal preschool and early school-aged children. Pediatrics 2006; 117(3):741–53.

94. Traeger N, Schultz B, Pollock AN, et al. Polysomnographic values in children 2–9 years old: additional data and review of the literature. Pediatr Pulmonol 2005; 40(1):22–30.

95. Verhulst SL, Schrauwen N, Haentjens D, et al. Reference values for sleep-related respiratory variables in asymptomatic european children and adolescents. Pediatr Pulmonol 2007;42(2):159–67.

96. Kheirandish-Gozal L. What is "abnormal" in pediatric sleep? Respir Care 2010; 55(10):1366–76.

97. Chervin RD, Fetterolf JL, Ruzicka DL, et al. Sleep stage dynamics differ between children with and without obstructive sleep apnea. Sleep 2009; 32(10):1325–32.

98. Chervin RD, Malhotra RK, Burns JW. Respiratory cycle-related EEG changes during sleep reflect esophageal pressures. Sleep 2008;31(12):1713–20.

99. Chervin RD, Weatherly RA, Ruzicka DL, et al. Subjective sleepiness and polysomnographic correlates in children scheduled for adenotonsillectomy vs other surgical care. Sleep 2006;29(4):495–503.

100. Chervin RD, Burns JW, Subotic NS, et al. Correlates of respiratory cycle-related EEG changes in children with sleep-disordered breathing. Sleep 2004;27(1): 116–21.

101. Kheirandish-Gozal L, Miano S, Bruni O, et al. Reduced NREM sleep instability in children with sleep disordered breathing. Sleep 2007;30(4):450–7.

102. Kirk VG, Bohn SG, Flemons WW, et al. Comparison of home oximetry monitoring with laboratory polysomnography in children. Chest 2003;124(5):1702–8.

103. Nixon GM, Kermack AS, McGregor CD, et al. Sleep and breathing on the first night after adenotonsillectomy for obstructive sleep apnea. Pediatr Pulmonol 2005;39(4):332–8.

104. Nixon GM, Kermack AS, Davis GM, et al. Planning adenotonsillectomy in children with obstructive sleep apnea: the role of overnight oximetry. Pediatrics 2004;113(1 Pt 1):e19–25.

105. Foo JY. Pulse transit time in paediatric respiratory sleep studies. Med Eng Phys 2007;29(1):17–25.

106. Tauman R, O'Brien LM, Mast BT, et al. Peripheral arterial tonometry events and electroencephalographic arousals in children. Sleep 2004;27(3):502–6.

107. Snow A, Gozal D, Valdes R Jr, et al. Urinary proteins for the diagnosis of obstructive sleep apnea syndrome. Methods Mol Biol 2010;641:223–41.

108. Gozal D, Jortani S, Snow AB, et al. Two-dimensional differential in-gel electrophoresis proteomic approaches reveal urine candidate biomarkers in pediatric obstructive sleep apnea. Am J Respir Crit Care Med 2009;180(12): 1253–61.

109. Jones DT, Yoon MJ, Licameli G. Effectiveness of postoperative follow-up telephone interviews for patients who underwent adenotonsillectomy: a retrospective study. Arch Otolaryngol Head Neck Surg 2007;133(11):1091–5.

110. Mitchell RB, Kelly J. Outcomes and quality of life following adenotonsillectomy for sleep-disordered breathing in children. ORL J Otorhinolaryngol Relat Spec 2007;69(6):345–8.

111. O'Brien LM, Sitha S, Baur LA, et al. Obesity increases the risk for persisting obstructive sleep apnea after treatment in children. Int J Pediatr Otorhinolaryngol 2006;70(9):1555–60.

112. Fung E, Cave D, Witmans M, et al. Postoperative respiratory complications and recovery in obese children following adenotonsillectomy for sleep-disordered breathing: a case-control study. Otolaryngol Head Neck Surg 2010;142(6): 898–905.

113. Kuhle S, Urschitz MS, Eitner S, et al. Interventions for obstructive sleep apnea in children: a systematic review. Sleep Med Rev 2009;13(2):123–31.

114. Fiorino EK, Brooks LJ. Obesity and respiratory diseases in childhood. Clin Chest Med 2009;30(3):601–8, x.

115. Bonuck KA, Freeman K, Henderson J. Growth and growth biomarker changes after adenotonsillectomy: systematic review and meta-analysis. Arch Dis Child 2009;94(2):83–91.

116. Marcus CL, Rosen G, Ward SL, et al. Adherence to and effectiveness of positive airway pressure therapy in children with obstructive sleep apnea. Pediatrics 2006;117(3):e442–51.

117. Koontz KL, Slifer KJ, Cataldo MD, et al. Improving pediatric compliance with positive airway pressure therapy: the impact of behavioral intervention. Sleep 2003;26(8):1010–5.

118. Kirk VG, O'Donnell AR. Continuous positive airway pressure for children: a discussion on how to maximize compliance. Sleep Med Rev 2006;10(2): 119–27.

119. Uong EC, Epperson M, Bathon SA, et al. Adherence to nasal positive airway pressure therapy among school-aged children and adolescents with obstructive sleep apnea syndrome. Pediatrics 2007;120(5):e1203–11.

120. O'Donnell AR, Bjornson CL, Bohn SG, et al. Compliance rates in children using noninvasive continuous positive airway pressure. Sleep 2006;29(5):651–8.

121. Archbold KH, Parthasarathy S. Adherence to positive airway pressure therapy in adults and children. Curr Opin Pulm Med 2009;16(6):585–90.

122. Singh GD, Garcia-Motta AV, Hang WM. Evaluation of the posterior airway space following biobloc therapy: geometric morphometrics. Cranio 2007; 25(2):84–9.

123. Villa MP, Bernkopf E, Pagani J, et al. Randomized controlled study of an oral jaw-positioning appliance for the treatment of obstructive sleep apnea in children with malocclusion. Am J Respir Crit Care Med 2002;165(1):123–7.

124. Villa MP, Malagola C, Pagani J, et al. Rapid maxillary expansion in children with obstructive sleep apnea syndrome: 12-month follow-up. Sleep Med 2007;8(2): 128–34.

125. Miano S, Rizzoli A, Evangelisti M, et al. NREM sleep instability changes following rapid maxillary expansion in children with obstructive apnea sleep syndrome. Sleep Med 2009;10(4):471–8.

126. Kheirandish-Gozal L, Serpero LD, Dayyat E, et al. Corticosteroids suppress in vitro tonsillar proliferation in children with obstructive sleep apnoea. Eur Respir J 2009;33(5):1077–84.

127. Kheirandish-Gozal L, Gozal D. Intranasal budesonide treatment for children with mild obstructive sleep apnea syndrome. Pediatrics 2008;122(1): e149–55.

128. Goldbart AD, Goldman JL, Veling MC, et al. Leukotriene modifier therapy for mild sleep-disordered breathing in children. Am J Respir Crit Care Med 2005; 172(3):364–70.

129. Dayyat E, Serpero LD, Kheirandish-Gozal L, et al. Leukotriene pathways and in vitro adenotonsillar cell proliferation in children with obstructive sleep apnea. Chest 2009;135(5):1142–9.
130. Kheirandish L, Goldbart AD, Gozal D. Intranasal steroids and oral leukotriene modifier therapy in residual sleep-disordered breathing after tonsillectomy and adenoidectomy in children. Pediatrics 2006;117(1):e61–6.
131. Khalyfa A, Gharib SA, Kim J, et al. Transcriptomic analysis identifies phosphatases as novel targets for adenotonsillar hypertrophy of pediatric obstructive sleep apnea. Am J Respir Crit Care Med 2010;181(10):1114–20.

Restless Legs Syndrome, Periodic Leg Movements, and Periodic Limb Movement Disorder in Children

Jeffrey S. Durmer, MD, PhD[a,b],*, Ghazala H. Quraishi, MD[a]

KEYWORDS

• Restless legs syndrome • Periodic leg movements
• Periodic limb movement disorder • Children

The characteristic symptoms of restless legs syndrome (RLS) have been known for hundreds of years and were first reported in medicine in the 1600s. The Swedish neurologist Karl Ekbom formally described the clinical, epidemiologic, and pathophysiologic correlates of the condition in 1945.[1] The syndrome, initially referred to as Ekbom's disease, has 4 well-known clinical criteria: (1) an uncomfortable sensation or unexplainable urge to move the legs or other affected body part, (2) increasing symptoms with rest or inactivity, (3) a reduction of symptoms with movement, and (4) a circadian enhancement of symptoms in the evening and/or at night. Although Ekbom clearly reported all aspects of RLS occurring in children, it was not until the mid 1990s that the first case reports of children with RLS were published.[2,3] Since the 1990s, much has been discovered with regards to the genetics, potential pathophysiology, and epidemiology of RLS. Most of these advances have not included specific information about children. Correlations between RLS and select pediatric populations such as attention-deficit/hyperactivity disorder (ADHD) and iron deficiency have helped generate new perspectives with regards to potential pathophysiology. The lack of pediatric-specific information about RLS in the literature has led to the use of age-adjusted adult criteria for the diagnosis of this condition in children. Caveats added to the adult diagnostic criteria are meant to increase the selectivity of these criteria for children; however, the inherent difficulties of relying on verbal

[a] Fusion Sleep Medicine Program, 4245 Johns Creek Parkway, Atlanta, GA 30024, USA
[b] School of Health Professions, Department of Respiratory Therapy, College of Health and Human Sciences, Georgia State University, Atlanta, GA 30302-3995, USA
* Corresponding author. Fusion Sleep Medicine Program, Atlanta, GA.
E-mail address: jdurmer@fusionsleep.com

Pediatr Clin N Am 58 (2011) 591–620
doi:10.1016/j.pcl.2011.03.005
0031-3955/11/$ – see front matter © 2011 Elsevier Inc. All rights reserved.

descriptions in a linguistically developing population to diagnose a largely subjective disorder increase the clinical complexity of this task. An accurate diagnosis of RLS is clearly the single most important aspect of treating children with this condition. Clinicians must consider potential mimics, comorbid, and associated conditions when evaluating children with RLS symptoms. In addition, the use of more objective findings such as periodic leg movements in sleep (PLMS) and a family history of RLS increase diagnostic certainty.

The traditional differentiation of RLS from periodic limb movement disorder (PLMD) is noted in children as well as adults. The diagnostic criteria for PLMD include increased PLMS for age (>5 per hour) and a clinical sleep disturbance that is not accounted for by another sleep disorder, including RLS. Although evidence is limited to clinical case studies, data suggest that children may manifest PLMD at a younger age and develop RLS later in childhood.[4] Observations such as these help researchers to postulate the biologic relationships between the sensory and motor components of these seemingly distinct but related disorders. In addition, clinicians can use this sort of information to assist them with cases in which diagnostic certainty is in question. Because current pediatric RLS research is sparse, this article provides the most up-to-date evidence-based as well as consensus opinion-based information on childhood RLS and PLMD. Prevalence, pathophysiology, diagnosis, treatment, and clinical associations are discussed.

DESCRIPTION AND PREVALENCE OF RLS AND PLMD IN CHILDREN

The adult literature suggests that RLS and PLMD is common in northern European populations and may be one of the most common inherited conditions known. Surveys indicate that between 4% and 15% of adults in the United States and Western Europe have symptoms consistent with RLS.[5–7] In addition, there is evidence that up to 40% of adult RLS sufferers report symptoms starting in childhood or adolescence.[8,9] Variation in prevalence figures may represent genetic heterogeneity as well as differences in survey tools used to detect RLS in large populations. In 1995, the International Restless Legs Syndrome Study Group developed standardized criteria for the diagnosis of RLS in adults.[10] The 4 essential features (noted earlier) and 5 additional clinical features of RLS were noted in this seminal paper, including (1) sleep disturbance or daytime result of sleep disturbance, (2) involuntary movements during sleep (PLMS) and when awake, (3) neurologic examination findings consistent with secondary RLS, (4) clinical course and exacerbating factors, and (5) family history. Idiopathic or primary RLS was also distinguished from reactive or secondary RLS and its many causes including uremia, neuropathy, medications, anemia, and other causes for motor restlessness.

In 2003, a National Institutes of Health (NIH) workshop produced expert consensus criteria for the diagnosis of RLS in children and special populations.[11] Categories of diagnostic certainty for RLS in children aged 2 to 12 years were established based on varying levels of clinical evidence (**Fig. 1**). The use of adult criteria for adolescents (13-year-olds to 18-year-olds) was retained for the "Definite" diagnosis with the addition of "Possible" and "Probable" criteria as noted.

The adoption of diagnostic criteria in adults and children has led to less methodological variation between more recent studies. In addition, validated RLS inventories such as the International Restless Legs Syndrome Study Group rating scale,[12] which uses a 10-question, 40-point format to detect and rate the severity of RLS symptoms, have allowed investigators to use common tools in adult studies. Aside from tools used to assess populations, prevalence rates vary based on the age and gender of

DIAGNOSTIC CRITERIA FOR RLS IN CHILDHOOD AND ADOLESCENCE

Adult essential criteria

1. An urge to move the legs, usually accompanied or caused by uncomfortable and unpleasant sensations in the legs. (Sometimes the urge to move is present without the uncomfortable sensations and sometimes the arms or other body parts are involved in addition to the legs).
2. The urge to move or unpleasant sensations begin or worsen during periods of rest or inactivity such as lying or sitting.
3. The urge to move or unpleasant sensations are partially or totally relieved by movement, such as walking or stretching, at least as long as the activity continues.
4. The urge to move or unpleasant sensations are worse in the evening or night than during the day or only occur in the evening or night. (When symptoms are very severe, the worsening at night may not be noticeable but must have been previously present).

Definite RLS in children (age 2 to 12 years)

  1) the child meets all 4 essential criteria for RLS and
  2) there is a description, in the child's own words, consistent with leg discomfort. — Definite 1

or

  1) the child meets all 4 essential criteria for RLS and
  2) 2 of 3 criteria supportive of the diagnosis are present (see below). — Definite 2

Terms such as "wiggly", "tickle", "bugs", "spiders", "hurt", "shaky", "boo-boos", "want to run" and "a lot of energy in my legs" may be used by the child to describe symptoms. Age-appropriate descriptors are encouraged.

Supportive of the diagnosis:

  1)   sleep disturbance for age
  2)   a biologic parent or sibling has definite RLS
  3)   the child has a PLMS index of $\geq$ 5/hour on polysomnography

Definite RLS in adolescents (age 13 to 18 years)

  The 4 essential criteria as above.

For pediatric and adult RLS: The condition is not better explained by another current sleep disorder, medical or neurological disorder, mental disorder, medication use, or substance use disorder.

RESEARCH CRITERIA (age 0 to 18 years)

Probable RLS

  1) the child meets all 4 essential criteria for RLS, except #4: "worse in the evening or at night" and
  2) the child has a biologic parent or sibling with definite RLS. — Probable 1

or*

  1) the child is observed to have behavior manifestations of lower-extremity discomfort when sitting or lying, accompanied by motor movement of the affected limbs, the discomfort has characteristics 2, 3, and 4 of the essential criteria and
  2) the child has a biologic parent or sibling with definite RLS. — Probable 2

*This last category is intended for young children or cognitively-impaired children, who do not have sufficient language to describe the sensory component of RLS.

Possible RLS

  1) the child has periodic limb movement disorder (PLMD) and
  2) the child has a biologic parent or sibling with definite RLS but the child does not meet definite or probable childhood RLS definitions (as above).

Fig. 1. NIH workshop diagnostic criteria for RLS in children (2003). (*From* Picchietti D, Allen RP, Walters AS, et al. Restless legs syndrome: prevalence and impact in children and adolescents–The Peds REST Study. Pediatrics 2008;120(2):255; with permission.)

the individuals included. The risk of RLS is notably increased in women compared with men, with an overall 3:2 female/male ratio. More than the age of 65 years the prevalence of RLS is reported to increase to 10% to 20%.[13]

Recent studies that use common standard RLS criteria show a prevalence of approximately 8% to 20% in adults of varying age when all severity levels are included.[14,15] Investigations that separate prevalence rates for RLS based on clinical severity report that moderate to severe RLS (episodes twice or more per week with moderate to severe distress) occurs in 2.7% to 3.9% of adults.[14,16] Clinical relevance of RLS symptoms is important because it helps to establish our understanding of how many individuals may require medical attention. Using the NIH consensus criteria for the diagnosis of definite RLS in children, Picchietti and colleagues[17] recently investigated the prevalence of RLS in a large population of US and UK children. These investigators showed that 1.9% of 8-year-olds to 11-year-olds and 2% of 12-year-olds to 17-year-olds fulfilled these criteria. The prevalence of moderately severe RLS was noted in 0.5% and 1% of 8-year-olds to 11-year-olds and 12-year-olds to 17-year-olds, respectively. Compared with adult prevalence studies, no gender preference has been noted in the pediatric population. In addition, these investigators reported a strong potential genetic component in this study, with 71% of children age 8 to 11 years and 80% of children age 12 to 17 years with RLS symptoms noted to have at least 1 parent with RLS. The development of an RLS symptom severity scale for children and adolescents was recently developed using a semistructured interview for the detection of symptoms and severity.[18] No large-scale studies have yet used this tool or validated it in larger more varied populations.

From the mid 1990s to the present, a higher prevalence of RLS and PLMD has been noted in children with ADHD and symptoms consistent with ADHD.[3,19] Although most of the available research in this area is limited by sample sizes (n between 19 and 98 individuals), estimates for RLS in the ADHD pediatric population range between 10.5% and 44%. The estimated prevalence of ADHD in the RLS population is similarly increased between 18% and 26%.[20] The recent US and UK population-based prevalence study by Picchietti and colleagues[17] also shows a clear relationship between ADHD and RLS. In the US sample, 23.9% of 8-year-olds to 11-year-olds and 28.6% of 12-year-olds to 17-year-olds with definite RLS also had attention-deficit disorder (ADD)/ADHD diagnoses by self-report. The relationship between these 2 disorders is complex because sleep deprivation in children may mimic hyperactivity and/or inattention noted with ADD and ADHD. In addition, physiologic and genetic investigations suggest that these 2 conditions may share similar features such as iron deficiency and dopamine (DA) dysfunction. The potential comorbidity of these 2 conditions is clinically relevant but also provides a unique opportunity for RLS researchers to determine the common mechanisms that may help us to understand the complex pathophysiology of both RLS and ADHD.

PLMD and Periodic Leg Movements

Although PLMD is delineated as its own sleep-related movement disorder in the *International Classification of Sleep Disorders (2nd edition), Diagnostic and Coding Manual* (American Academy of Sleep Medicine, 2005),[21] many experts in the field consider PLMD as existing on a continuum with RLS. Clinically, both disorders are associated with low ferritin levels, respond to dopaminergic medications and share similar genetics. Both RLS and PLMS are noted predominately in White children versus other racial groups (odds ratio = 9.5).[22] With the recent discovery of the dose-dependent association between the BTBD9 gene on chromosome 6p and the presence of PLMS and low serum ferritin in RLS, there remains little doubt that the motor and sensory features of RLS are related.[23] Clinically, most RLS sufferers are noted to have PLMS on polysomnography (PSG) testing (reports vary from 80% to 100%), which suggests a common neural mechanism.[24] However, it is clear that PLMS occurs in other disorders such as narcolepsy, Parkinson disease and Tourette syndrome as well as in situations such as pregnancy and as a result of medications (eg, elective serotonin reuptake inhibitors [SSRIs] and tricyclic antidepressants [TCAs]).[25-27] Thus, although PLMS are clearly linked to RLS both clinically and genetically, they also represent a common neural pattern that can be activated in multiple ways.

Given the common and nonspecific nature of PLMS, some authorities question whether or not PLMS, and thus PLMD, should be considered abnormal. Speculation that PLMS are not necessarily pathologic is further supported by the fact that they are noted in association with other sleep disorders such as obstructive sleep apnea (OSA),[28,29] as a result of OSA treatment with continuous positive airway pressure,[30] and are noted to occur with sleep deprivation.[31] PLMS are also well known to increase with age and may be noted in up to 30% of adults more than 50 years old.[8]

Counter to the argument that PLMS represent normal motor activity are data that show the effect of PLMS and RLS on both health and psychological well-being. In adults, sympathetic overactivation is hypothesized to be at the heart of the association between PLMS and chronic cardiovascular conditions such as congestive heart failure and hypertension.[32] This relationship also is believed to increase the risk for stroke and may even increase the risk for insulin resistance and type II diabetes.[33] In addition, the effect of age on sympathetic hyperactivity suggests that younger individuals may show a more dramatic swing in autonomic response associated with PLMS, thus potentially predisposing them to even higher risks for cardiovascular and neurovascular complications.[34] With regards to the psychological and potential developmental effect of RLS and PLMD, several adult and pediatric studies show a strong relationship with ADHD, behavioral disorders, and cognitive deficits as well as depression and anxiety.[19,35-37] Overall, between 25% and 30% of children with RLS have symptoms consistent with ADHD and a similar number of children with ADHD fulfill the criteria for RLS.[17,38-41] Adults with RLS are noted to carry a 4-fold to 5-fold and 13-fold increased risk for depression and panic disorder, respectively.[42-45] In addition, multiple patient-reported outcome measures have shown the significant effect of RLS in adults, which is often noted as worse than the effects of hypertension, diabetes, and arthritis.[46-50] Although studies showing causation are lacking in the pediatric population and there are notably few in adults, the strikingly significant overlap with medical and psychological conditions as well as reduced quality-of-life measures should not be ignored by clinicians.

A critical component to the diagnosis of PLMD aside from increased PLMS (more than 15/h in adults and 5/h in children) is a noted sleep disturbance (eg, insomnia or fragmented sleep) and/or daytime dysfunction (eg, excessive daytime sleepiness or behavioral problem). The diagnosis of PLMD in children and adolescents is made by (1) PLMS documented by PSG and exceeding a periodic limb movement index (PLMi) of 5 per hour, (2) clinical sleep disturbance, and (3) the absence of another primary sleep disorder or reason for the PLMS (including RLS). Standardized criteria commonly used to score PLMS measured via bilateral anterior tibialis electromyography[31] were recently modified such that 4 movements must be scored in a row to qualify as periodic leg movements and each movement must be greater than 8 μV in amplitude, occur at a frequency of at least 5 seconds and no more than 90 seconds between movements, and individual movements must last at least 0.5 seconds and no longer than 10 seconds (**Fig. 2**).[51]

Despite the small number of investigations concerning PLMD and/or PLMS in children, there is ample evidence to support that PLMS in children, especially with RLS, are common. Studies suggest that between 8.4% and 11.9% of children may have PLMD.[52] In addition, substantial normative data in children from studies that record PLMS via PSG and/or accelerometry show that few children or adolescents have PLMi greater than 5/h.[22,52-55] Children with RLS are also noted to have similar rates

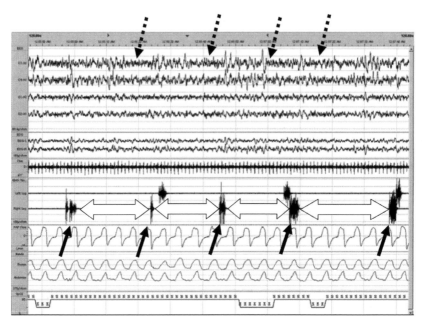

Fig. 2. PLMS depicted on 2-minute PSG recording page. Each solid arrow shows an individual PLM in a sequence of PLMS recorded with right and left anterior tibialis EMG. Block arrows denote the intermovement interval, which is consistent as noted in RLS. Also, note cortical arousals (*dashed arrows*) associated with PLMS, which are believed to confer excessive autonomic activity and sleep fragmentation.

of increased PLMS as noted in adults. One recent study of parent-child RLS pairs reported that 74% of children with definite RLS had PLMS in excess of 5/h.[56] Thus, when PLMS are noted in children clinicians are obligated to investigate the possibility of RLS.

When PLMS is measured, the PLMi represents only the number of specific leg movements that fulfill scoring criteria per hour of sleep (eg, 5/h). Another line of investigation with regards to PLMS is the variability of intermovement intervals rather than just the overall number of PLMS.[57] Studies of adults and children with RLS and other conditions in which PLMS are noted such as narcolepsy and ADHD show that subjects with RLS-related PLMS (and likely PLMD) have less intermovement interval variability that tends to cluster on average between 24 and 28 seconds between movements.[58–60] Speculation as to the cause of this particular frequency range includes potential neural pattern generators in the spinal cord and/or diencephalon. Differentiation of RLS-related PLMS from other PLMS that fulfill the classic periodic leg movement (PLM) criteria requires further research and may not only aid in the identification of children with RLS but also help us understand the physiologic relationship between RLS and PLMS.

Another important clinical point to consider is that PLMS show marked night-to-night variability in children, as well as adults, and may preclude diagnosis on a single-night PSG.[61]

Multiple-night testing may be necessary to quantify PLMS. Accelerometry has been found to correlate with PLMS on PSG in adults, and may be useful in the clinical evaluation of a child suspected of PLMD or RLS.[62,63] Accelerometry (also referred to as actigraphy and actometry) uses a small three-dimensional electronic gravitational force detector that is strapped to the ankle during sleep. It is well tolerated by children and can be used to sample movements in a continuous fashion for a predetermined number of hours or days. When used together with a sleep log and sleep question-naire, accelerometry data can reveal night-to-night variability, the effectiveness of therapy over time, and may also provide a more naturalistic measure of PLMS frequency and effect (**Fig. 3**).

An intriguing area of research that further shows the PLMD-RLS continuum comes from clinical evidence that some children manifest PLMD and/or PLMS years before the symptoms of RLS develop.[4] This retrospective longitudinal study of 18 children (mean age = 10.3 years) described the initial diagnosis of PLMD or probable/possible RLS and subsequent diagnosis of definite RLS at an average of 11.6 years later. In addition, the cohort had many of the comorbidities commonly associated with RLS such as ADHD, parasomnias, and a low serum ferritin level. Thus, despite the differen-tiation of RLS from PLMD on clinical grounds, it is clear that these disorders share much in terms of potential pathophysiology, comorbid conditions, and treatment. With additional research we may find that PLMD is not only on a continuum with RLS, but may represent a forme fruste of RLS.

PATHOPHYSIOLOGY AND GENETICS OF RLS/PLMD

The mechanisms leading to the motor and sensory symptoms of RLS/PLMD are unclear. Years of clinical observation show that almost all idiopathic cases of RLS

A

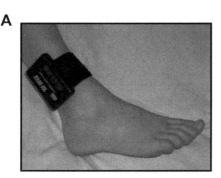

B

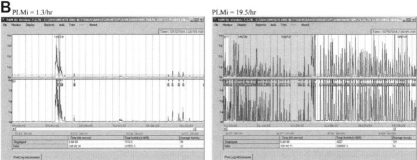

Fig. 3. Ambulatory accelerometry for the detection of PLMS. (*A*) A commercially available accelerometer on the right ankle of a 10-year-old girl. (*B*) Representative downloaded accel-erometry data from the same child after 2 nights of sleep. Note the significant difference in PLMS from 1 night to the next as depicted by increased number of vertical forces lines on the second night. Both data screens represent 30 minutes of acquired data, and the overall PLMi for that night of sleep is noted above each image. (*B*) PLMi = 1.3/h. PLMi = 19.5/h.

respond to dopaminergic medications such as levodopa (L-DOPA)/carbidopa, ropinir-ole, and pramipexole. This finding suggests a common monoaminergic mechanism within the central nervous system. Neuroanatomic and physiologic models of dience-phalic and spinal cord dopaminergic systems support an intriguing hypothesis that the sole source of DA to the spinal cord, the A11 hypothalamic cell group, may be a major contributor to the development of RLS.[64] In addition, animal models of DA receptor knockout mice (D_2-like receptors) suggest that loss of spinal cord gating of sensory input and motor output may also confer the symptoms of RLS/PLMD (**Fig. 4**).[65]

The association of iron deficiency with RLS was first noted by Nordlander in 1954.[66] Impairment of brain iron availability is now hypothesized to play a role in the pathogen-esis of RLS and PLMD based on several studies in animals and humans. Serum iron indices such as total iron, hemoglobin, and hematocrit values are usually within the normal ranges for age and gender in patients with RLS. Despite normal serum iron tests, brain iron deficiency has been implicated in human investigations using cerebro-spinal fluid analysis of iron and ferritin,[67,68] magnetic resonance imaging and ultra-sound of the substantia nigra,[69–71] and autopsy examination of brain tissue from patients with RLS.[72,73] The potential mechanistic link between iron deficiency and dysfunction of central dopaminergic systems is based on evidence that iron is a cofactor for the rate-limiting enzyme, tyrosine hydroxylase, in DA synthesis. It also plays a major role in the proper functioning of postsynaptic D_2 receptors, and iron defi-ciency has been noted to cause downregulation of striatum and nucleus accumbens DA receptors as well as dysregulation of DA vesicular release.[74–76] Correlations between peripheral serum ferritin levels and cerebrospinal ferritin levels in patients with RLS show that there is an association between the two, and that serum ferritin levels less than 50 ng/mL correlate with relative body iron storage deficiency.[67,68] Recent evidence suggests that lower ferritin status in RLS may not only correlate with alterations in DA metabolism and neural transmission but may also be associated with an inability to retain intracellular ferritin.[77] In a study of 24 women with early-onset RLS and a control group of 25 women without RLS, Earley and colleagues[77] reported that despite equivalent serum iron indices between the 2 groups (serum ferritin, hemo-globin, total iron-binding capacity, and percent saturation) marked differences were noted in 2 proteins associated with iron trafficking into cells (soluble transferrin receptor [TfR] and divalent metal transporter 1 protein [DMT-1]) and movement out of cells (ferroportin protein). As expected, patients with RLS had higher TfR and DMT-1 levels consistent with an increased cellular need for iron. Paradoxically, they also had higher ferroportin protein levels, which would normally signify high intracel-lular iron levels because this protein regulates iron efflux. This finding adds another dimension to the RLS-iron story in that patients with RLS seem to have an intracellular need for iron yet the proteins responsible for regulating cellular iron content create a situation tantamount to a leaky bucket.

Genetic investigations of RLS using twin concordance, family association, familial linkage, and genomic association methods over the past 10 years have created a more complex picture. Twin studies suggest a heritability of approximately 54% for RLS.[78] Additional genomic and linkage studies suggest that different sensorimotor phenotypes may be linked to different genetic loci.

Evidence from familial segregation analysis in Germany first showed that early-onset RLS (<30 years old) supported a single major gene model with an autosomal-dominant mode of inheritance.[79] Late-onset RLS did not have this effect and on further analysis 2 distributions of RLS were identified based on age of onset, with 26.3 years of age as the pivotal point. Conclusions from these studies suggest that RLS is primarily genetic in younger-onset groups but also includes an environmental

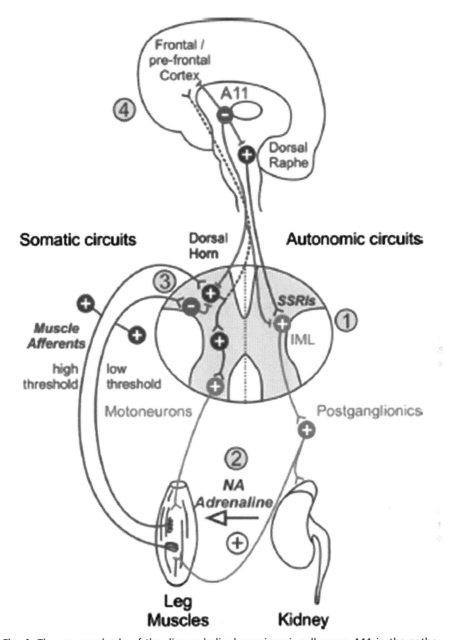

Fig. 4. The proposed role of the diencephalic dopaminergic cell group A11 in the patho-physiology of RLS. A11 neurons project caudally to inhibit the serotonergic dorsal raphe nucleus. This situation results in less sympathetic (autonomic) excitation via the spinal cord intermediolateral cell column (IML). A11 neurons also project to every level of the spinal cord and inhibit dorsal horn sensory transmission as well as the afferent projections of the IML (1). Loss of A11 dopaminergic inhibition (as proposed in RLS) results in increased sensory input to cortex (experienced as the uncomfortable sensation or urge to move), increased sensory activation of the spinal cord reflex arc (3) (causing PLMS), and increased sympathetic activity (2) (accentuating PLMS and associated medical conditions such as hypertension and proinflammatory states). The loss of rostral A11 projections also enhances cortically mediated sensory discomfort associated with RLS (4). (*From* Clemens S, Rye D, Hochman S. RLS revisiting the dopamine hypothesis from the spinal cord perspective. Neurology 2006;67:127; with permission.)

component for expression, which may be more relevant to the later-onset groups.[80] In addition, multiple studies report genetic anticipation, whereby subsequent generations show earlier and earlier age of symptom onset similar to trinucleotide repeat disorders such as spinocerebellar ataxia and Huntington disease.[81–83] No evidence supports a trinucleotide repeat mechanism in RLS.[84]

Familial linkage studies have identified 5 different genetic loci thus far. The power of these types of studies is that they are able to detect rare disease alleles but also they are limited by the specific nature of the phenotype used, small sample size, genetic heterogeneity, phenocopy, penetrance, and marker allele frequencies. The first genetic locus (RLS1) was discovered in French Canadian families. It is on chromosome 12p and shows a pseudodominant pattern of inheritance, with a high allele frequency and recessive inheritance pattern.[85,86] The second locus (RLS2) was found on chromosome 14q in a 3-generation Italian pedigree. Variable phenotypes or RLS with and without PLMS were included, and a common allele haplotype was identified for all positive family members.[87] Two separate familial linkage studies did not find this association in other multifamily studies, suggesting a rare allele in this case. The third RLS linkage locus (RLS3) was described in 2 extended US family pedigrees on chromosome 9p using the phenotype of early-onset RLS.[88] Subsequent transmission disequilibrium tests showed low significance in association with this loci and RLS in 2 other European populations.[89] RLS4 was discovered in a South Tyrolean population on chromosome 2q. This isolated population reduced the genetic and environmental heterogeneity inherent in other multicultural studies. An autosomal-dominant mode of inheritance with a founder effect was described in 3 of 18 families.[90] RLS5 was noted in French Canadian families on chromosome 20p in association with early age of RLS onset (<26.6 years). The autosomal-dominant pattern of inheritance in this study also pointed to a single common gene.[91] Thus, the nature of the numerous genetic loci (12p, 14q, 9p, 2q, and 20p) identified in these studies with varying RLS phenotypes suggests that RLS/PLMD is a complex genetic trait that interacts with environmental factors.

Given the number of different and possibly rare alleles discovered in familial linkage studies or RLS, it is essential to understand if there exist more common disease-associated alleles with particular RLS phenotypes. Genomic association studies using single-nucleotide polymorphisms are able to compare multiple phenotypes in a large genetic sample. The results of 2 major genomic RLS association studies were reported in 2007. An Icelandic investigation of 306 cases and 15,664 controls[23] reported that 3 genes (BTBD9, GLO1, and DNAH8) on chromosome 6p were associated with patients with RLS who had PLMS as a major component of their phenotype. This study showed a dose-dependent genetic association with PLMS and serum ferritin levels. Individuals with heterogenous alleles showed twice the risk for RLS with PLMS, whereas those homozygous for this variant had 4 times the risk. Serum ferritin levels were also lower in those with the addition of each BTBD9 allele. The second genomic study[92] was performed in a German cohort of 401 familial RLS sufferers and 1644 controls. The study was replicated in 2 separate French Canadian and German populations. Four genes (MEIS1-ch. 2p, BTBD9-ch 6p, MAP2K5-ch15q, and LBXCOR1-ch 15q) were associated with RLS. In both studies, BTBD9, which is widely distributed in the brain and body, was found to be associated with RLS.

Replication of these findings using all-adult RLS-related genomic genes and RLS1–5 loci in children have not shown any clear associations. One study specifically looking at gene variants in 23 children found an 87% positive family history of RLS and a trend toward association with MEIS1 and MAP2K/LBX-COR1 variants, but not BTBD9.[94] Another study looking at 386 children with ADHD and RLS did not find a genetic prevalence.[94] Additional genetic research focused on children and parents with varying RLS/PLMD phenotypes may help to elucidate pathophysiologic mechanisms associated with pediatric and early-onset RLS. In particular the use of enriched samples, such as ADHD, may add much to our understanding of the underlying biology.

DIAGNOSING RLS/PLMD IN CHILDREN

The consensus criteria for the diagnosis of RLS in children established by the NIH expert panel in 2003 include that a child should be able to state in their own words their experience of the symptoms. By raising the threshold for the RLS diagnosis in children, these criteria not only reduce potential misdiagnosis, but they also make the job of the clinician more challenging given the hurdles presented by the developmental process of verbal fluency. As previously discussed, up to 40% of adults first experience RLS symptoms in childhood and/or adolescence. In addition, PLMS and PLMD may precede the diagnosis of RLS in children by on average 11 to 12 years. Thus, clinicians must be prepared to take a careful nonleading history to elicit the salient features of RLS in children.

Recent evidence from the development of a multidimensional, self-administered, patient-reported outcome questionnaire to assess pediatric RLS symptom severity and effect has set the stage for a more systematic approach to diagnosing RLS in childhood.[18] The outcomes of this study show that children experience RLS symptoms within multiple domains including day and night RLS sensations, associated countermeasures (ie, rubbing or moving), and pain. In addition, the study provides a measure of effect on sleep and wake activities, as well as on emotions and tiredness. Although additional validation of this tool is needed, it is believed to provide a valid clinical measure of RLS symptoms in children 9 years of age or older, but should be used with some caution in children 6 to 8 years old. As part of this project children also communicated many nonverbal descriptions of their symptoms using a visual analogue scale and free-hand drawings of their experiences.[95]

Although drawings can be interpreted in many ways, this format may be of particular use in younger or less fluent children to provide a starting point for elaboration and description with a clinician or parent (**Fig. 5**).

When clinicians engage children in a discussion of RLS sensations it is important to provide a nonleading introduction to allow the child to express their experience. Given the genetic nature of RLS it is common that 1 or more adult family members may have noted similar symptoms or even have an RLS diagnosis themselves. For this reason clinicians should direct their inquiry first toward the child to help them recreate the last time they experienced something that "made it difficult to fall asleep" or "made it difficulty to lie in bed." Often the presenting complaint from the child or parent may not seem to be related to restlessness or kicking, which may prompt further RLS/PLMD questions. Complaints are generally related to difficulty falling asleep, not wanting to go to sleep, and occasionally difficulty remaining asleep. In some cases young children may not recall any RLS symptoms at all because they may not be experiencing them at the moment of the interview. When this occurs, clinicians can direct the conversation to the routine that precedes getting into bed, what happens on a typical night when the child gets into bed, and what happens on a typical night after they fall asleep. It is helpful to have the child describe their surroundings to contextualize the sleep-onset experience because this is one of the most common times for symptoms to emerge. If a complaint is noted at other times during the day, such as sitting in class at a desk, or while doing homework after school, the

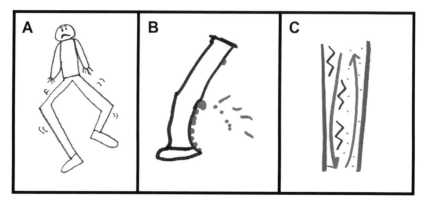

Fig. 5. Drawings of RLS symptoms in children of different ages. Diagnostic criteria for RLS in children requires a description of the symptoms from the child's perspective. This task is often difficult for adults as well as children, thus drawings may enhance diagnostic accuracy. (*A*) The RLS symptoms of an 8-year-old boy: "It's like my legs are wiggly...". (*B*) An 11-year-old girl describing her symptoms: "Well this picture shows like, see like it's ant bites that's kind of showing you that it's really hurting me like in those areas.". (*C*) The RLS symptoms of a 14-year-old girl: "I feel stuff going up and down my legs where it just tingles. And that's more when it starts feeling like a little numb and then these represent my tingles. And then the red would be just when it hurts." (*From* Picchietti DL, Arbuckle R, Abetz L et al. Pediatric restless legs syndrome: analysis of symptom descriptions and drawings. J Child Neurol 2011; 26, in press.)

clinician can use the same techniques to recreate the context in order help the child to remember how they felt and to provide their own description. Children use many imaginative ways to describe RLS symptoms such as "soda bubbles in my legs" and "ants biting my leg." However, it is more common that children are unable to describe a sensation, and like adults they may use descriptions such as "just want to move" or "got to kick."[17,96] The terms used by children to describe the sensory experience of RLS can be further elaborated on by many forms of nonverbal communication such as drawings (see earlier discussion). It is not common for children to use the term "urge to move" in relationship to their description of RLS symptoms, but it is helpful to allow them to physically demonstrate compensatory maneuvers such as wiggling, rubbing, kicking, hitting, and even "constantly moving to find the cool spot." After exhausting direct inquiry with a child it is sometimes helpful to incorporate the parent into the discussion to remind the child of bedtime rituals and activities that may jar the child's recall. It is a complex medical art to direct the discussion toward understanding if the cause for a sleep disturbance is related to a sensory discomfort; however, it is more common for children and parents to complain of the secondary effects of RLS than the primary sensory discomfort required for the diagnosis.

The remaining diagnostic criteria including timing of the symptoms, exacerbating conditions, and compensatory maneuvers can be elicited by focusing on the bad-feeling symptom that the child describes. With regards to timing, it is common to note some degree of classroom difficulty as noted by the child, the child's teacher, or parent. Difficulty sitting quietly at a desk and paying attention, as well as irritability and hyperactivity, may be notable symptoms of children with RLS. The overlap with ADHD-like symptoms is often brought up in this context and a helpful clinical pearl is to remember that the hyperactivity noted with RLS is related to an internal sensory discomfort resulting in excessive motor activity. The child with ADHD may also experience RLS, but the hyperactivity noted with ADHD is related to an external reaction to the environment resulting in variable attention. There is much overlap between these 2 clinical populations and it is important to consider the basis for excessive motor activity given that treatment strategies may be dramatically different.

Whether using the NIH consensus criteria or a semistructured interview clinicians must be aware of conditions that can mimic RLS symptoms in children. Identifiable causes of RLS symptoms are well described in the literature (often referred to as secondary RLS) and it is important to eliminate these as potential causes because treatment may vary widely. Some of the more commonly associated conditions in adults such as diabetes and pregnancy are not so common in children. Therefore, it is important to recognize other causes including joint pain associated with Osgood-Schlatter disease and arthritis, dysasthesias related to peripheral neuropathy or radiculopathy, akathesia related to antidopaminergic medications, and cutaneous pain related to dermatitis or rashes. As mentioned earlier, there is a large overlap between children with ADHD and RLS, and identification of one should prompt clinicians to ask about symptoms of the other. Another commonly associated condition with RLS is well known as growing pains. Studies of children diagnosed with growing pains unrelated to any other identifiable disorder commonly report a strong family history of RLS, and in most cases fulfill the diagnostic criteria for RLS.[97] The prevalence of growing pains in children aged 4 to 6 years measured with validated instruments is as high as 37%.[98] Thus, a description of typical growing pains in children with either a family history of growing pains or RLS should provide a cue for clinicians (**Box 1**).

Children with RLS may also present with symptoms of other sleep or medical/psychiatric disorders. Irritability, depression, anxiety, and hyperactivity may be noted in children with RLS and may be secondary to sleep deprivation. They may also be symptoms of comorbid conditions such as panic disorder, generalized anxiety disorder, ADHD, oppositional defiant disorder, and depression. Parasomnias such as sleep walking and sleep terrors, sleep-related movement disorders such as rhythmical movement disorders, and behavioral and psychophysiologic insomnias also may be the presenting symptoms in some cases of childhood RLS.[4,96,99] It is the clinician's task to determine if a sleep disorder is at the heart of the primary presenting symptoms or if another disorder is in play. The effects of sleep deprivation whether caused by RLS/PLMD or another sleep or medical disorder can exacerbate mood and behavioral symptoms in children. As part of the workup and treatment of RLS/PLMD it is important to make note of mood and behavioral symptoms. By doing this any therapy can be judged with regards to its effects on both primary and secondary symptoms.

A critical component in the diagnosis of both RLS and PLMD is the use of objective information. Reliance on subjective sensory-motor descriptions from a child, or adult, may suffice in straightforward cases. However, when there is a question of diagnostic certainty or the possibility of comorbid conditions, it is appropriate to collect data that are less subject to interpretation. In the future genetic testing may become a reality for RLS, but currently the most objective evidence for this diagnosis is family history and sleep testing. As noted earlier, RLS shows genetic anticipation and a pseudodominant mode of transmission. Thus, the idiopathic form of pediatric RLS is likely to occur in families with a history of this or similar symptoms. Clinicians should probe for a family history of RLS, PLMD, or other sleep-related complaints, which can sometimes lead to the discovery that a previously noted family trait is unrecognized RLS.

Although the clinical symptoms of RLS may be readily diagnosed without testing, it is not possible to determine the presence or effect of PLMS on a child's sleep without a test. Parental reports and even clinical evaluation by trained sleep clinicians is not adequate to predict the presence of PLMS. In addition, sleep testing is required

Box 1
Potential identifiable causes of RLS symptoms

Musculoskeletal

    Osgood-Schlatter

    Muscle soreness

    Injury (eg, sprain, bruise, strain)

    Cramps

    Arthritis

    Connective-tissue disorders (eg, plantar fasciitis)

    Myopathy

Neurovascular

    Positional discomfort (eg, pins and needles)

    Peripheral neuropathy

    Radiculopathy

    Myelopathy

    Sickle cell disease

    Multiple sclerosis

    Neoplasm

Cutaneous

    Dermatitis

    Dry skin

Endocrine

    Diabetes

    Thyroid disease

Substances

    Antidopaminergic medications

    SSRI medications

    Tricyclic medications

    Caffeine

    Alcohol

Other

    ADHD

    Iron deficiency

    Oppositional defiant disorder

    Pregnancy

    Celiac disease

    Uremia

when symptoms suggest other sleep disorders such as sleep-disordered breathing (SDB) or parasomnias.[100,101] Traditionally, the use of PSG testing with bilateral anterior tibialis electromyography (EMG) is used to detect PLMS. As noted earlier, because of night-to-night variability as well as the limitations of testing young or neurobehaviorally impaired children in a laboratory setting, the usefulness of PSG for the detection of PLMS can be difficult. In some cases the use of accelerometry may be preferred, or used in addition to PSG testing. Provided that the testing team has technical and clinical expertise using accelerometry, the application of this technology can be helpful in the diagnosis and monitoring of therapy over time.

RLS AND ADHD

The noted clinical relationship of RLS with ADHD in children provides an important connection for researchers and clinicians interested in both of these disorders. ADHD is a common childhood behavioral disorder. The estimated worldwide prevalence is about 5% in school-aged children. According to the *Diagnostic and Statistical Manual of Mental Disorders (Fourth edition-text revised)* ADHD is characterized by developmentally inappropriate symptoms of inattention, hyperactivity, and/or impulsivity, with the onset before age 7 years, and impaired functioning in 2 or more settings (ie, home and school). Sleep disturbances are more prevalent in children with ADHD compared with normal subjects including nonrapid eye movement sleep parasomnias, rhythmical movement disorders, insomnia, and RLS. Other than stimulant-related insomnia, children treated for ADHD do not suffer significant medication-related sleep problems. Studies using subjective parental reports indicate that children with ADHD commonly have more bedtime resistance, sleep-onset difficulties, night awakenings, restlessness, excessive movement, difficulties with waking in the mornings, and daytime sleepiness compared with controls. Objective sleep measures show increased sleep disruption in children with ADHD including PLMS, SDB, increases in sleep-onset latency, and the number of stage shifts per total hours of sleep.[102,103]

Several theories are postulated concerning the high correlation between RLS/PLMD and ADHD. The typical symptoms of sleep-deprived children can mimic the symptoms of hyperactivity and inattention noted in ADHD. This finding may help to explain why the higher incidence of other sleep disorders, such as SDB, in ADHD as well. In terms of SDB there is also the added possibility that the intermittent hypoxia or increased number of central nervous system arousals induced by upper airway collapse may also contribute to DA dysfunction during development. Experiments using episodic intermittent hypoxia performed briefly during the neonatal period in animals show consistent long-term deficits consistent with ADHD, including reductions in executive function and working memory as well as increased hyperactivity. Immunohistochemical studies of these animals show significant increases in D_1 receptor and antivesicular monoamine transporter 2 labeling in the striatum, which is consistent with depressed DA signaling.[104] In addition, this same manipulation has also been noted to result in decreases in extracellular DA and increased intracellular sequestration of DA in nigrostriatal neurons. This finding provides an important neuropharmacologic model to help explain the noted responsiveness of ADHD-like symptoms to amphetamine stimulants.[105] Although it is difficult to generalize the results from an animal model to a clinical population, it is , an intriguing hypothesis to suggest that mild changes consistent with SDB may contribute to dopaminergic dysfunction and disorders dependent on DA systems such as ADHD and RLS.

The DA connection between ADHD and RLS is further supported by converging areas of genetic evidence that the DA system may play a major role in both disorders.

ADHD, like RLS, is a complex neurodevelopmental disorder with multiple subtypes that likely represent dysfunction within several neural systems. The most frequently associated candidate genes with ADHD are those in the DA system. This relationship is further supported by evidence that: (1) the most effective treatments for ADHD are stimulants that block DA transport, (2) neural imaging findings in ADHD show neuro-anatomic and physiologic dysfunction of the frontostriatal system, and (3) executive function deficits noted in ADHD are secondary to dopaminergic transmission abnormalities. Genes associated with ADHD include the D_4 DA reception gene (*DRD4*), D_5 DA receptor gene (*DRD5*), D_1 DA receptor gene (*DRD1*), and the DA transporter gene (*DAT1*).[106–112] Additional genetic associations are also noted within DA metabolic pathways including the *DDC* gene, which catalyzes the conversion of DOPA to DA, the *DβH* gene, which regulates an enzyme responsible for the conversion of DA to norepinephrine, a polymorphism of the catechol-*O*-methyl transferase (COMT) gene, and the *MAOA* gene.[113] There are also associations between ADHD and other monoaminergic genes responsible for noradrenergic and serotonergic activity. In terms of phenotype-genotype relationships, it is notable that despite the increasing body of ADHD candidate genes, no studies have attempted to determine the relationship of RLS-ADHD phenotypes with any of the known ADHD genetic markers.

Another common factor linking RLS and ADHD is the association of iron deficiency in both conditions. Studies of children with RLS, ADHD, or both have shown a relationship with low iron states, as determined by serum ferritin measures when compared with age-matched and gender-matched controls.[38,103,114,115] Deficits in serum ferritin are often missed even on testing because the normal ranges occur well below the levels at which RLS and PLMD symptoms tend to emerge or worsen (<50 ng/mL). Treatment of relative iron deficiency using oral iron repletion in children with ADHD has been studied in a small, randomized, double-blind, placebo-controlled trial.[116] Iron treatment shows benefits in both clinical global impression scales and ADHD rating scales. Because of the limited size of the trial (n = 23) additional studies are required to understand the applicability of this therapy in various subpopulations of children with ADHD. In terms of children with RLS and ADHD, a separate study by the same group[115] showed that children with RLS and ADHD have lower ferritin levels than children with ADHD alone, and they have more severe symptoms of ADHD. Clinical application of iron therapy for ADHD and/or RLS based on these small samples should be considered, but only on a case-by-case basis. These data coupled with evidence from iron/DA pathophysiology, DA genetics, and pharmacotherapy with dopaminergic agents suggest that ADHD and RLS may not only co-occur in specific subpopulations, but actually represent a comorbid condition resulting from the same neural system dysfunction.

TREATMENT AND MANAGEMENT OF RLS/PLMD

Along with the diagnosis of RLS or PLMD, many children and parents report symptoms of behavioral sleep disorders that may have become ingrained in the family's or child's approach to sleep. Behavioral insomnias (including the sleep-onset association type and limit-setting type) and inadequate sleep hygiene as well as insufficient sleep can all result in symptomatic worsening, and reduce the effectiveness of treatments for RLS/PLMD. Therefore, the initial approach to treating RLS/PLMD revolves around education to establish the proper behaviors (sleep-wake routines and preparation), environment (reduced noise, light, novelty, and temperature), avoid exercise and excitement before bed, and control food and drink at bedtime. The use of cognitive and physical countermeasures for RLS symptoms such as physical relaxation techniques, warm baths, and cognitive restructuring may be helpful during the sleep-onset routine. In addition to behavioral strategies clinicians should focus on removing activators of RLS symptoms such as sleep deprivation, specific medications (such as SSRIs, TCAs, antiemetics, and antihistamines) and substances like caffeine and nicotine. The more structure that can be instituted with regards to the dos and don'ts of sleep-wake behavior, the easier it is for a child and a family to become successful.

Given the evidence of relative iron body storage deficits in children with RLS, it is practical to obtain serum tests before embarking on any particular therapy. Studies of familial RLS show that aside from an earlier age of onset, patients typically have lower serum ferritin levels, which predict therapeutic challenges such as augmentation to dopaminergic therapies.[117,118] Typical serum tests include ferritin, total iron-binding capacities, transferrin, complete blood count (CBC), and soluble TfR. At a minimum the serum ferritin with a CBC should be obtained. Whenever testing serum ferritin levels it is important to remember that infection, liver disease, cancer, or significant stress (eg, if the patient is postoperative) can increase ferritin levels, creating an inaccurate result. In addition, serum ferritin levels may be decreased without overt iron deficiency anemia, as manifested by a low hemoglobin or hematocrit level. Current recommendations for iron supplementation in children with RLS symptoms include any child with a serum ferritin less than 50 ng/mL.[119] The basis of this recommendation is partially related to the finding that in adult patients with RLS a serum ferritin less than 50 ng/mL is associated with significantly worse RLS symptoms.[120,121] In addition, it seems that the effect of iron therapy is related to the ferritin level before treatment begins. Patients with lower ferritin levels (<50 ng/mL) are noted to be significantly more responsive to iron repletion therapy. The goal of therapy is to achieve a level of 80 to 100 ng/mL because saturation of peripheral iron stores typically occurs in this range. Before iron repletion clinicians should obtain a history of any hemachromatosis in the family and consider genetic testing for this condition if applicable.

Iron repletion therapy has been shown to treat both RLS and PLMS symptoms in children.[99,122,123] Although extensive clinical data are lacking with regards to this therapy, both oral and intravenous (IV) iron repletion for RLS is available. Oral supplementation may take 3 or more months to result in adequate ferritin increases. Dosing is usually 3 to 6 mg/kg/d and should be taken on an empty stomach with vitamin C for improved absorption. Many different oral iron supplements are available for children, including liquids and tablets, with the most common side effect being gastrointestinal symptoms. To help reduce side effects and maximize absorption supplements should be taken without calcium-containing foods or drinks. Repeat serum iron testing is recommended within 2 to 3 months to ensure iron levels do not become excessively high and that therapy is working. Once serum ferritin levels reach 80 to 100 ng/mL iron therapy may be discontinued or tapered. Some clinicians continue a low-maintenance iron supplementation with vitamins, but no data regarding the effectiveness of this strategy are available.

Studies using IV iron preparations show significant effects on serum ferritin levels and in some cases complete amelioration of RLS symptoms in adults.[124–126] There are no similar studies in children with IV iron therapy. The effects of serial iron infusions have been studied and illustrate an important point of iron therapy. With each infusion there is a reliable increase in ferritin levels, followed by a progressively longer decrease in ferritin level over successive treatments (**Fig. 6**). This finding is clinically relevant with any form of iron therapy because a return to previously low ferritin levels may follow the initial weeks of therapy. Therefore, serum ferritin retesting should be considered if a child reports a return of RLS symptoms or over time to ensure that ferritin levels remain more than 50 ng/mL. Clinically, the use of IV iron dextran compounds is noted

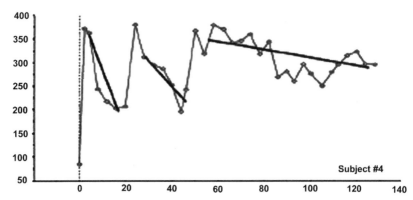

Fig. 6. Serum ferritin response to 3 serial IV ferrous dextran infusions over a 130-week period. Infusions were performed at approximately week 1, 24, and 50. With serial treatments there is a more prolonged response, as noted by the average slope line for the 3 post-infusion periods. (*From* Early CJ, Heckler D, Allen RP. Repeated IV doses of iron provide effective supplemental treatment of restless legs syndrome. Sleep Med 2005;6:304; with permission.)

to result in a superior outcome versus other formulations. In addition, with the advent of low-molecular-weight IV dextran many of the previously noted hypersensitivity and allergic reactions to the dextran molecule can be avoided. Because IV iron infusion does require close monitoring for allergic reactions, a standardized protocol in an infusion unit that includes a test dose and pretreatment to avoid complications is suggested.

Given the time period required for ferritin levels to improve, particularly with oral iron repletion, additional treatments may be required for children if their symptoms affect their sleep and daytime activities on a regular basis. The use of pharmacotherapy in children for RLS is left to the clinician, parent, and child because no medications approved by the US Food and Drug Administration (FDA) are available. The usefulness of medication depends on the nature of the symptom frequency and intensity. Much like migraine headache therapy, occasional symptoms, occurring less than weekly, may be treated on an as-needed basis rather than with daily prophylactic treatment. Studies that implement a daily medical therapy in adults with RLS do so in moderately severe RLS (2 or more d/wk). This suggests that prophylactic use should be reserved for cases in which at least 2 or more days per week are affected by symptoms. Another important factor when considering medical intervention is the intensity of symptoms. Symptoms that are painful, intrusive in sleep, or that cause daytime dysfunction are more likely to engender a medical response than those that can be controlled with nonpharmacologic countermeasures. Because there are no FDA-approved medical interventions for children with RLS, it is important for clinicians to understand the features of medical therapy that can be gleaned from adult studies to help parents and children make as much of an informed decision as possible.

There are 5 general categories of medications commonly prescribed for RLS: dopaminergic agents, antiadrenergics, opioids, anticonvulsants, and benzodiazepines.

Dopaminergics

The most widely used and successful medical therapies for RLS are dopaminergic medications. The diagnostic criteria for adult RLS even include the response to a dopaminergic medication as a supportive feature. Treatment with DA therapy results in control of both sensory and motor symptoms. Also, the use of dopaminergic medications has proved successful in numerous case reports and small open-label studies of children with RLS with and without ADHD.[4,93,127–134] No large-scale double-blind, placebo-controlled trial with dopaminergic medications in children has been performed.

L-DOPA was the first DA agent shown to be effective for both the sensory and motor symptoms of RLS.[135] Because of the short half-life of L-DOPA (1.5–2 hours) it is usually reserved as an abortive or diagnostic agent and is not routinely used for prophylaxis.[24] In addition to the short-action of L-DOPA there is also a higher reported rate of augmentation, which may affect up to 60% to 73% of users.[136,137] Because RLS augmentation is noted to occur only with the use of dopaminergic agents it is important to understand this concept before prescribing it to patients.

As defined by the Max Plank Institute criteria, augmentation includes 3 basic features and 2 additional features (**Box 2**). Augmentation is a shift of RLS symptoms in time (earlier), location (other body parts), and/or intensity (severity or quality) during pharmacologic therapy, and which is reversible after withdrawal of the therapy. The

---

Box 2
The Max Plank Institute criteria for augmentation

PREAMBLE

Augmentation is a worsening of RLS symptom severity experienced by patients undergoing treatment of RLS. The RLS symptoms in general are more severe than those experienced at baseline.

1. Basic features (all of which need to be met):

    a. The increase in symptom seventy was experienced on 5 out of 7

    b. The increase in symptom severity is not accounted for by other factors such as a change in medical status, lifestyle, or the natural progression of the disorder

    c. It is assumed that there has been a previous positive response to treatment.

In addition, either B or C or both have to be met:

2. Persisting (although not immediate) paradoxic response to treatment: RLS symptom severity increases some time after a dose increase, and improves some time after a dose decrease

3. Earlier onset of symptoms:

    a. An earlier onset by at least 4 hours

    OR

    b. An earlier onset (between 2 and 4 hours) occurs with one of the following compared with symptom status before treatment:

        i. Shorter latency to symptoms when at rest

        ii. Spreading of symptoms to other body parts

        iii. Intensity of symptoms is greater (or increase in periodic limb movements [PLM] if measured by polysomnography [PSG] or the suggested immobilization test [SIT])

        iv. Duration of relief from treatment is shorter

    Augmentation requires criteria A + B or A + C or A + B + C to be met

From Garcia-Borreguero D, Williams A. Dopaminergic augmentation of restless legs syndrome. Sleep Med Rev 2010;14:340; with permission.

occurrence of augmentation is related to lower serum ferritin levels, extended time on a therapy, and the use of dopaminergic medications.[138] It is important to distinguish augmentation from tolerance, early-morning rebound, neuroleptic-induced akathesia, and RLS disease progression.[137] Tolerance, also referred to as tachyphylaxis, is a reduction in medication effectiveness that necessitates an increase in dose. It is unclear if this is related to the development of augmentation, but it has been reported to precede some cases of augmentation in adults. Early-morning rebound occurs in up to 35% of adult patients with RLS because of a wearing-off effect and shorter half-life medications. Neuroleptic-induced akathesia is distinguished from augmentation by the inner sense of restlessness rather than discrete limb restlessness. Also it is usually caused by DA-blocking agents rather than dopamimetics and does not follow a circadian rhythm like RLS. The progression of RLS symptoms may also seem similar to augmentation, but generally they occur on a time scale of many years as opposed to several weeks or months. The addition of medication results in benefits if symptoms are related to natural progression, which is the opposite response with augmentation.

When augmentation is diagnosed the first course of action is to determine the serum ferritin level and treat accordingly. In addition, the immediate reduction of dopaminergic therapy to the lowest tolerated dose should not only result in symptomatic improvement but also serves to confirm the diagnosis of augmentation. Changes in medications, other health and sleep disorders, and sleep-wake routines should be noted and addressed because they may also be responsible for worsening RLS. The final approach to treating augmentation is discontinuation of the DA agent in favor of an alternative medical therapy such as an opiate, an α_2-δ agonist, or benzodiazepine.[137]

The most widely used and FDA-approved dopaminergic agents are nonergot selective D_2, D_3, and D_4 agonists. Ropinirole was first in this class approved for the treatment of moderate to severe primary RLS in 2005. Pramipexole followed with the same indication in 2006. The longer half-lives of these agents (6–8 hours for ropinirole and 8–10 hours for pramipexole), lower total daily dose, and lower augmentation rate (20%–30%) make these medications the preferred prophylactic therapy for RLS. Common side effects in adults include nausea, vomiting, nasal congestion, headaches, insomnia, hypersomnia, fluid retention, and augmentation. The developmental effects of DA agonists are not known, and given the well-known plasticity of the dopaminergic system it is difficult to predict if children have higher or lower rates of side effects and augmentation than adults. Clinical observation suggests that classic augmentation may not be common in children, but in some cases, particularly with co-occurring ADHD or obsessive-compulsive disorder, children may manifest increased impulsive behaviors and even obsessive thinking with dopaminergic therapy. The long-term effects of childhood DA agonist therapy on the symptomatic progression of RLS are also unknown, and longitudinal research is required to understand the complex interaction between therapy and the course of disease progression from childhood into adulthood.

Antiadrenergics

Developed and generally used as an antihypertensive because of its α_2-receptor agonist properties, clonidine can be used in the treatment of RLS and comorbid ADHD-related insomnia.[139,140] Clonidine has been shown in a small, randomized, double-blind, placebo-controlled trial to effectively treat RLS sensory symptoms in adults without any significant side effects.[141] Clonidine is reported to be the most commonly used pediatric sleep aid,[142] and has pharmacologic attributes that make it particularly useful with children who show hyperactivity. In addition, a reduction in adrenergic activity may also have benefits by reducing an overactive sympathetic nervous system, which is believed to contribute to excessive motor activity and associated medical conditions such as cardiovascular disease. Because clonidine is well tolerated by children, soporific, and is rapidly effective, it is appropriate for as-needed use and can be used routinely, although clinical tachyphylaxis is noted. The most common side effects include sedation and hypotension.

Opioids

Opioids are less commonly prescribed as prophylactic therapy and usually are reserved for painful refractory RLS, or cases of dopaminergic augmentation. Double-blind, placebo-controlled trials and case reports in adults have shown the effective nature of oral and intrathecal opioids for RLS, including methadone, morphine, and oxycodone.[143–147] The pharmacologic action of opioids with regards to RLS is believed to be medicated through interactions with the DA system.[148] The successful use of opioids as a bridging agent after the withdrawal from dopaminergic therapy may be due in part to this activity and also the effective control of refractory pain-related symptoms that can occur in more severe RLS or as a result of augmentation. Polysomnographic studies also show that opioids do not consistently reduce PLMS but do reduce arousals associated with them.[144] The use of opioids in children with chronic pain syndromes and acute pain related to sickle cell crisis has been shown and may be appropriate for select cases of pediatric RLS; however, issues of dependence, tolerance, sedation, and neuromuscular relaxation must be considered before use in children.

The centrally acting, nonnarcotic analgesic tramadol may offer an alternative to opioid use in children given its lower abuse potential and fewer adverse side effects. Small open-label studies show the effectiveness of this medication in treating the subjective complaints associated with RLS in adults,[149] but no similar studies have been conducted in children.

Anticonvulsants

Several studies in adults show the acute and long-term benefits of the α_2-δ agonist gabapentin[150–152] and the prodrug gabapentin enacarbilin[153–155] in the management of RLS-related symptoms. It seems that the major effect of this class of drug is amelioration of sensory symptoms, but data also suggest a significant reduction in PLMS.[150,151] Because these medications have few adverse side effects (emotional liability and edema are most notable) and may enhance slow-wave sleep and help to reduce sleep-onset latency, gabapentin is often considered a first choice for children requiring RLS therapy. In addition, because there is no appreciable metabolism of gabapentin in humans, resulting in circulatory renal excretion, it can be used safely in combination with many other medications. The half-life is 5 to 7 hours and is unaltered by dose or after multiple doses. Gabapentin and gabapentin enacarbilin have not yet been approved by the FDA for the treatment of RLS despite approval for other conditions including epilepsy in children more than 3 years old, and postherpetic neuralgia in adults.

Benzodiazepines

Before FDA approval of DA agonists for the treatment of RLS in adults, clonazepam was the most commonly used medication because of its noted effects in controlling myoclonic jerks and myoclonus after anoxia. The first published use of clonazepam for RLS was case reports in 1979 and 1980.[156,157] Subsequent reports include double-blind, placebo-controlled trials showing significant benefits in objective sleep efficiency, subjective sleep quality but no effects on PLMS[158] The benefits of clonazepam include its long half-life of 18 to 50 hours, which may be required because of prolonged sleeping time in children. In addition it has a well-described soporific effect that tends to eliminate insomnia-based symptoms. Clonazepam is approved by the FDA for use in children with epilepsy and adults with panic attacks. The side effects include mental confusion, muscle relaxation, and depression, but in context with RLS and ADHD it may also aggravate hyperactivity in some children. In addition, the benefits of other benzodiazepines such as temazepam and nonbenzodiazepine sedative hypnotics in the imidazopyridine class such as zolpidem are documented in the adult literature.[159,160]

Other Agents

Bupropion inhibits DA and noradrenaline reuptake and is typically used as an antidepressant. A few small studies in the adult literature show the beneficial effects of bupropion use for RLS sensory symptoms and sleep-quality outcomes.[161,162] Evidence also supports the use of bupropion for the control of PLMS and PLMD.[161,163] The use of bupropion for patients with RLS with coincidental depression may be considered. The side effects of bupropion include the potentiation of seizures in patients with epilepsy and hypomania because of heightened dopaminergic function. Another potentially important pharmacotherapy for children is rotigotine. This drug is a nonergot selective D_1, D_2, D_3 DA agonist that is available in a transdermal patch form in Europe and is awaiting FDA reapproval for use in Parkinson disease and adult RLS in the United States. Studies in children with RLS may also be forthcoming because the use of transdermal therapy has multiple advantages for children, as noted with transdermal methylphenidate in ADHD.

REFERENCES

1. Ekbom KA. Restless legs: a clinical study. Acta Med Scand Suppl 1945;158: 1–122.
2. Walters AS, Picchietti DL, Ehrenberg BL, et al. Restless legs syndrome in childhood and adolescence. Pediatr Neurol 1994;11(3):241–5.
3. Picchietti DL, Walters AS. Restless legs syndrome and periodic limb movement disorder in children and adolescents comorbidity with attention-deficit hyperactivity disorder. Child Adolesc Psychiatr Clin N Am 1996;5:729–40.
4. Picchietti DL, Stevens HE. Early manifestations of restless legs syndrome in childhood and adolescence. Sleep Med 2008;9(7):770–81.
5. Lavigne GJ, Montplaisir JY. Restless legs syndrome and sleep bruxism: prevalence and association among Canadians. Sleep 1994;17:739–43.
6. Berger K, Luedemann J, Trenkwalder C, et al. Sex and the risk of restless legs syndrome in the general population. Arch Intern Med 2004;164:196–202.
7. Ulfberg J, Nystrom B, Carter N, et al. Prevalence of restless legs syndrome among men aged 18 to 64 years: an association with somatic disease and neuropsychiatric symptoms. Mov Disord 2001;16:1159–63.
8. Montplaisir J, Boucher S, Poirier G, et al. Clinical, polysomnographic, and genetic characteristics of restless legs syndrome: a study of 133 patients diagnosed with new standard criteria. Mov Disord 1997;12(1):61–5.
9. Walters AS, Hickey K, Maltzman J, et al. A questionnaire study of 138 patients with restless legs syndrome: the "Night-Walkers" survey. Neurology 1996; 46(1):92–5.

10. Walters AS. The International Restless Legs Syndrome Study Group. Toward a better definition of the restless legs syndrome. Mov Disord 1995;10: 634–42.

11. Allen RP, Picchietti D, Henning WA, et al. Restless legs syndrome: diagnostic criteria, special considerations, and epidemiology. A report from the RLS diagnosis and epidemiology workshop at the NIH. Sleep Med 2003;4:101–19.

12. The International RLS Study Group. Validation of the International Restless Legs Syndrome Study Group rating scale for restless legs syndrome. Sleep Med 2003;4:121–32.

13. Zucconi M, Ferini-Strambi L. Epidemiology and clinical findings of restless legs syndrome. Sleep Med 2004;5:293–9.

14. Allen RP, Walters AS, Montplaisir J, et al. Restless legs syndrome prevalence and impact: REST general population study. Arch Internal Med 2005;156: 1286–92.

15. Juuti AK, Laara E, Rajala U, et al. Prevalence and associated factors of restless legs in a 57-year-old urban population in northern Finland. Acta Neurol Scand 2009;10:1111.

16. Henning W, Walters AS, Allen RP, et al. Impact, diagnosis and treatment of restless legs syndrome (RLS) in a primary care population: the REST (RLS epidemiology, symptoms and treatment) primary care study. Sleep Med 2004;5(3): 237–46.

17. Picchietti D, Allen RP, Walters AS, et al. Restless legs syndrome: prevalence and impact in children and adolescents–the Peds REST study. Pediatrics 2007; 120(2):253–66.

18. Arbuckle R, Abetz L, Durmer JS, et al. Development of the pediatric restless legs syndrome severity scale (P-RLS-SS): a patient-reported outcome measure of pediatric RLS symptoms and impact. Sleep Med 2010;11:897–906.

19. Picchietti DL, England SJ, Walters AS, et al. Periodic limb movement disorder and restless legs syndrome in children with attention-deficit hyperactivity disorder. J Child Neurol 1998;13(12):588–94.

20. Cortese S, Konofal E, Lecendreux M, et al. Restless legs syndrome and attention-deficit/hyperactivity disorder: a review of the literature. Sleep 2005; 28(8):1007–13.

21. American Academy of Sleep Medicine. International classification of sleep disorders. 2nd edition. Diagnostic and coding manual. Westchester (IL): AASM; 2005.

22. O'Brien LM, Holbrook CR, Jones F, et al. Ethnic difference in periodic limb movements in children. Sleep Med 2007;8(3):240–6.

23. Stephansson H, Rye DB, Hicks A, et al. A genetic risk factor for periodic limb movements in sleep. NEJM 2007;357:639–47.

24. Gamaldo CE, Earley CJ. Restless legs syndrome: a clinical update. Chest 2006; 130(5):1596–604.

25. Benes H, Walters AS, Allen RP, et al. Definition of restless legs syndrome, how to diagnose it, and how to differentiate it from RLS mimics. Mov Disord 2007; 22(Suppl 18):S401–8 [review. Erratum in Mov Disord 2008;23(8):1200].

26. Yang C, White DP, Winkelman JW. Antidepressants and periodic leg movements of sleep. Biol Psychiatry 2005;58:510–4.

27. Hoque R, Chesson AL Jr. Pharmacologically induced/exacerbated restless legs syndrome, periodic limb movements of sleep, and REM behavior disorder/REM sleep without atonia: literature review, qualitative scoring, and comparative analysis. J Clin Sleep Med 2010;6(1):79–83.

28. Shraf SM, Tubman A, Smale P. Prevalence of concomitant sleep disorders in patients with obstructive sleep apnea. Sleep Breath 2005;9:50–6.
29. Al-Alawi A, Mulgrew A, Tench E, et al. Prevalence, risk factors and impact on daytime sleepiness and hypertension of periodic leg movements with arousals in patients with obstructive sleep apnea. J Clin Sleep Med 2006;2(3):281–7.
30. Baran AS, Richert AC, Douglass AB, et al. Change in periodic limb movement index during treatment of obstructive sleep apnea with continuous positive airway pressure. Sleep 2003;26(6):717–20.
31. Walters AS, Lavigne G, Hening W, et al. The scoring of movements in sleep. J Clin Sleep Med 2007;3(2):155–67.
32. Sforza E, Pichot V, Barthelemy JC, et al. Cardiovascular variability during periodic leg movements: a spectral analysis approach. Clin Neurophysiol 2005; 116:1096–104.
33. Walter AS, Rye DB. Review of the relationship of restless legs syndrome and periodic limb movements in sleep to hypertension, heart disease and stroke. Sleep 2009;32(5):589–97.
34. Gosselin N, Lanfranchi P, Michaud M, et al. Age and gender effects on heart rate activation associated with periodic leg movements in patients with restless legs syndrome. Clin Neurophysiol 2003;114:2188–95.
35. Chervin RD, Archbold KH, Dillon JE, et al. Associations between symptoms of inattention, hyperactivity, restless legs and periodic leg movements. Sleep 2002;25(2):213–8.
36. Chervin RD, Dillon JE, Archbald KH, et al. Conduct problems and symptoms of sleep disorders in children. J Am Acad Child Adolesc Psychiatry 2003;42(2):201–8.
37. Pearson VE, Allen RP, Dean T, et al. Cognitive deficits associated with restless legs syndrome (RLS). Sleep Med 2006;7:25–30.
38. Oner P, Dirik EB, Taner Y, et al. Association between low serum ferritin and restless legs syndrome in patients with attention deficit hyperactivity disorder. Tohoku J Exp Med 2007;213(3):269–76.
39. Silvestri R, Gagliano A, Arico I, et al. Sleep disorders in children with attention-deficit/hyperactivity disorder (ADHD) recorded overnight by video-polysomnography. Sleep Med 2009;10(10):1132–8.
40. Wagner ML, Walters AS, Fisher BC. Symptoms of attention-deficit/hyperactivity disorder in adults with restless legs syndrome. Sleep 2004;27(8):1499–504.
41. Wiggs L, Montgomery P, Stores G. Actigraphic and parent reports of sleep patterns and sleep disorders in children with subtypes of attention-deficit hyperactivity disorder. Sleep 2005;28(11):1437–45.
42. Sevim S, Dogu O, Kaleagasi H, et al. Correlation of anxiety and depression symptoms in patients with restless legs syndrome: a population based survey. J Neurol Neurosurg Psychiatry 2004;75(2):226–30.
43. Picchietti D, Winkelman JW. Restless legs syndrome, periodic limb movements in sleep, and depression. Sleep 2005;28(7):891–8.
44. Winkelmann J, Prager M, Lieb R, et al. "Anxietas tibiarum". Depression and anxiety disorders in patients with restless legs syndrome. J Neurol 2005; 252(1):67–71.
45. Lee HB, Hening WA, Allen RP, et al. Restless legs syndrome is associated with DSM-IV major depressive disorder and panic disorder in the community. J Neuropsychiatry Clin Neurosci 2008;20(1):101–5.
46. Allen RP, Walters AS, Montplaisir J, et al. Restless legs syndrome prevalence and impact: REST general population study. Arch Intern Med 2005;165(11): 1286–9.

47. Winkelman JW, Redline S, Baldwin CM, et al. Polysomnographic and health-related quality of life correlates of restless legs syndrome in the sleep heart health study. Sleep 2009;32(6):772–8.

48. Happe S, Reese JP, Stiasny-Kolster K, et al. Assessing health-related quality of life in patients with restless legs syndrome. Sleep Med 2009;10(3):295–305.

49. Allen RP, Burchell BJ, MacDonald B, et al. Validation of the self-completed Cambridge-Hopkins questionnaire (CH-RLSq) for ascertainment of restless legs syndrome (RLS) in a population survey. Sleep Med 2009;10(10):1097–100.

50. Rothdach AJ, Trenkwalder C, Haberstock J, et al. Prevalence and risk factors of RLS in an elderly population: the MEMO study. Memory and Morbidity in Augsburg Elderly. Neurology 2000;54(5):1064–8.

51. Iber C, Ancoli-Israel A, Chesson AI, et al. The AASM manual for the scoring of sleep and associated events; rules, terminology and technical specifications. 1st edition. Westchester (IL): AASM; 2007.

52. Crabtree VM, Ivanenko A, O'Brien LM, et al. Periodic limb movement disorder of sleep in children. J Sleep Res 2003;12:73–81.

53. Montgomery-Downs HE, O'Brien LM, Gulliver TE, et al. Polysomnographic characteristics in normal preschool and early school-aged children. Pediatrics 2006; 117:741–53.

54. Pennestri MH, Whittom S, Adam B, et al. PLMS and PLMW in healthy subjects as a function of age: prevalence and interval distribution. Sleep 2006;29:1183–7.

55. Traeger N, Schultz B, Pollock AN, et al. Polysomnographic values in children 2-9 years old: additional data and review of the literature. Pediatr Pulmonol 2005;40: 22–30.

56. Picchietti DL, Picchietti MA. Pediatric restless legs syndrome and periodic limb movement disorder: parent-child pairs. Sleep Med 2009;10:925–31.

57. Ferri R, Zucconi M, Manconi M, et al. New approaches to the study of periodic leg movements during sleep in restless legs syndrome. Sleep 2006;29(6):759–69.

58. Ferri R, Manconi M, Lanuzza B, et al. Age-related changes in periodic leg movements during sleep in patients with restless legs syndrome. Sleep Med 2008; 9(7):790–8.

59. Ferri R, Franceschini C, Zucconi M, et al. Sleep polygraphic study of children and adolescents with narcolepsy/cataplexy. Dev Neuropsychol 2009;34(5): 523–38.

60. Bruni O, Ferri R, Verrillo E, et al. New approaches to the study of leg movements during sleep in ADHD children. In: Proceedings of the 20th meeting of the Associated Sleep Societies. Salt Lake City (UT), June 17–22, 2006. Sleep 2006;29(Suppl 2006). p. 259.

61. Trotti LM, Bliwise DL, Greer SA, et al. Correlates of PLMs variability over multiple nights and impact upon RLS diagnosis. Sleep Med 2009;10:668–71.

62. Sforza E, Johannes M, Bassetti C. The PAM-RL ambulatory device for detection of periodic leg movements: a validation study. Sleep Med 2005;6:407–13.

63. Morrish E, King MA, Pilsworth SN, et al. Periodic limb movement in a community population detected by a new actigraphy technique. Sleep Med 2002;3:489–95.

64. Rye DB. Parkinson's disease and RLS: the dopaminergic bridge. Sleep Med 2004;5:317–28.

65. Clemens S, Rye D, Hochman S. RLS revisiting the dopamine hypothesis from the spinal cord perspective. Neurology 2006;67:125–30.

66. Nordlander NB. Restless legs. Br J Phys Med 1954;17:160–2.

67. Earley CJ, Connor JR, Beard JL, et al. Abnormalities in CSF concentrations of ferritin and transferrin in restless legs syndrome. Neurology 2000;54:1698–700.

68. Mizuno S, Mihara T, Miyaoka T, et al. CSF iron, ferritin and transferrin levels in restless legs syndrome. J Sleep Res 2005;14:43–7.
69. Earley CJ, Barker PB, Horska A, et al. MRI-determined regional brain iron concentrations in early- and late-onset restless legs syndrome. Sleep Med 2006;7:459–61.
70. Allen RP, Barker PB, Wehrl F, et al. MRI measurement of brain iron in patients with restless legs syndrome. Neurology 2001;56:263–5.
71. Schmidauer C, Sojer M, Seppi K, et al. Transcranial ultrasound shows nigral hypoechogenicity in restless legs syndrome. Ann Neurol 2005;58:630–4.
72. Connor JR, Boyer PJ, Menzies SL, et al. Neuropathological examination suggests impaired brain iron acquisition in restless legs syndrome. Neurology 2003;61:304–9.
73. Connor JR, Wang XS, Patton SM, et al. Decreased transferrin receptor expression by neuromelanin cells in restless legs syndrome. Neurology 2004;62:1563–7.
74. Erikson KM, Jones BC, Beard JL. Iron deficiency alters dopamine transporter functioning in rat striatum. J Nutr 2000;130:2831–7.
75. Erikson KM, Jones BC, Hess EJ, et al. Iron deficiency decreases dopamine D1 and D2 receptors in rat brain. Pharmacol Biochem Behav 2001;69:409–18.
76. Wang X, Wiesinger J, Beard J, et al. Thy1 expression in the brain is affected by iron and is decreased in Restless Legs Syndrome. J Neurol Sci 2004;220:59–66.
77. Early CJ, Ponnuru P, Wang X, et al. Altered iron metabolism in lymphocytes from subjects with restless legs syndrome. Sleep 2008;31(6):847–52.
78. Desai AV, Cherkas LF, Spector TD, et al. Genetic influences in self-reported symptoms of obstructive sleep apnoea and restless legs: a twin study. Twin Res 2004;7(6):589–95.
79. Winkelmann J, Muller-Myhsok B, Wittchen HU, et al. Complex segregation analysis of restless legs syndrome provides evidence for an autosomal dominant mode of inheritance in early age at onset families. Ann Neurol 2002;52(53):297–302.
80. Mathias RA, Hening W, Washburn M, et al. Segregation analysis of restless legs syndrome: possible evidence for a major gene in a family study using blinded diagnoses. Hum Hered 2006;62(3):157–64.
81. Lazzarini A, Walters AS, Hickey K, et al. Studies of penetrance and anticipation in five autosomal-dominant restless legs syndrome pedigrees. Mov Disord 1999;14:111–6.
82. Trenkwalder C, Seidel VC, Gasser T, et al. Clinical symptoms and possible anticipation in a large kindred of familial restless legs syndrome. Mov Disord 1996;11:389–94.
83. Vogl FD, Pichler I, Adel S, et al. Restless legs syndrome: epidemiological and clinicogenetic study in a South Tyrolean population isolate. Mov Disord 2006;21:1189–95.
84. Konieczny M, Bauer P, Tomiuk J, et al. CAG repeats in Restless Legs syndrome. Am J Med Genet B Neuropsychiatr Genet 2006;141:173–6.
85. Desautels A, Turecki G, Montplaisir J, et al. Identification of a major susceptibility locus for restless legs syndrome on chromosome 12q. Am J Hum Genet 2001;69:1266–70.
86. Desautels A, Turecki G, Montplaisir J, et al. Restless legs syndrome: confirmation of linkage to chromosome 12q, genetic heterogeneity, and evidence of complexity. Arch Neurol 2005;62:591–6.
87. Bonati MT, Ferini-Strambi L, Aridon P, et al. Autosomal dominant restless legs syndrome maps on chromosome 14q. Brain 2003;126:1485–92.

88. Chen S, Ondo WG, Rao S, et al. Genomewide linkage scan identifies a novel susceptibility locus for restless legs syndrome on chromosome 9p. Am J Hum Genet 2004;74:876–85.

89. Winkelmann J, Lichtner P, Putz B, et al. Evidence for further genetic locus heterogeneity and confirmation of RLS-1 in restless legs syndrome. Mov Disord 2006;21:28–33.

90. Pichler I, Marroni F, Volpato CB, et al. Linkage analysis identifies a novel locus for restless legs syndrome on chromosome 2q in a South Tyrolean population isolate. Am J Hum Genet 2006;79:716–23.

91. Levchenko A, Provost S, Montplaisir JY, et al. A novel autosomal dominant restless legs syndrome locus maps to chromosome 20p13. Neurology 2006;67:900–1.

92. Winkelmann J, Schormair B, Lichtner P, et al. Genomewide association study of restless legs syndrome identifies common variants in three genomic regions. Nat Genet 2007;39:1000–6.

93. Muhle H, Neumann A, Lohmann-Hedrich K, et al. Childhood-onset restless legs syndrome: clinical and genetic features of 22 families. Mov Disord 2008;23(8):1113–21.

94. Young JE, Vilariño-Güell C, Lin SC, et al. Clinical and genetic description of a family with a high prevalence of autosomal dominant restless legs syndrome. Mayo Clin Proc 2009;84(2):134–8.

95. Picchietti DL, Arbuckle R, Abetz L, et al. Pediatric restless legs syndrome: analysis of symptom descriptions and drawings. J Child Neurol Proc 2011;26, in press.

96. Mohri I, Kato-Nishimura K, Tachibana N, et al. RLS: an unrecognized cause for bedtime problems and insomnia in children. Sleep Med 2008;9:701–2.

97. Rajaram A, Walters AS, England SJ, et al. Some children with growing pains may actually have restless legs syndrome. Sleep 2004;27(4):767–73.

98. Evans AM, Scutter SD. Prevalence of growing pains in young children. J Pediatr 2004;145:255–8.

99. Kryger MH, Otake K, Foerster J. Low body stores of iron and restless legs syndrome: a correctable cause of insomnia in adolescents and teenagers. Sleep Med 2002;3:127–32.

100. Martin BT, Williamson BD, Edwards N, et al. Parental symptom report and periodic limb movements of sleep in children. J Clin Sleep Med 2008;4(1):57–61.

101. Chervin RD, Hedger KM. Clinical prediction of periodic leg movements during sleep in children. Sleep Med 2001;2:501–10.

102. Silvestri R, Gagliano A, Arico I, et al. Sleep disorders in children with ADHD recorded overnight by video-polysomnography. Sleep Med 2009;10:1132–8.

103. Konofal E, Lecendreux M, Cortese S. Sleep and ADHD. Sleep Med 2010;11:652–8.

104. Decker MJ, Hue GE, Caudle WM, et al. Episodic neonatal hypoxia evokes executive dysfunction and regionally specific alterations in markers of dopamine signaling. Neuroscience 2003;117:417–25.

105. Decker MJ, Jones KA, Solomon IG, et al. Reduced extracellular dopamine and increased responsiveness to novelty: neurochemical and behavioral sequelae of intermittent hypoxia. Sleep 2005;28(2):169–78.

106. Faraone SV, Doyle AE, Mick E, et al. Meta-analysis of the association between the 7-repeat allele of the dopamine D(4) receptor gene and attention deficit hyperactivity disorder. Am J Psychiatry 2001;158(7):1052–7.

107. Li D, Sham PC, Owen MJ, et al. Meta-analysis shows significant association between dopamine system genes and attention deficit hyperactivity disorder (ADHD). Hum Mol Genet 2006;15(14):2276–84.

108. Lowe N, Kirley A, Hawi Z, et al. Joint analysis of the DRD5 marker concludes association with attention deficit/hyperactivity disorder confined to the predominately inattentive and combined subtypes. Am J Hum Genet 2004;74(2):348–56.

109. Misener VL, Luca P, Azeke O, et al. Linkage of the dopamine receptor D1 gene to attention deficit/hyperactivity disorder. Mol Psychiatry 2004;9(5):500–9.

110. VanNess SH, Owens MJ, Kilts CD. The variable number of tandem repeats element in DAT1 regulates in vitro dopamine transporter density. BMC Genet 2005;6:55.

111. Cook EH, Stein MA, Krasowski MD, et al. Association of attention-deficit disorder and the dopamine transporter gene. Am J Hum Genet 1995;56:993–8.

112. LaHoste GJ, Swanson JM, Wigal SB, et al. Dopamine D4 receptor gene polymorphism is associated with attention deficit hyperactivity disorder. Mol Psychiatry 1996;1:21–124.

113. Coghill D, Banaschewski T. The genetics of ADHD. Expert Rev Neurother 2009; 9(10):1547–65.

114. Konofal E, Lecendreux M, Arnulf I, et al. Iron deficiency in children with attention-deficit/hyperactivity disorder. Arch Pediatr Adolesc Med 2004;158: 1113–5.

115. Konofal E, Cortese S, Marcahnd M, et al. Impact of restless legs syndrome and iron deficiency on attention-deficit/hyperactivity disorder in children. Sleep Med 2007;8:711–5.

116. Konofal E, Lecendreux M, Deron J, et al. Effects of iron supplementation on attention deficit hyperactivity disorder in children. Pediatr Neurol 2008;38:20–6.

117. Frauscher B, Gschliesser V, Brandauer E, et al. The severity of RLS and augmentation in a prospective patient cohort: association with ferritin levels. Sleep Med 2009;10(6):611–5.

118. Whittom S, Dauvilliers Y, Pennestri MH, et al. Age-at-onset in restless legs syndrome: a clinical and polysomnographic study. Sleep Med 2007;9(1):54–9.

119. Earley CJ. Restless legs syndrome. N Engl J Med 2003;348(21):2103–9.

120. Sun ER, Chen CA, Ho G, et al. Iron and the restless legs syndrome. Sleep 1998; 21:371–7.

121. O'Keeffe ST, Gavin K, Lavan JN. Iron status and restless legs syndrome in the elderly. Age Ageing 1994;23(3):200–3.

122. Simakajornboon N, Gozal D, Vlasic V, et al. PLMS and iron status in children. Sleep 2006;26(6):735–8.

123. Davis BJ, Rajput A, Rajput ML, et al. A randomized double-blind placebo controlled trail of iron in restless legs syndrome. Eur Neurol 2000;43:70–5.

124. Early CJ, Heckler D, Allen RP. Repeated IV doses of iron provide effective supplemental treatment of restless legs syndrome. Sleep Med 2005;6:301–5.

125. Ondo WG. IV iron dextran for severe refractory RLS. Sleep Med 2010;11:494–6.

126. Grote L, Leissner L, Hedner J, et al. A randomized, double-blind, placebo controlled, multi-center study of intravenous iron sucrose and placebo in the treatment of restless legs syndrome. Mov Disord 2009;24(10):1445–52.

127. Walters AS, Mandelbaum DE, Lewin DS, et al. Dopaminergic Study Group. Dopaminergic therapy in children with restless legs/periodic limb movements in sleep and ADHD. Pediatr Neurol 2000;22:182–6.

128. Konofal E, Arnulf I, Lecendreux M, et al. Ropinirole in a child with ADHD and RLS. Pediatr Neurol 2005;32:350–1.

129. Kotagal S, Silber MH. Childhood-onset restless legs syndrome. Ann Neurol 2004;56(6):803–7.
130. Starn AL, Udall JN Jr. Iron deficiency anemia, pica, and restless legs syndrome in a teenage girl. Clin Pediatr (Phila) 2008;47(1):83–5.
131. Cortese S, Konofal E, Lecendreux M. Effectiveness of ropinirole for RLS and depressive symptoms in an 11-year-old girl. Sleep Med 2009;10(2):259–61.
132. Picchietti DL, Walters AS. Moderate to severe periodic limb movement disorder in childhood and adolescence. Sleep 1999;22(3):297–300.
133. Guilleminault C, Palombini L, Pelayo R, et al. Sleepwalking and sleep terrors in prepubertal children: what triggers them? Pediatrics 2003;111(1):e17–25.
134. Martinez S, Guilleminault C. Periodic leg movements in prepubertal children with sleep disturbance. Dev Med Child Neurol 2004;46(11):765–70.
135. Conti CF, de Oliveira MM, Andriolo RB, et al. Levodopa for idiopathic restless legs syndrome: evidence-based review. Mov Disord 2007;22(13):1943–51.
136. Allen RP, Earley CJ. Augmentation of the restless legs syndrome with carbidopa/levodopa. Sleep 1996;19:205–13.
137. Garcia-Borreguero D, Williams A. Dopamine augmentation of restless legs syndrome. Sleep Med Rev 2010;14:339–46.
138. Paulus W, Trenkwalder C. Less is more: pathophysiology of dopaminergic related augmentation in restless legs syndrome. Lancet Neurol 2006;5:878–86.
139. Newcorn JH, Schulz K, Harrison M, et al. Alpha 2 adrenergic agonists. Neurochemistry, efficacy, and clinical guidelines for use in children. Pediatr Clin North Am 1998;45(5):1022–99 [viii].
140. Prince JB, Wilens TE, Biederman J, et al. Clonidine for sleep disturbances associated with attention-deficit hyperactivity disorder: a systematic chart review of 62 cases. J Am Acad Child Adolesc Psychiatry 1996;35(5):599–605.
141. Wager ML, Walters AS, Coleman RG, et al. Randomized double-blind placebo-controlled study of clonidine in restless legs syndrome. Sleep 1996;19(1):52–8.
142. Owens JA, Rosen CL, Mindell JA. Medication use in the treatment of pediatric insomnia: results of a survey of community-based pediatricians. Pediatrics 2003;111(5 Pt 1):e628–35.
143. Walters AS, Wagner ML, Hening WA, et al. Successful treatment of the idiopathic restless legs syndrome in a randomized double-blind trial of oxycodone versus placebo. Sleep 1993;16:327–32.
144. Kaplan PW, Allen RP, Buchholz DW, et al. A double-blind, placebo-controlled study of the treatment of periodic limb movements in sleep using carbidopa/levodopa and propoxyphene. Sleep 1993;16(8):717–23.
145. Ross DA, Narus MS, Nutt JG. Control of medically refractory RLS with intrathecal morphine: case report. Neurosurgery 2008;62(1):e263.
146. Jakobsson B, Ruuth K. Successful treatment of RLS with an implanted pump for intrathecal drug delivery. Acta Anaesthesiol Scand 2002;46:114–7.
147. Ondo WG. Methadone for refractory RLS. Mov Disord 2005;20(3):345–8.
148. Walters AS. Review of receptor agonist and antagonist studies relevant to the opiate system in restless legs syndrome. Sleep Med 2002;3:301–30.
149. Laurma H, Markkula J. Treatment of restless legs syndrome with tramadol: an open study. J Clin Psychiatry 1999;60:241–4.
150. Garcia-Borreguero D, Larrosa O, de la Llave Y, et al. Treatment of restless legs syndrome with gabapentin: a double-blind, cross-over study. Neurology 2002;59(10):1573–9.

151. Happe S, Klosch G, Saletu B, et al. Treatment of idiopathic restless legs syndrome (RLS) with gabapentin. Neurology 2001;57(9):1717–9.
152. Happe S, Sauter C, Klosch G, et al. Gabapentin versus ropinirole in the treatment of idiopathic restless legs syndrome. Neuropsychobiology 2003;48(2): 82–6.
153. Cundy KC, Sastry S, Luo W, et al. Clinical pharmacokinetics of XP13512, a novel transported prodrug of gabapentin. J Clin Pharmacol 2008;48(12):1378–88.
154. Kushida CA, Becker PM, Ellenbogan AL, et al. XP052 Study Group. A randomized, double-blind, placebo-controlled trial of XP13512/GSK1838262 in patients with RLS. Neurology 2009;72(5):439–46.
155. Bogan R, Bornemann MA, Kushida CA, et al, XP060 Study Group. Long-term maintenance treatment of RLS with gabapentin enacarbil: a randomized control study. Mayo Clin Proc 2010;85(7):693–4.
156. Matthews WB. Treatment of restless legs syndrome with clonazepam. Br Med J 1979;1:751.
157. Oshtory MA, Vijayan N. Clonazepam treatment of insomnia due to sleep myoclonus. Arch Neurol 1980;37:119–20.
158. Saletu M, Ander P, Saletu-Zyhlarz G, et al. RLS and PLMD acute placebo-controlled sleep laboratory studies with clonazepam. Eur Neuropsychopharmacol 2001;11:153–61.
159. Silber MH, Ehrenberg BL, Allen RP, et al. An algorithm for the management of restless legs syndrome. Mayo Clin Proc 2004;79(7):916–22.
160. Hening W, Allen R, Earley C, et al. The treatment of restless legs syndrome and periodic limb movement disorder. An American Academy of Sleep Medicine review. Sleep 1999;22(7):970–99.
161. Kim SW, Shin IS, Kim JM, et al. Bupropion may improve restless legs syndrome. A report of three cases. Clin Neuropharmacol 2005;28:298–301.
162. Lee JJ, Erdos J, Wilkosz MF, et al. Bupropion as a possible treatment option for restless legs syndrome. Ann Pharmacother 2009;43:370–4.
163. Nofzinger EA, Fasiczka A, Berman S, et al. Bupropion SR reduces periodic limb movements associated with arousals from sleep in depressed patients with periodic limb movement disorder. J Clin Psychiatry 2000;61:858–62.

Circadian Rhythm Sleep Disorders

James K. Wyatt, PhD, D.ABSM

KEYWORDS

- Sleep disorders • Circadian rhythm
- Circadian rhythm sleep disorders
- Sleep homeostasis • Melatonin • Phototherapy

When seeing pediatric patients in clinic, there are many presenting complaints that could lead to the diagnosis of a circadian rhythm sleep disorder. Parents may report their teenager has sleep-onset insomnia and extreme difficulty awakening for school on weekdays, yet manages to sleep in on weekends until past the noon hour. Parents of a child with autism may report their child has delayed sleep onset and frequent, unintentional daytime napping. A child with severe visual impairment may be noted to fall asleep at a progressively later time each day. On pulling the focus back one frame from the child to the parents, the clinician may note the appearance of significant daytime sleepiness that negatively affects caregiving, perhaps related to night-shift work or frequent episodes of jet lag.

As a brief preview, the International Classification of Sleep Disorders, 2nd edition[1] (ICSD-2) details the diagnostic criteria for 6 circadian rhythm sleep disorders. Of these, 2 are primarily related to voluntarily moving sleep and wake episodes significantly earlier or later relative to the previous sleep-wake schedule (jet lag and shift work disorder). Another 2 circadian sleep disorders are related to a misalignment of the patient's circadian phase with his or her desired sleep-wake schedule (delayed and advanced sleep phase disorders). A fifth disorder, free-running type, is related to a circadian system that cannot synchronize ("entrain") to the 24-hour light-dark cycle, and hence drifts (typically) later or (more rarely) earlier each day. The sixth circadian rhythm sleep disorder, irregular sleep-wake type, is thought to result from dysfunction of the circadian pacemaker itself, resulting in suboptimal-to-nil impact on the consolidation of sleep and wake bouts.

This article begins with a review of the major central nervous system (CNS) functional systems that allow for optimal alertness during the waking day, and the rapid initiation and good maintenance of sleep at night. Subsequent sections discuss each of the 6 primary circadian rhythm sleep disorders. Attention is paid to known or suspected pathophysiology, diagnostic criteria and assessment methodology, and treatment

Sleep Disorders Service and Research Center, Rush University Medical Center, 1653 West Congress Parkway, Chicago, IL 60612-3833, USA
E-mail address: jwyatt@rush.edu

Pediatr Clin N Am 58 (2011) 621–635
doi:10.1016/j.pcl.2011.03.014
0031-3955/11/$ – see front matter © 2011 Elsevier Inc. All rights reserved.

pediatric.theclinics.com

options. The article concludes with a discussion of challenges that must be met to improve the recognition and treatment of these quite-impactful sleep disorders.

MODULATION OF SLEEP AND WAKEFULNESS

Among myriad functional systems within the CNS, the 2 best studied in terms of sleep-wake regulation are the sleep homeostatic system and the intrinsic circadian time-keeping system. These 2 critical brain systems, when working together under optimal conditions (eg, a regular sleep-wake schedule, optimal durations of sleep and wake, no confounding effects of alerting or sedating medications or substances) allow for the consolidation of a sustained bout of wakefulness during the daytime hours and a nocturnal sleep episode of good depth and duration. This discussion will assume the development and functioning of the circadian system, which occurs during the first year of life, and will not discuss early infancy. Similarly, there are massive changes in the first few years of life in total sleep time per 24 hours, in part related to development of the sleep homeostatic system. Thus, again, this article pertains more to preschoolers, school-aged children, and teenagers, as opposed to infants and toddlers.

Sleep Homeostasis

A common observation is that once children try to maintain alertness beyond the usual 12 to 16 hours of the habitual waking day, each passing hour makes it more and more difficult to fend off sleep. Indeed, just as appetite grows in the hours subsequent to eating, the brain keeps track of each hour of sustained wakefulness, commonly referred to as the homeostatic drive for sleep or sleep homeostasis. The concept of "homeostasis" is often credited to the work of American physiologist Walter Bradford Cannon in the early 1900s, who wrote that the body actively modulates physiology to maintain internal constancy in the face of environmental and other challenges that may offset that balance.[2]

Perhaps the easiest way to understand sleep homeostasis is to begin at morning wake time, in a child who has obtained a full night of sleep and is free of sleep disorders. Being fully rested, there is essentially no sleep homeostatic drive at wake time, although it begins a slow and persistent buildup with each subsequent hour of wakefulness. Near evening bedtime, great accumulation of sleep homeostatic pressure is the primary process allowing for rapid sleep initiation, as well as the prominence of deep or "slow-wave sleep" seen typically in the first third to half of the nocturnal sleep episode. A much-studied marker of the strength of sleep homeostatic drive during sleep is the amount of electroencephalogram (EEG) power in the slower frequencies (eg, "slow-wave activity" or "SWA," the 0.75-Hz to 4.50-Hz band). After sleep deprivation, recovery sleep shows a significant increase in SWA particularly in the first few non–rapid eye movement (NREM) cycles.[3] In normal sleep, with each passing NREM cycle, sleep homeostatic drive dissipates, as reflected in less and less SWA in subsequent NREM cycles.[4] During naps, sleep homeostatic drive is rapidly dissipated,[5] which is thought to explain the great restorative benefit experienced after a nap. Of the possible markers for the accumulation of sleep homeostatic drive during sustained wakefulness, frontal EEG power in the 0.75-Hz to 4.50-Hz band has also shown great promise.[6,7]

When moving from models and markers to actual physiologic substrates of sleep homeostasis, the science quickly becomes more complex. Without attempting to decipher this biologic enigma in this article, several key observations are noted. Much work has been published on the role of adenosine as a pharmacologic substrate of sleep homeostasis. In animal models, increase and decrease in adenosine is observed during sustained wake and sleep, respectively.[8] Perhaps easier to appreciate is the human preference for drinking a caffeinated beverage as a legal, relatively inexpensive, nonprescription wake-promoting substance, owing to caffeine's ability to attenuate the expression of sleep homeostatic drive because of its function as an adenosine receptor antagonist.[9,10] However, there are likely many neurotransmitters and neuromodulators functioning within the sleep homeostatic system. Orexin, a substance nearly absent in narcolepsy, is likely an endogenous wake-promoting substance (reviewed in ref.[11]). Histamine has wake-promoting properties (reviewed in ref.[12]), known to anyone who has taken an antihistaminergic medication perhaps for allergies or motion sickness.

Given that sleep homeostatic drive increases with every hour of sustained wakefulness, questions can be raised. How can a young child skip a nap and manage to remain awake as long as 12 hours? How can a teenager remain awake for 18 to 20 hours? Why do well-rested teenagers typically note a relatively stable level of alertness for the entire waking day instead of a progressive, linear increase in daytime sleepiness? Consolidation of wakefulness during the daytime, and indeed sleep at night, is possible owing to the interaction of the aforementioned sleep homeostatic system with the intrinsic circadian timekeeping system.

Circadian Rhythms

In mammals, including humans, the primary, CNS circadian oscillator is found in the suprachiasmatic nucleus (SCN) of the hypothalamus.[13,14] Extirpation of the SCN results in a lack of 24-hour rest-activity and sleep-wake rhythms, as well as greatly decreased durations of individual sleep and wake episodes.[15] In mammals, the SCN gets its primary time cue (or "zeitgeber") needed to properly synchronize internal biology to the 24-hour day from the external light-dark cycle, transduced by a special class of retinal ganglion cells and transmitted to the SCN via the retinohypothalamic tract.[16] Without daily time cues or "zeitgebers" forcing small phase shifts to "entrain" to the 24-hour light-dark cycle, the circadian system "free runs" or expresses its intrinsic period length, which is approximately 24.2 hours.[17] But with proper entrainment, the circadian system uses its many output pathways to coordinate the daily oscillation of many biologic functions (eg, sleep-wake, core body temperature, pineal melatonin production). As with the description of sleep homeostasis given previously, this is indeed a dramatic oversimplification of the richness and complexity of the circadian timekeeping system, which has myriad neurophysiological and pharmacologic input and output pathways, allowing communication with other hypothalamic nuclei as well as other structures within the brain and body.

Shared Homeostatic and Circadian Modulation of Sleep and Wake

There are a host of graphical and mathematical models of simple or complex interactions of the homeostatic and circadian systems and their modulation of sleep and wakefulness. One such model is the "2-process model" of Borbély,[18] which has served as the basis of decades of subsequent work by many research groups. Recent research studies using the "forced desynchrony" protocol[19-21] have greatly advanced our understanding of the modulatory effects of each process on sleep and wakefulness, as well as their complex interaction. We now know that the low level of sleep homeostatic drive existing after a sufficient duration of nocturnal sleep allows an individual with normal sleep to have good alertness for the first half of the normal waking day. The active promotion of wakefulness by the circadian system opposes the buildup of sleep homeostatic drive during the second half of the waking day, maintaining alertness at high levels.[22] Following the "wake maintenance zone"[23] (also called the "forbidden zone for sleep"[24]) located approximately 2 hours before habitual bedtime, the circadian system ceases its drive for wakefulness and the accumulated homeostatic sleep pressure allows for swift onset of the nocturnal sleep episode, as well as consolidation of approximately the first half to two-thirds of the sleep episode. However, as sleep pressure is satiated during sleep and is no longer sufficient to maintain uninterrupted sleep, the circadian system actively promotes sleep. The circadian system in fact strongly promotes sleep in the second half of the night, reaching peak sleep promotion at and for 2 hours after one's habitual, morning wake time—the "circadian sleep maintenance zone."[25] Thus, proper functioning of the sleep homeostatic and circadian systems, as well as maintenance of a nocturnal sleep schedule, avoiding durations of sustained wakefulness beyond 14 to 16 hours, and keeping a consistent sleep-wake cycle set the conditions for optimal consolidation of sleep and wake. Alternatively, violation of one or more of these conditions can set the stage for the emergence (or maintenance) of a circadian rhythm sleep disorder.

CIRCADIAN RHYTHM SLEEP DISORDERS
Circadian Rhythm Sleep Disorder: Delayed Sleep Phase Type

From the perspective of pediatrics, the most common of the circadian rhythm sleep disorders seen in the clinic is the delayed sleep phase type. This disorder can also be called delayed sleep phase disorder (DSPD), and in the past was called delayed sleep phase syndrome (DSPS). Formally reported in 1981,[26] this disorder is typified by complaints of difficulty falling asleep until much later than preferred, accompanied by difficulty or frank inability to arise in the morning at the desired hour. When permitted to go to bed and awaken on a later sleep schedule, however, sleep initiation is rapid, sleep consolidation is good, and final awakening is easier. Per the ICSD-2,[1] at least 1 week of a sleep diary alone or accompanied by wrist actigraphy is required to confirm the diagnosis. Ideally, the sleep diary would capture an "early" sleep schedule such as one requiring an early bedtime and wake time for school or a day-shift job, and a "late" ad lib sleep schedule over a weekend. Thus, the early sleep schedule would demonstrate increased sleep latency and decreased total sleep time, and the late sleep schedule would demonstrate resolution of symptoms. However, the American Academy of Sleep Medicine's (AASM) 2007 practice parameter[27] found moderate-strength evidence justifying the use of sleep diaries or wrist actigraphy for diagnosing DSPD. Although chronotype questionnaires such as the "Owl and Lark" or "Morningness-Eveningness Questionnaire"[28] make sense as a diagnostic questionnaire for DSPD, the practice parameter[27] cited insufficient evidence for such instruments, as well as for actual measurement of biologic circadian parameters.

The pathophysiology of DSPD has been a source of much speculation, without great supporting evidence. It has been proposed that for unknown reasons, the intrinsic circadian system is "stuck" at a later phase (and hence a later clock hour) in a patient with DPSD, and thus the wake maintenance zone makes it difficult to fall asleep at the desired, socially appropriate bedtime. Similarly, the circadian sleep maintenance zone occurs at a later clock time, greatly increasing the difficulty arising at the morning wake time. There have been reports that the trough of core body temperature, a marker of circadian phase, occurs abnormally early in the sleep episode in patients with DSPD,[29,30] although a more recent report found no difference in the timing of the presleep release of melatonin by the circadian system relative to the habitually timed sleep wake cycle.[31] Other proposed mechanisms for the genesis of DSPD include an abnormally long intrinsic circadian period or "tau," an impaired ability to make the small, daily phase advances required to entrain the circadian system to the 24-hour light-dark cycle, and even contributions of psychological or other factors (see Wyatt[32] for review). The prevalence estimates for DSPD vary widely, from slightly above 0.1% to as high as 3.0%.[33,34]

Treatment options for DSPD include sleep scheduling, exogenous melatonin, and properly timed exposure to light and darkness. According to the recent standard of practice paper from the AASM, the use of sleep scheduling, including chronotherapy, has only weak evidence supporting treatment efficacy, exogenous melatonin has moderate strength evidence, and phototherapy has moderate strength evidence.

The first treatment proposed for DSPD was chronotherapy. In the original model, the patient was instructed to maintain a reasonable time-in-bed per sleep episode (eg, 8 hours) but to delay each successive bedtime and wake time by 3 hours per day. Thus, the patient would sleep "around the clock," ceasing the delaying sleep schedule on reaching their desired, earlier clock times for bedtime and morning wake time. The original case series reported good efficacy and continued resolution of symptoms months later.[35] Further reports of chronotherapy have been published, although typically as part of a multicomponent treatment (eg, Yamadera and colleagues[36] and Okawa and colleagues[37]). A curious facet of chronotherapy was that it was devised as a treatment before the demonstration that artificial bright light could phase shift the human circadian system. Given our current understanding of circadian physiology, it is unlikely that chronotherapy as a stand-alone treatment actually causes the circadian system to phase delay 3 hours each day, and hence, the actual mechanism whereby chronotherapy treats DSPD remains unknown.

Exogenous melatonin administration causes a phase advance or a phase delay of the circadian rhythm depending on the timing of administration relative to circadian phase, which can be graphically depicted as a "phase response curve for melatonin."[38–41] For DSPD, melatonin would be delivered in the phase advance region of the circadian phase response curve (PRC) to melatonin to pull the circadian rhythm earlier. In individuals with normal sleep, Burgess and colleagues[41] showed that maximal phase advancing comes from exogenous melatonin administration at 9 to 11 hours before the middle of the habitual sleep episode for a 0.5-mg dose, and 11 to 13 hours before the middle of the sleep episode for a 3.0-mg dose. To the contrary, there was no difference in the direct, sleep-promoting effect of 0.3 mg versus 5.0 mg melatonin on sleep episodes that were scheduled before the normal nocturnal release of melatonin.[42] There are numerous reports of 5.0 mg (or lower dose) melatonin successfully phase advancing the clock time of sleep onset and/or circadian markers in DPSD patients, with ingestion typically being anywhere from 5 hours before bedtime or simply before bedtime at a time of the patient's choosing.[43–46] However, it appears that relapse may be quite high after exogenous melatonin discontinuation,[47] raising the possibility that this may be a chronic treatment. There is also concern over giving a hormone, with demonstrated importance to the reproductive endocrine system in seasonal breeding mammals, to children with maturing reproductive systems. The risk-benefit ratio takes on paramount importance in consideration of exogenous melatonin administration in children. Although not always formally diagnosed with DSPD, there are numerous reports of successful treatment of DSPD-like sleep problems in children with significant neurodevelopmental disorders (eg, autism[48] and Angelman syndrome[49]).

Phototherapy has also been reported as a treatment for DSPD. Artificial bright light is delivered during the phase advance portion of the phase response curve (PRC) to light,[50–52] repeated daily, with gradual scheduled or ad lib advancement of the sleep schedule. Studies have varied in the light source (light visor[53] vs traditional light box[54]), light intensity (up to several thousand lux), duration of light exposure, and timing of light exposure relative to circadian phase and/or the timing of sleep. Given the lack of a PRC to light derived specifically in patients with DSPD, the precision of treatment recommendations is lacking. However, it does seem that preventing bright light exposure for several hours before bedtime is important to minimize the potential for phase-delaying light exposure. After awakening, daily, scheduled exposure to bright light of 2000 to 8000 lux appears to gradually phase advance the circadian system and allows earlier timing of the major sleep episode. Without requiring a laboratory assessment of circadian phase, a conservative approach would be to begin the first day's phototherapy treatment at the habitual, late wake time, and to gradually advance the sleep schedule by 15 to 30 minutes per day.[55] Phototherapy is recommended at the "guideline" level as a treatment for DSPD in the AASM's 2007 practice parameter.[27]

In summary, although chronotherapy is perhaps the easiest treatment for DSPD, it has the least empirical support to document efficacy. Exogenous melatonin and phototherapy have equivalent, moderate levels of supporting evidence. In this author's opinion, phototherapy is favored as a first-line approach over melatonin treatment, given that phototherapy yields larger phase advances per day of treatment and lacks the potential adverse consequences on reproductive endocrine systems.

Circadian Rhythm Sleep Disorder: Free-running Type (or) Nonentrained Type

As noted earlier, in the absence of time cues required to align the circadian system with Earth's 24-hour light-dark cycle, the SCN free runs with a period of approximately 24.2 hours.[17] Many individuals who are retinally blind also cannot transmit light-dark information from the retina to the SCN, and hence, their circadian systems free run at their intrinsic period, which is typically close to but not exactly 24 hours (reviewed in Sack and Lewy[56]). Hence, they may have a presenting complaint of a progressive (typically later each day) daily shift of their sleep-wake cycle in synchrony with the drifting circadian phase. Alternatively, they may present with episodic insomnia every few weeks to few months, during periods where their circadian system has drifted sufficiently such that the patient is attempting to sleep at night but the circadian system has drifted to a phase where it is actively promoting alertness instead of sleep at night. For unknown reasons, there have been documented cases of free running in individuals who are not blind (eg, Hashimoto and colleagues[57]), suggesting that there may be more than one subtype of free-running disorder, each with different causes. Further, there are some blind patients who appear to retain integrity of the circadian visual pathway.[58] There are also case reports (eg, Boivin and colleagues[59]) of patients alternating between DSPD and free-running type symptoms, suggesting possible overlap of these disorders. In addition to the presenting complaints noted previously, the ICSD-2 requires at least 1 week of a daily sleep diary with or without wrist actigraphy confirming the complaint (eg, a progressively delaying sleep schedule).[1]

Treatment options include trying to strengthen the light-dark cycle, particularly in sighted individuals but also in blind individuals who may lack conscious light perception but still have an intact circadian visual pathway. Keeping a regular sleep-wake schedule is also recommended, as sleep itself or the rest-activity cycle may act as a zeitgeber helping to entrain the circadian system. Napping should be discouraged, as it will lessen homeostatic sleep drive and could delay nocturnal sleep onset. The strongest treatment evidence comes from studies demonstrating the efficacy of nightly exogenous melatonin administration as a phase-entraining agent, essentially stopping progressive circadian drifting or free running. Doses initially studied were in the multi-milligram range,[60] but efficacy has more recently been demonstrated with melatonin doses of 0.3 to 0.5 mg.[61,62]

Circadian Rhythm Sleep Disorder: Irregular Sleep-Wake Rhythm

The fundamental observation in irregular sleep-wake rhythm disorder is a lack of consolidation of major sleep and wake episodes. Hence, across the 24-hour day there are 3 or more sleep episodes, and this must be verified with at least 1 week of a daily sleep diary with or without wrist actigraphic monitoring. Although sleep is polyphasic, total sleep time per 24 hours is typically within normal limits. Obviously, this disorder should not be diagnosed in an infant or a very young child who has not yet reached the developmental stage when sleep could be expected to be consolidated into a major nocturnal sleep episode with no or only one daytime nap. The presenting complaint can be of insomnia, excessive daytime sleepiness, or both.[1]

Pathophysiology of this disorder could be either an entirely absent or dysfunctional circadian system, which cannot exert its normal functions, to actively promote daytime alertness in service of consolidating a single major wake episode, and consolidating nocturnal sleep to allow for a normal-duration sleep episode. In fact, this deranged sleep-wake pattern is similar to what is observed in an animal model when the SCN has been removed. This absence of consolidated sleep and wake bouts can be observed in children with severe neurodevelopmental disorders. In the pediatrics literature, it is often difficult to discern if the patients had circadian problems suggestive of delayed sleep phase type, free-running type, irregular sleep-wake rhythm type, or a combination. Unfortunately, most of the research in the irregular sleep-wake rhythm type has been conducted on older adults, particularly in patients with neurodegenerative diseases such as Alzheimer's.

Caveats aside, presleep melatonin administration has been shown to decrease daytime sleep duration and increase nighttime sleep duration in children with severe psychomotor retardation[63] and in other clinical populations where irregular sleep-wake rhythm may have been a factor (eg, Jan and colleagues[64]). Prescribing a regular sleep-wake schedule with active parental involvement is also recommended at the "option" level by the AASM practice parameter,[27] although the supporting evidence base is relatively weak.

Circadian Rhythm Sleep Disorder: Jet Lag Type

With an understanding of the shared modulation of sleep and wakefulness from the sleep homeostatic and circadian systems, the easiest circadian rhythm sleep disorders to understand are jet lag and shift work. These two disorders share much in common, in terms of symptomatology, the "voluntary" circumstances that initiate them, and the treatment alternatives.

Developments in aviation over the past century have occurred in many areas. Speed nears the sound barrier, owing first to turbojet and now turbofan engines found on modern commercial aircraft. The efficiency of turbofan engines and increased fuel capacity allow aircraft to travel distances up to halfway around the world, in fact more than 12,000 miles. To achieve high speed and fuel efficiency requires travel at high altitudes where the air density is extremely low, typically in the 30,000-ft to 45,000-ft range above sea level, requiring cabin pressurization. Unfortunately, cabin pressurization is typically well below the air pressure found at ground elevation, resulting in a condition similar to acute mountain sickness.[65] Also, to avoid premature deterioration of the aircraft cabin's aluminum skin, cabin humidity is kept very low, which leads to further physical discomfort (eg, dry skin, eyes, and nasal passages, as well as dehydration). Stress and/or time spent in preparation for travel before a flight can lead to curtailment of the sleep episode preceding travel, and hence the traveler has excessive daytime (or nighttime) sleepiness and fatigue. Many seek the aid of caffeine to maintain alertness before or during the flight, perhaps impairing subsequent sleep and causing further dehydration in flight. Alcohol is commonly used (by adults and hopefully not by children) as a sleep aid[66] and/or anxiolytic,[67] yet alcohol further compounds dehydration, and risks rebound alerting and even anxiety.[68] These are many of the features commonly encountered in jet travel that have nothing to do with crossing time zones.[69] In essence, much of the constellation of symptoms noted after crossing time zones have nothing to do with adaptation to the new time zone, but are rather attributable to the previously listed contributing factors. However, behavioral treatments can address many of these threats, such as keeping the child hydrated, avoiding dehydrating substances, and minimizing stress and optimizing sleep before travel.

The "true" pathophysiology of the circadian features of jet lag are attributable to the attempt to sleep and be awake in a new time zone, and hence, at different circadian phases than in one's home time zone. Travel eastward, such as the 4 to 8 hours encountered from the United States to the European Union forces the traveler to attempt to initiate sleep much earlier than normal, during the wake-promoting region of the circadian system's "daytime." Sleep onset may be further delayed because the new "bedtime" on arrival occurs hours earlier than the previous sleep episode, and hence not as much sleep homeostatic pressure may have accumulated during the wake episode preceding the first sleep attempt on arrival. Similarly, the circadian system will lag many hours behind the new, earlier sleep schedule and hence for up to the first half of the daytime hours in the new time zone, the circadian system will still be promoting sleep, impairing alertness and concentration. Travel westbound, such as from the East Coast to the West Coast or Hawaii is typically accompanied by milder symptoms of circadian misalignment. It is typically easier to extend the duration of wake by several hours and build additional sleep homeostatic drive, which will further increase ease of sleep initiation and sleep consolidation. However, an early morning awakening may occur, because the circadian system will begin its "morning" stimulation of wakefulness too early for the new "later" time zone.

The official diagnosis of jet lag per the ICSD-2[1] requires a complaint of insomnia and/or excessive daytime sleepiness following crossing 2 or more time zones, accompanied by physical or other consequences within 2 days of arrival. Sequelae are many and vary across individuals, and can include gastrointestinal complaints, general malaise, and impaired cognitive functioning. No objective testing is required to make the diagnosis.

Treatments for jet lag can be divided up many ways: homeostatic versus circadian, behavioral versus pharmacologic, or preflight versus in flight versus postflight. The last model will be used here. Before the flight, many behavioral strategies will be important, not only for children but for adults as well. Optimization of sleep on the nights leading up to travel is critical to avoid sleep deprivation before flight. If the flight is to be of sufficient duration to permit sleep, then it will be best to have the child avoid caffeine intake before flight, minimizing dehydration and also the sleep-impairing effects of caffeine. Finally, many children experience anxiety surrounding travel, and hence, strategies to minimize this anticipatory (and subsequent real-time) anxiety will be helpful.

During the flight, as noted earlier, adequate fluid intake is important to avoid dehydration and associated tissue irritation. Optimization of opportunity for sleep is important, particularly on longer flights or if sleep loss occurred before flight. Just as sleep hygiene[70,71] is recommended for optimal sleep at home, measures can be taken to improve sleep in flight, such as the use of an eye mask or sunglasses, ear plugs or noise-cancelling headphones, and adding or removing layers of clothing for temperature regulation. On arrival at the destination, recommendations for sleep depend on the direction and the number of time zones crossed. For shorter flights and minimal time zone difference, such as a westbound flight crossing 3 time zones, it may be enough to supplement with an in-flight nap, allowing children sufficient sleep to remain awake 3 hours "later" that evening to maintain their "at home" bedtime in the new time zone (eg, even though it might be midnight at home in New York, the child can remain awake until their normal "9 PM bedtime" in Los Angeles).

The most sophisticated treatments for jet lag involve increasing the rate of circadian phase shifting on arrival, or in more recent advances, even "preadapting" by partially or fully shifting circadian phase before travel. Most of the phase-shifting literature on jet lag involves the use of exogenous melatonin, which unfortunately is not typically recommended for use in young children or adolescents, given potential effects on the reproductive endocrine system. But because of the high quality of evidence showing efficacy of exogenous melatonin as a treatment for jet lag, it is recommended at the "standard of practice" level in the AASM's 2007 practice parameter.[27] However, the use of properly timed, artificial bright light is an effective treatment to preadapt before jet lag, although the studies have typically involved only adult participants. For an extremely comprehensive description of multicomponent (eg, sleep schedule shifting, exogenous melatonin, and both sunlight and artificial bright light) protocols to preadapt before jet travel, the reader is referred to the work of Charmane Eastman and colleagues.[72–74]

Circadian Rhythm Sleep Disorder: Shift Work Type

Given child labor laws and the fact that most are attending daytime school, it is extremely rare to encounter shift work disorder in children or adolescents. However, many adolescents are involved in after-school jobs to supplement their or their family's income, many of these jobs going well into the evening hours, such as the traditional "second shift." Further, the pediatrician could be the first to note significant daytime sleepiness in a parent who works rotating or night-shift work. Thus, indirectly, by encouraging the parent to note the significance of their sleepiness and the ability to seek treatment for shift work disorder, caregiving of the child may improve in the balance. Thus, shift work disorder will be covered briefly in this article.

Typically, the patient reports difficulty obtaining sufficient total sleep time (insomnia) during a sleep episode falling outside of the typical nocturnal hours, inability to maintain optimal alertness during work hours that fall outside of a normal day shift, or both. The shift work schedule has to have been worked for at least 1 month, and accompanying physical or other seqeulae must be reported, as with jet lag. At least 1 week of a daily sleep diary with or without actigraphic monitoring must suggest sleep episodes are attempted at an adverse circadian phase, although circadian phase itself does not have to be objectively measured.[1] Just as with jet lag, the symptoms of shift work disorder are multifactorial, and caused by similar factors. Behavioral and pharmacologic factors come into play, such as unintentional dehydration owing to ingestion of caffeine in an attempt to minimize excessive sleepiness during the work shift, or side effects experienced from alcohol or drugs used to self-medicate insomnia. As a general note, and across the circadian rhythm (and other) sleep disorders, the clinician is advised to ask in the clinical history about recreational or self-medication use of alcohol and/or illicit substances.

Pharmacologic strategies have shown great promise for increasing on-the-job alertness and performance during real or simulated shift work in adult research subjects, such as the planned use of caffeine before or during work,[25,75,76] or ingestion of the wake-promoting substances modafinil[77,78] and armodafinil before the work shift.[79] Although many would be hesitant to prescribe a wake-promoting medication for a child, it is a reality that caffeine is commonly used in the pediatric population,[80,81] perhaps for a variety of biologic, social, and psychological factors. Melatonin has also shown great promise as a sleep-promoting substance for daytime sleep episodes in shift work or when given to shift circadian phase into proper alignment with the new sleep-wake schedule required by the shift work.[82–84] It is likely the case that a sleep-promoting effect of exogenous melatonin does not occur with ingestion before night-time sleep episodes, and that the hypnotic effect is present only during daytime administration, at times when endogenous melatonin from the pineal is at very low levels or even absent.[42] But as noted earlier, exogenous melatonin is not typically recommended for children, and the efficacy and safety of many of the wake-promoting substances have not been studied in children. Scheduled exposure to artificial bright light, phototherapy, has been demonstrated in numerous publications to effectively shift circadian phase into proper alignment in night-shift workers[85,86] to increase nighttime alertness and increase daytime sleep duration. Phototherapy is in fact recommended at the "guideline" level as a treatment for shift work disorder in the AASM's 2007 practice parameter.[27] However, this approach is not practical for young children and adolescents who essentially are not part of the night-shift working population. Sleep scheduling is recommended at the "standard of practice" level for shift work disorder.[27] Scheduled, prophylactic naps[87–89] are of particular utility for teenagers or adults working into the evening hours, and can be critical for those working the night shift to supplement their typically shortened daytime sleep episode.

Circadian Rhythm Sleep Disorder: Advanced Sleep Phase Type

Advanced sleep phase disorder is nearly the opposite of DSPD; the primary complaints in ASPD are difficulty remaining awake until the desired evening bedtime and early morning awakening. Sleep is of reasonable duration and quality when initiated at this earlier hour. As with DSPD, the diagnosis of ASPD requires at least 1 week of a daily sleep diary with or without accompanying wrist actigraphic monitoring that verifies the earlier or advanced timing of sleep.[1] The suspected pathophysiology of ASPD is that for reasons unknown, the patient's circadian phase has shifted too early relative to the desired sleep-wake schedule, and thus the circadian promotion of wakefulness ceases too far in advance of the desired bedtime, resulting in the advanced timing of sleep onset. Further, the circadian sleep maintenance zone ends too early to sustain the nocturnal sleep episode until the desired wake time, leading to the early morning awakening. There may also be contributions of changes in how the circadian system engages in sleep regulation; it is noted that even healthy older adults are more likely to describe themselves as "morning larks" are less "phase tolerant" of sleeping in late (they awaken at an earlier circadian phase and hence an earlier clock hour). Treatment options for ASPD include hypnotics to extend sleep duration, afternoon or evening bright light exposure to cause a circadian phase delay, and chronotherapy. Given the observation that ASPD is not a disorder typically found in young children or adolescents and hence is not relevant to the theme of this book, readers are encouraged to consult any of a number of excellent reviews for further information.

Clinical Challenges

The reader is encouraged to think about the circadian rhythm sleep disorders as having been well-specified in terms of clinical presentation, but highly variable in terms of degree of certainty of pathophysiology (eg, DSPS and ASPD). Thus, objective and subjective measures should be used to make the diagnosis and/or measure response to treatment, as well as the efficacy and effectiveness of treatments. A particular problem in pediatrics and pediatric sleep medicine is that although commonly prescribed, there is a lack of data in children for efficacy and safety for most hypnotic and wake-promoting medications.[90,91] Another challenge is appreciating that in certain clinical populations, such as in severe neurodevelopmental disorders, there may be diffuse sleep complaints from the patient and/or by proxy from the parents that do not fit neatly within a single ICSD-2 insomnia or circadian rhythm sleep disorder diagnosis, but nonetheless may be responsive to single or multicomponent treatment approaches.

REFERENCES

1. American Academy of Sleep Medicine. International classification of sleep disorders. Diagnostic and coding manual. 2nd edition. Westchester (IL): American Academy of Sleep Medicine; 2005.
2. Cannon WB. The wisdom of the body (revised). New York: W.W. Norton and Company, Inc; 1963.
3. Brunner DP, Dijk DJ, Tobler I, et al. Effect of partial sleep deprivation on sleep stages and EEG power spectra: evidence for non-REM and REM sleep homeostasis. Electroencephalogr Clin Neurophysiol 1990;75:492–9.
4. Dijk DJ, Brunner DP, Beersma DG, et al. Electroencephalogram power density and slow wave sleep as a function of prior waking and circadian phase. Sleep 1990;13:430–40.
5. Dijk DJ, Beersma DG, Daan S. EEG power density during nap sleep: reflection of an hourglass measuring the duration of prior wakefulness. J Biol Rhythms 1987;2: 207–19.
6. Cajochen C, Khalsa SB, Wyatt JK, et al. EEG and ocular correlates of circadian melatonin phase and human performance decrements during sleep loss. Am J Physiol 1999;277:R640–9.
7. Cajochen C, Wyatt JK, Czeisler CA, et al. Separation of circadian and wake duration-dependent modulation of EEG activation during wakefulness. Neuroscience 2002;114:1047–60.
8. Porkka-Heiskanen T, Strecker RE, Thakkar M, et al. Adenosine: a mediator of the sleep-inducing effects of prolonged wakefulness. Science 1997;276: 1265–8.
9. Snyder SH, Katims JJ, Annau Z, et al. Adenosine receptors and behavioral actions of methylxanthines. Proc Natl Acad Sci U S A 1981;78:3260–4.
10. Nehlig A, Daval JL, Debry G. Caffeine and the central nervous system: mechanisms of action, biochemical, metabolic and psychostimulant effects. Brain Res Brain Res Rev 1992;17:139–70.
11. Nishino S, Mignot E. Narcolepsy and cataplexy. Handb Clin Neurol 2011;99: 783–814.
12. Thakkar MM. Histamine in the regulation of wakefulness. Sleep Med Rev 2011; 15(1):65–74.
13. Moore RY, Eichler VB. Loss of a circadian adrenal corticosterone rhythm following suprachiasmatic lesions in the rat. Brain Res 1972;42:201–6.
14. Stephan FK, Zucker I. Circadian rhythms in drinking behavior and locomotor activity of rats are eliminated by hypothalamic lesions. Proc Natl Acad Sci U S A 1972;69:1583–6.
15. Mosko SS, Moore RY. Neonatal suprachiasmatic nucleus lesions: effects on the development of circadian rhythms in the rat. Brain Res 1979;164:17–38.
16. Berson DM, Dunn FA, Takao M. Phototransduction by retinal ganglion cells that set the circadian clock. Science 2002;295:1070–3.

17. Czeisler CA, Duffy JF, Shanahan TL, et al. Stability, precision, and near-24-hour period of the human circadian pacemaker [see comments]. Science 1999;284: 2177–81.
18. Borbély AA. A two process model of sleep regulation. Hum Neurobiol 1982;1: 195–204.
19. Dijk DJ, Czeisler CA. Paradoxical timing of the circadian rhythm of sleep propensity serves to consolidate sleep and wakefulness in humans. Neurosci Lett 1994; 166:63–8.
20. Dijk DJ, Czeisler CA. Contribution of the circadian pacemaker and the sleep homeostat to sleep propensity, sleep structure, electroencephalographic slow waves, and sleep spindle activity in humans. J Neurosci 1995;15:3526–38.
21. Wyatt JK, Ritz-De Cecco A, Czeisler CA, et al. Circadian temperature and melatonin rhythms, sleep, and neurobehavioral function in humans living on a 20-h day. Am J Physiol 1999;277:R1152–63.
22. Czeisler CA, Dijk DJ, Duffy JF. Entrained phase of the circadian pacemaker serves to stabilize alertness and performance throughout the habitual waking day. In: Ogilvie RD, Harsh JR, editors. Sleep onset: normal and abnormal processes. Washington, DC.: American Psychological Association; 1994. p. 89–110.
23. Strogatz SH, Kronauer RE, Czeisler CA. Circadian pacemaker interferes with sleep onset at specific times each day: role in insomnia. Am J Physiol 1987; 253:R172–8.
24. Lavie P. Ultrashort sleep-waking schedule. III. 'Gates' and 'forbidden zones' for sleep. Electroencephalogr Clin Neurophysiol 1986;63:414–25.
25. Wyatt JK, Cajochen C, Ritz-De CA, et al. Low-dose repeated caffeine administration for circadian-phase-dependent performance degradation during extended wakefulness. Sleep 2004;27:374–81.
26. Weitzman ED, Czeisler CA, Coleman RM, et al. Delayed sleep phase syndrome. A chronobiological disorder with sleep- onset insomnia. Arch Gen Psychiatry 1981;38:737–46.
27. Morgenthaler TI, Lee-Chiong T, Alessi C, et al. Practice parameters for the clinical evaluation and treatment of circadian rhythm sleep disorders. An American Academy of Sleep Medicine report. Sleep 2007;30(11):1445–59.
28. Horne JA, Ostberg O. A self-assessment questionnaire to determine morningness-eveningness in human circadian rhythms. Int J Chronobiol 1976; 4(2):97–110.
29. Watanabe T, Kajimura N, Kato M, et al. Sleep and circadian rhythm disturbances in patients with delayed sleep phase syndrome. Sleep 2003;26:657–61.
30. Uchiyama M, Okawa M, Shibui K, et al. Altered phase relation between sleep timing and core body temperature rhythm in delayed sleep phase syndrome and non-24-hour sleep-wake syndrome in humans. Neurosci Lett 2000;294: 101–4.
31. Wyatt JK, Stepanski EJ, Kirkby J. Circadian phase in delayed sleep phase syndrome: predictors and temporal stability across multiple assessments. Sleep 2006;29:1075–80.
32. Wyatt JK. Delayed sleep phase syndrome: pathophysiology and treatment options. Sleep 2004;27:1195–203.
33. Yazaki M, Shirakawa S, Okawa M, et al. Demography of sleep disturbances associated with circadian rhythm disorders in Japan. Psychiatry Clin Neurosci 1999; 53:267–8.
34. Ando K, Kripke DF, Ancoli-Israel S. Delayed and advanced sleep phase symptoms. Isr J Psychiatry Relat Sci 2002;39:11–8.

35. Czeisler CA, Richardson GS, Coleman RM, et al. Chronotherapy: resetting the circadian clocks of patients with delayed sleep phase insomnia. Sleep 1981;4:1–21.
36. Yamadera H, Takahashi K, Okawa M. A multicenter study of sleep-wake rhythm disorders: therapeutic effects of vitamin B12, bright light therapy, chronotherapy and hypnotics. Psychiatry Clin Neurosci 1996;50:203–9.
37. Okawa M, Uchiyama M, Ozaki S, et al. Circadian rhythm sleep disorders in adolescents: clinical trials of combined treatments based on chronobiology. Psychiatry Clin Neurosci 1998;52:483–90.
38. Lewy AJ, Ahmed S, Jackson JML, et al. Melatonin shifts human circadian rhythms according to a phase-response curve. Chronobiol Int 1992;9:380–92.
39. Lewy AJ, Bauer VK, Ahmed S, et al. The human phase response curve (PRC) to melatonin is about 12 hours out of phase with the PRC to light. Chronobiol Int 1998;15:71–83.
40. Burgess HJ, Revell VL, Eastman CI. A three pulse phase response curve to three milligrams of melatonin in humans. J Physiol 2008;586:639–47.
41. Burgess HJ, Revell VL, Molina TA, et al. Human phase response curves to three days of daily melatonin: 0.5 mg versus 3.0 mg. J Clin Endocrinol Metab 2010;95: 3325–31.
42. Wyatt JK, Dijk DJ, Ritz-De Cecco A, et al. Sleep facilitating effect of exogenous melatonin in healthy young men and women is circadian-phase dependent. Sleep 2006;29:609–18.
43. Kayumov L, Brown G, Jindal R, et al. A randomized, double-blind, placebo-controlled crossover study of the effect of exogenous melatonin on delayed sleep phase syndrome. Psychosom Med 2001;63:40–8.
44. Nagtegaal JE, Kerkhof GA, Smits MG, et al. Delayed sleep phase syndrome: a placebo-controlled cross-over study on the effects of melatonin administered five hours before the individual dim light melatonin onset. J Sleep Res 1998;7: 135–43.
45. Dahlitz M, Alvarez B, Vignau J, et al. Delayed sleep phase syndrome response to melatonin. Lancet 1991;337:1121–4.
46. Mundey K, Benloucif S, Harsanyi K, et al. Phase-dependent treatment of delayed sleep phase syndrome with melatonin. Sleep 2005;28:1271–8.
47. Dagan Y, Yovel I, Hallis D, et al. Evaluating the role of melatonin in the long-term treatment of delayed sleep phase syndrome (DSPS). Chronobiol Int 1998;15: 181–90.
48. Giannotti F, Cortesi F, Cerquiglini A, et al. An open-label study of controlled-release melatonin in treatment of sleep disorders in children with autism. J Autism Dev Disord 2006;36:741–52.
49. Zhdanova IV, Wurtman RJ, Wagstaff J. Effects of a low dose of melatonin on sleep in children with Angelman syndrome. J Pediatr Endocrinol Metab 1999;12:57–67.
50. Khalsa SB, Jewett ME, Cajochen C, et al. A phase response curve to single bright light pulses in human subjects. J Physiol 2003;549:945–52.
51. Minors DS, Waterhouse JM, Wirz-Justice A. A human phase-response curve to light. Neurosci Lett 1991;133:36–40.
52. Honma K, Honma S. A human phase response curve for bright light pulses. Jpn J Psychiatry Neurol 1988;42:167–8.
53. Cole RJ, Smith JS, Alcala YC, et al. Bright-light mask treatment of delayed sleep phase syndrome. J Biol Rhythms 2002;17:89–101.
54. Rosenthal NE, Joseph-Vanderpool JR, Levendosky AA, et al. Phase-shifting effects of bright morning light as treatment for delayed sleep phase syndrome. Sleep 1990;13:354–61.

55. Wyatt JK. Circadian rhythm sleep disorders in children and adolescents. Sleep Med Clin 2007;2:387–96.
56. Sack RL, Lewy AJ. Circadian rhythm sleep disorders: lessons from the blind. Sleep Med Rev 2001;5:189–206.
57. Hashimoto S, Nakamura K, Honma S, et al. Free-running circadian rhythm of melatonin in a sighted man despite a 24-hour sleep pattern: a non-24-hour circadian syndrome. Psychiatry Clin Neurosci 1997;51:109–14.
58. Czeisler CA, Shanahan TL, Klerman EB, et al. Suppression of melatonin secretion in some blind patients by exposure to bright light [see comments]. N Engl J Med 1995;332:6–11.
59. Boivin DB, Caliyurt O, James FO, et al. Association between delayed sleep phase and hypernyctohemeral syndromes: a case study. Sleep 2004;27:417–21.
60. Sack RL, Lewy AJ, Blood ML, et al. Melatonin administration to blind people: phase advances and entrainment. J Biol Rhythms 1991;6(3):249–61.
61. Lewy AJ, Emens JS, Lefler BJ, et al. Melatonin entrains free-running blind people according to a physiological dose-response curve. Chronobiol Int 2005;22: 1093–106.
62. Hack LM, Lockley SW, Arendt J, et al. The effects of low-dose 0.5-mg melatonin on the free-running circadian rhythms of blind subjects. J Biol Rhythms 2003;18: 420–9.
63. Pillar G, Shahar E, Peled N, et al. Melatonin improves sleep-wake patterns in psychomotor retarded children. Pediatr Neurol 2000;23:225–8.
64. Jan JE, Hamilton D, Seward N, et al. Clinical trials of controlled-release melatonin in children with sleep- wake cycle disorders. J Pineal Res 2000;29:34–9.
65. Muhm JM, Rock PB, McMullin DL, et al. Effect of aircraft-cabin altitude on passenger discomfort. N Engl J Med 2007;357:18–27.
66. Johnson EO, Roehrs T, Roth T, et al. Epidemiology of alcohol and medication as aids to sleep in early adulthood. Sleep 1998;21:178–86.
67. Bolton J, Cox B, Clara I, et al. Use of alcohol and drugs to self-medicate anxiety disorders in a nationally representative sample. J Nerv Ment Dis 2006;194: 818–25.
68. Castaneda R, Sussman N, Levy R, et al. A review of the effects of moderate alcohol intake on psychiatric and sleep disorders. Recent Dev Alcohol 1998; 14:197–226.
69. Graeber RC. Jet lag and sleep disruption. In: Kryger MH, Roth T, Dement WC, editors. Principles and practice of sleep medicine. Philadelphia: Saunders; 1994. p. 463–70.
70. Hauri PJ. Sleep hygiene, relaxation therapy, and cognitive interventions. In: Hauri PJ, editor. Case studies in insomnia. New York: Plenum; 1991. p. 65–84.
71. Stepanski EJ, Wyatt JK. Use of sleep hygiene in the treatment of insomnia. Sleep Med Rev 2003;7:215–25.
72. Burgess HJ, Crowley SJ, Gazda CJ, et al. Preflight adjustment to eastward travel: 3 days of advancing sleep with and without morning bright light. J Biol Rhythms 2003;18:318–28.
73. Eastman CI, Gazda CJ, Burgess HJ, et al. Advancing circadian rhythms before eastward flight: a strategy to prevent or reduce jet lag. Sleep 2005;28:33–44.
74. Eastman CI, Burgess HJ. How to travel the world without jet lag. Sleep Med Clin 2009;4:241–55.
75. Walsh JK, Muehlbach MJ, Humm TM, et al. Effect of caffeine on physiological sleep tendency and ability to sustain wakefulness at night. Psychopharmacology (Berl) 1990;101:271–3.

76. Muehlbach MJ, Walsh JK. The effects of caffeine on simulated night-shift work and subsequent daytime sleep. Sleep 1995;18:22–9.
77. Czeisler CA, Walsh JK, Roth T, et al. Modafinil for excessive sleepiness associated with shift-work sleep disorder. N Engl J Med 2005;353:476–86.
78. Grady S, Aeschbach D, Wright KP Jr, et al. Effect of modafinil on impairments in neurobehavioral performance and learning associated with extended wakefulness and circadian misalignment. Neuropsychopharmacology 2010;35:1910–20.
79. Czeisler CA, Walsh JK, Wesnes KA, et al. Armodafinil for treatment of excessive sleepiness associated with shift work disorder: a randomized controlled study. Mayo Clin Proc 2009;84:958–72.
80. NSF. 2006 Sleep in America Poll [report]. Washington, DC, National Sleep Foundation 2006.
81. Mindell JA, Meltzer LJ, Carskadon MA, et al. Developmental aspects of sleep hygiene: findings from the 2004 National Sleep Foundation Sleep in America Poll. Sleep Med 2009;10:771–9.
82. Sharkey KM, Eastman CI. Melatonin phase shifts human circadian rhythms in a placebo-controlled simulated night-work study. Am J Physiol Regul Integr Comp Physiol 2002;282:R454–63.
83. Burgess HJ, Sharkey KM, Eastman CI. Bright light, dark and melatonin can promote circadian adaptation in night shift workers. Sleep Med Rev 2002;6:407–20.
84. Sharkey KM, Fogg LF, Eastman CI. Effects of melatonin administration on daytime sleep after simulated night shift work. J Sleep Res 2001;10:181–92.
85. Eastman CI, Boulos Z, Terman M, et al. Light treatment for sleep disorders: consensus report. VI. Shift work. J Biol Rhythms 1995;10:157–64.
86. Eastman CI, Stewart KT, Mahoney MP, et al. Dark goggles and bright light improve circadian rhythm adaptation to night-shift work. Sleep 1994;17:535–43.
87. Akerstedt T, Torsvall L. Napping in shift work. Sleep 1985;8:105–9.
88. Bonnet MH, Arand DL. The use of prophylactic naps and caffeine to maintain performance during a continuous operation. Ergonomics 1994;37:1009–20.
89. Rosekind MR, Smith RM, Miller DL, et al. Alertness management: strategic naps in operational settings. J Sleep Res 1995;4:62–6.
90. Owens JA, Rosen CL, Mindell JA, et al. Use of pharmacotherapy for insomnia in child psychiatry practice: a national survey. Sleep Med 2010;11:692–700.
91. Owens JA, Rosen CL, Mindell JA. Medication use in the treatment of pediatric insomnia: results of a survey of community-based pediatricians. Pediatrics 2003;111:e628–35.

Sleep in Adolescents: The Perfect Storm

Mary A. Carskadon, PhD

KEYWORDS

- Adolescence • Circadian rhythms • Sleep regulation
- Homeostatic pressure • Melatonin • Mood

The perfect storm metaphor applies to sleep patterns of adolescents in the sense that developmental trajectories of biopsychosocial factors conspire to limit the quantity of sleep for many adolescents, resulting in a number of negative consequences. A reduction in sleep amount from late childhood through the second decade has long been known; however, the weight of current evidence holds that sleep need does not decline across this span. Nevertheless, parents, pediatricians, and schoolteachers, it seems, long assumed that this sleep decline was an inevitable part of growing up and a normative expectation. This article will describe how the loss of sleep through adolescence is not driven by lower need for sleep but arises from a convergence of biologic, psychological, and socio-cultural influences.

SLEEP PATTERNS OF ADOLESCENTS

Adolescent sleep patterns have been surveyed by investigators in many countries from virtually every continent around the world, and a consistent finding is that the timing of bedtime on school nights gets later across the middle school and high school years (roughly ages 11 through 17 years).[1-15] Rise times on school mornings, by contrast, tend to stay relatively consistent except in countries such as the United States where the starting time of school moves to an earlier hour at the transition to high school. Weekend sleep for teenagers tends to delay further, and the difference in amount of sleep reported for school days versus weekends becomes more pronounced as children pass into higher grades (ie, greater reported sleep on weeknights than school nights).

The most recent US poll of sleep patterns in adolescents was reported by the National Sleep Foundation in 2006, and collected self- and parent-reported sleep patterns from grades 6 through 12.[16] These data serve as a good example of these general trends, as shown in **Table 1**. The young people interviewed in this telephone poll reported that average bedtime on the nights before school days were approximately 1.5 hours later from grade 6 to grade 12, and reported weekend bedtime delayed from 10:31 PM to 12:45 AM across this same grade span. Sixth graders

Bradley Hospital Sleep Lab, E.P. Bradley Hospital, 300 Duncan Drive, Providence, RI 02906, USA
E-mail address: mary_carskadon@brown.edu

Pediatr Clin N Am 58 (2011) 637–647
doi:10.1016/j.pcl.2011.03.003
0031-3955/11/$ – see front matter © 2011 Elsevier Inc. All rights reserved.

pediatric.theclinics.com

Table 1
Sleep patterns reported by adolescent school children: National Sleep Foundation 2006 Sleep in America Poll

	Grade in School						
Sleep Variable	6th	7th	8th	9th	10th	11th	12th
School Nights							
Bedtime (24-h)	2124	2152	2153	2215	2232	2251	2302
Rise Time (24-h)	0642	0635	0636	0628	0623	0623	0631
Average Sleep (Hours)	8.4	8.1	8.1	7.6	7.3	7.0	6.9
Weekend Nights							
Bedtime (24-h)	2231	2305	2326	2353	0003	0025	0045
Rise Time (24-h)	0853	0912	0921	0954	0954	1006	0951
Average Sleep (Hours)	9.2	8.9	9.0	8.8	8.9	8.8	8.4
School Night– Weekend Hours Slept Difference	0.8	0.8	0.9	1.2	1.6	1.9	1.5

Data from National Sleep Foundation. 2006 Sleep in America Poll Summary Findings. Available at: http://www.sleepfoundation.org/site/c.huIXKjM0IxF/b.2419037/k.1466/2006_Sleep_in_America_Poll. htm. Accessed February 14, 2007.

reported going to bed about an hour later on weekend nights, and for 12th graders, the weekend bedtime delay was about an hour and 45 minutes. The average reported rise time on school mornings was 6:42 AM in grade 6 and 6:31 AM in grade 12. The reported number of hours slept on school nights declined from 8.4 hours in the 6th grade students to 6.9 hours in the 12th graders; reported weekend sleep was more consistent from grades 6 through 11—about 9 hours—falling to 8.4 hours in grade 12. The weekend extension of sleep time in this report was nearly an hour in the middle school children (grades 6–8) and approached 2 hours for grade 11 students.

Amounts of sleep reported by adolescents vary across countries and regions; however, the overall patterns of later sleep timing and diminished sleep across adolescence is reported by most investigators. Reports of Korean youth, for example, indicate they begin and end grades 6 to 12 with later school night bedtimes and less sleep than those in the United States.[15] Children were assessed with a survey administered in the classroom querying usual sleep schedule. On average, the children reported:

- School night bedtime: grades 5–6 = 10:42 PM, grades 7–8 = 11:12 PM; grades 9–10 = 12 AM; grades 11–12 = 12:54 AM
- School morning rise time: grades 5–6 = 7:18 AM; grades 7–8 = 7 AM; grades 9–10 = 6:48 AM; grades 11–12 = 6:18 AM
- School night hours slept: grades 5–6 = 8.3; grades 7–8 = 7.6; grades 9–10 = 6.6; grades 11–12 = 5.4
- Weekend night bedtime: grades 5–6 = 11 PM, grades 7–8 = 11:30 PM; grades 9–10 = 11:46 PM; grades 11–12 = 11:54 PM
- Weekend morning rise time: grades 5–6 = 8:06 AM; grades 7–8 = 8:54 AM; grades 9–10- = 9:30 AM; grades 11–12 = 9:18 AM
- Weekend night hours slept: grades 5–6 = 9.0; grades 7–8 = 8.8; grades 9–10 = 9.0; grades 11–12 = 8.4.

An apparent difference in the older Korean children from the 11th and 12th graders in the US poll[16] was that the reported weekend bedtime was earlier than on school nights. The authors note that many students (71.1%) took additional course work in the evening, with classes lasting until midnight or later for 54.5% of the older students.

This pattern of late night classes on school days likely also explains why the Korean high school students reported earlier weekend than school-night bedtime on average.[15] It should also be noted that the standard deviation for reported weekend bedtime was 3 to 4 hours, much greater than for other variables.

The issue of determining the sleep need of adolescents is challenging, since the definition of sleep need itself is in dispute. Early work by Carskadon[4] started from a questionnaire assessment of school children in which the discrepancy between school day and weekend reported amount slept was zero, and the average amount was 10 hours a night. Of interest is the parallel finding of Iglowstein and colleagues[17] showing a concurrence of weekend and weekday sleep amounts at about 10 hours from reports by mothers of Swiss children.[17] In the longitudinal study of adolescents by Carskadon, time in bed was fixed at 10 hours a night, and the data showed that youngsters across the span of ages 10 to 17 slept about 9 hours and 20 minutes.[18] The younger children were more likely to waken spontaneously in the laboratory, whereas the older children took a bit longer to fall asleep and were rarely spontaneously awake at the end of the 10 hours. Furthermore, assessment with the multiple sleep latency test (MSLT, an objective measure of sleepiness) showed that the younger children were more alert across the day, whereas the pubertal and postpubertal adolescents showed a midday trough of alertness in spite of the same amount of nocturnal sleep.[19] In another study that may bear on the issue of sleep need of adolescents, Carskadon and colleagues[20] showed that adolescents (ages 11 to 14.6 years) given a 10-hour sleep schedule for 10 to 14 nights and then studied in the laboratory for 3 consecutive 18-hour nights, slept nearly 12.5 hours on average the first night and by night 3 still slept 10.1 hours on average (standard deviation about 1 hour).

ADOLESCENT DEVELOPMENT AND SLEEP REGULATION

In describing the biologic regulation of sleep, current thinking uses the 2-process model, first proposed by Borbély.[21] The 2 processes that comprise the model include a daily (circadian) rhythm of sleep propensity, thought to originate from the suprachiasmatic nucleus of the hypothalamus in mammals, and a sleep–wake pressure (homeostatic) system, for which a neuroanatomical locus has not been identified. In the case of the former process, the signal from the brain's central clock is thought to affect sleep and arousal systems to help gate the timing of sleep. The sleep homeostatic system favors sleep as the hours of wakefulness are extended and favors waking as sleep is prolonged, thus transducing information about the length and amount of prior sleep or wake, rather than the time of day. The role of these two processes can be distinguished independent from one another under certain experimental conditions,[22] but work interactively to regulate sleep from day to day.

Developmental changes in the circadian timing system were inferred by some from the delay in the timing of sleep onset, and 2 studies published in 1993 gave initial evidence for the hypothesis that a phase delay occurs in association with puberty. For example, Andrade and colleagues[23] found in a longitudinal study that later sleep times occurred for adolescents at a more mature Tanner stage[24] than others. Carskadon and colleagues[25] reported in a cross-sectional study using self-reported sleep and pubertal stage that 6th grade girls who rated themselves more mature had a more evening type score on a measure of circadian phase preference. A subsequent follow-up cross-sectional study in which adolescents' sleep–wake schedules were constrained for 2 weeks confirmed that circadian phase as evaluated with the objective measure of dim light melatonin onset (DLMO) phase was positively correlated with Tanner stage. In other words, the DLMO was later for participants rated more mature, indicating that the onset of the biologic night is later for more mature teens.

Several hypotheses have been put forward to explain the features of the circadian timing system that may underlie this developmental change. A review of adolescent changes in sleep and circadian rhythms by Hagenauer and colleagues[26] noted that signs of a juvenile phase delay were found in several mammalian species in addition to humans. **Table 2** highlights these findings. The occurrence of a circadian delay around the time of puberty for a number of species lends credence to the hypothesis that this phenomenon arises from intrinsic biologic processes rather than as a response to social/behavioral exposures. Whether or how the phase delay is linked to reproductive development is unknown.

If the adolescent phase delay is inherent, what mechanisms might explain the phenomenon? One hypothesis is that circadian period (ie, the internal day length) may become longer during adolescence. Pubertal male rats were found in 1 study to have longer intrinsic periods than adults,[27] and data from people show a longer period in teens than in adults.[28] An alternate explanation is that the circadian timing system manifests an altered sensitivity to phase-dependent effects of light; in particular, the pacemaker may become more sensitive to evening light's phase-delaying effects during adolescence than in childhood.[26] One animal study that offers support for this hypothesis showed an exaggerated delay of rhythms to light occurring at the phase-delaying time in pubertal mice compared with adult mice.[29] This hypothesis depends on an underlying biologic change that is then affected by behavioral exposures that arise during adolescence (ie, staying awake later, thus experiencing more evening light). A converse to this hypothesis is that adolescents become less sensitive to phase-advancing (morning) light or experience a change in the shape of the phase response curve. Preliminary data from one study of human adolescents provide a bit of evidence supporting this hypothesis.[30]

The influence of the sleep–wake homeostasis system is well understood, although specific neuroanatomical or neurochemical constituents are not yet fully established, nor has a link between adolescent maturation and this physiologic process been identified. Thus, whether the homeostatic process might be influenced by hormonal input, physical growth, brain maturation, or other factor(s) is unknown. On the other hand,

Table 2
Mammals with a juvenile phase delay[a]

Species	Amount of Delay	Rhythms Delayed	Sex Difference
Human (*Homo sapiens*)	1–3 h	Sleep, melatonin	Males>females
Rhesus monkey (*Macaca mulatta*)	2 h	Activity	Only females studied
Degu (*Octodon degus*)	3–5 h	Activity, sleep(?)	Males>females
Laboratory rat (*Rattus norvegicus*)	1–4 h	Activity	Males>females
Laboratory mouse (*Mus musculus*)	1 h (?)	Activity, corticosterone	Only females studied
Fat sand rat (*Psammomys obesus*)	0–3 h to 10–14 h (photoperiod dependent)	Oxygen consumption, temperature	Sex unspecified

[a] See Hagenauer and colleagues[26] for more information about these adolescent phase delays.

several evaluations of adolescent sleep physiology provide evidence for developmental changes in this sleep regulatory process. The theoretical model of sleep–wake homeostasis has a long history and a significant amount of experimental data supporting the model, based on sleep slow frequency electroencephalogram (EEG) data from animal and human models.[31] As waking is prolonged across a day or longer, slow-frequency EEG amplitude and incidence increase; as sleep unfolds across the night, slow-frequency EEG amplitude and incidence decay. Several studies have shown that adolescent development is not associated with a change in the decay of sleep homeostatic pressure (indexed by EEG slow-wave activity in sleep) but remains stable across early adolescent development (ages about 9–10 through ages about 14–15 years)[32] and up to age 18 years in another study.[33] On the other hand, preliminary data from a recent analyses of sleep EEG slow-wave activity in another adolescent cohort (ages 15–16 through about ages 17–19 years) demonstrate a longer time constant for the decay across the night in several brain regions.[34] One interpretation of the latter findings is that the sleep recovery process is unchanged in early adolescents and that certain parts of the brain may require more sleep to recover in older teens than when younger. This set of findings reinforces the likelihood that sleep need does not decline in adolescents.

Whereas the dissipation of sleep homeostatic pressure may speak to the recovery function of sleep, the other limb of the homeostatic process describes how the pressure to sleep or sleep propensity builds across the waking day. Jenni and colleagues[35] modeled the accumulation of sleep homeostasis in early adolescent humans (ages 9–14 years) who were either pre-/early pubertal or postpubertal. This analysis showed a longer time course for the build up of sleep pressure in the more mature group, indicating that the more mature adolescents may find it easier to stay awake longer than the less mature. This hypothesis was confirmed by analyzing speed of falling asleep on the multiple sleep latency test in a group of pre-/early pubescent versus a group of postpubertal adolescents across 36 hours of extended waking. The less mature adolescents fell asleep faster than the more mature on the tests occurring 14.5 and 16.5 hours after waking.[36]

In summary, current data on the maturation of the biologic regulation of sleep during adolescence show that

- The circadian timing system undergoes a phase delay
- The dissipation of sleep homeostatic pressure does not change until late adolescence when it shows evidence of slowing
- The accumulation of sleep homeostatic pressure slows during puberty.

These findings support the notion that the need for sleep is stable (or increases) across adolescent development and that the delay of sleep timing is supported by the circadian shift as well as the slowing of sleep homeostatic pressure accumulation.

PSYCHOSOCIAL FACTORS AFFECTING ADOLESCENT SLEEP

Many psychosocial factors affect sleep patterns in adolescents and contribute to the phase delay and the decline of time slept. A few examples will follow, as well as an examination of how they interact with these biologic regulatory processes. A primary psychodevelopmental task of adolescents is to achieve independence in many areas of their lives. One area where this striving for autonomy is displayed is the decision of when to go to sleep. One sleep habits surveys from the early 1980s showed that a significantly higher percentage of children ages 12 or 13 years reported setting their own bedtime on school nights (eg, 19% of 13-year-olds) than did younger children (eg, 50% of 10-year-olds) 10- to 12-year-old children and that reported bedtimes were later for the older children.[37] The other end of school night sleep—waking up—showed an opposite trend: more older children reported needing a parent or alarm to wake them than did the younger children, who were likelier to report that they "just wake up." Thus, the adolescents who actualize autonomy by staying up late seem to ride the wave of the circadian phase delay and to avail themselves of the relative emancipation from rapid sleep pressure accumulation. Yet, they were sleeping less, and rising early required external intervention to wake up.

Two recent studies highlight the importance of parental-set bedtimes. Gangwisch and colleagues[38] examined data in a large epidemiologic data set gathered from adolescents (grades 7–12) in the United States during the mid-1990s. The analysis showed that young people whose parent set their bedtime at midnight or after relative to those with bedtimes set at 10 PM or earlier, were significantly more likely to suffer from depression or suicidal ideation. The authors also found that this association was mediated by total sleep time; thus, those with earlier bedtimes reported sleeping more and were less likely to be depressed or experience suicidal ideation. A smaller, focused study of South Australian adolescents found that adolescents who reported a parental-set bedtime versus those without a set bedtime reported earlier bedtimes, more sleep, and less daytime fatigue experienced.[39] These 2 studies provide evidence that parental intervention by setting a bedtime results in extended sleep and that the combination of earlier bedtime and extended sleep contribute to more positive outcomes for depression, sleepiness, and fatigue. These findings may also indicate that such behavioral interventions as having a fixed, earlier bedtime may help mitigate the circadian phase delay associated with adolescent maturation, likely through preventing light to the circadian timing system at the delay-sensitive evening phase.

Screen time, technology use, and social engagement in the evening become more available as youngsters pass through adolescence. The US National Sleep Foundation poll of adolescents[16] reported that electronic devices (ie, electronic music devices, television, electronic/video games, cell phone, telephone, computer, Internet access) in the bedroom become more common for students from grade 6 to grade 12; the median number of such devices in bedrooms of younger adolescents was 2 versus a median of 4 in the older teens. A recent review by Cain and Gradisar[40] notes that the preponderance of studies report shorter, later, and/or more disrupted sleep, as well as such daytime consequences as sleepiness or disruptive behavior, for children and adolescents as TV watching, computer/Internet/electronic games use, or mobile phone use in the evening before bedtime is greater. These activities are arousing in and of themselves and usually more easily accessed by the older adolescents, taking advantage of increased accessibility of technology and of the changes to the sleep regulatory systems that make it easier to stay away later. Indeed, to the extent that the activities involve light exposure—perhaps particularly blue-spectrum light exposure to which the circadian clock may have greater sensitivity[41,42]—evening light has the phase-specific effect of delaying circadian rhythms, thus pushing sleep timing later.[43]

The impact of school schedules of adolescents is most often to restrict sleep by requiring an early rising time. As noted previously, however, school schedules can delay sleep further, such as described for Korean adolescents enrolled in evening classes to improve preparation for academic placement tests.[15] Evening homework assignments often carry a similar challenge for adolescents in the United States. More attention has been directed toward school starting times because of the tendency for many school systems in the United States to start the school day earlier as children get older, thus requiring teens to arise at an early hour relative to their typical bedtimes, circadian phases, and need for sleep.

One study examined sleep, sleepiness, and circadian rhythms in teens for whom the transition from 9th grade to 10th grade involved an advance of the school start time from 8:25 AM to 7:20 AM.[44] **Table 3** highlights findings from this study. Actigraphically monitored sleep data across 2 weeks confirmed that, although the students woke up significantly earlier on school days in tenth than ninth grade, they did not go to sleep earlier and consequently experienced less sleep on average. The general level of sleepiness in these students is shown with the daytime sleep latency data, showing a moderate level of sleepiness in 9th grade, and a significant change in 10th grade to a level considered severely sleepy for the sleep latency at 0830. The 0830 assessment was also associated with the occurrence of rapid eye movement (REM) sleep within 10 or 15 minutes of sleep onset, (a finding often used to aid in the diagnosis of narcolepsy) in about one half of the participants. The study also showed that the time of the DLMO was nearly 30 minutes later on average in the students when assessed in 10th grade; indeed, the DLMO time in the 10th graders was significantly later (2146 vs 2036) for those with the short sleep latency and REM sleep in the morning nap, interpreted as evidence that the circadian timing system of these teens was phase delayed relative to the early start time and favored sleep during the morning hours they were scheduled to attend school.[44] The association of a circadian phase delay, excessive morning sleep tendency, and REM sleep in morning trials for one-half of the adolescents studied is remarkable and raises the level of concern for early morning classes.

THE PERFECT STORM: SLEEP BEHAVIOR AND TROUBLING OUTCOMES

Fig. 1 illustrates the confluence of factors that combine for adolescents in the 21st century to reduce time spent sleeping on school nights below a healthful amount, with waking and expected school performance timed to occur at an inappropriate circadian phase. As reviewed previously, bioregulatory and psychosocial forces collude to push sleep onset later, yet schools are timed to begin earlier across adolescence, and sleep time is compressed as a consequence. The list of negative outcomes associated with insufficient sleep is lengthy and includes sleepiness and mood disturbances noted previously, as well as inattention, poor grades, behavior problems, substance use, driving crashes, overweight, and immune system compromise. For some

Table 3
Sleep, sleepiness, and circadian rhythms at a transition to early school days (mean [standard deviation])

	School Nights		Weekend Nights	
Actigraph Sleep Data	9th Grade	10th Grade	9th Grade	10th Grade
Sleep onset	2242 (36)	2238 (44)	2338 (56)	2344 (53)
Sleep offset	0626 (28)	0601 (19)[a]	0828 (69)	0832 (66)
Time slept	429 (47)	410 (42)[a]	485 (57)	478 (67)
Daytime Sleep Latency				
0830	10.9 (6.5)	5.1 (4.1)[a]	—	—
1030	10.7 (5.9)	9.2 (6.4)	—	—
1230	11.0 (5.5)	9.8 (5.5)	—	—
1430	11.5 (6.1)	11.0 (7.2)	—	—
Melatonin onset time	2024 (57)	2102 (77)[a]	—	—

[a] Statistically significant difference between 9th and 10th grade[4]

Adolescent Development & Sleep: The Perfect Storm

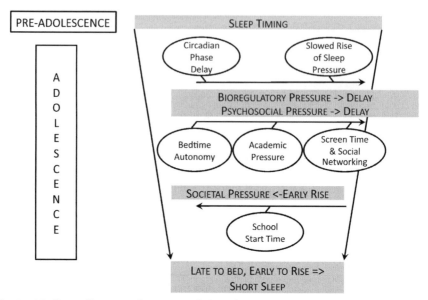

Fig. 1. This figure illustrates the timing of sleep from preadolescence through adolescent development, highlighting the factors that affect sleep as described in the text. Thus, sleep is relatively long and timed at an early hour for preadolescents, but maturational changes to intrinsic bioregulatory factors—the circadian phase delay arising from the circadian timing system and a slowed rise of sleep pressure stemming from sleep-wake homeostasis—push for a delay of the timing of sleep. Such psychosocial factors as self-selected bedtimes, response to academic pressure, and the availability and use of technology and social networking in the evening also push for a delay in the timing of sleep. Note that the length of sleep is not affected by these processes. Societal pressures that push for an early rise time—most notably an early start to the school day—are the forces that limit amount of time available for sleep. As a consequence, adolescents sleep too little and are asked to be awake at an inappropriate circadian phase.

adolescents, the issue can present as sleep-onset insomnia that may be associated with the circadian phase delay. When combined with lack of motivation, depressed mood, and fatigue, a depressive disorder is often the initial assumption. An approach that targets sleep timing and phase adjustment is likely to be ameliorative.

At the end of the day, the pediatrician can have positive impact by intervening in any of a number of levels:

- Encourage local school districts to consider starting the school day later for adolescents
- Recommend that the local school district also limit late-evening activities
- Galvanize schools to provide instructional information about sleep and circadian rhythms
- Support and encourage parents to identify and set an appropriate bedtime
- Encourage teens to avoid light and stimulating activities in the evening and to get light exposure in the morning
- Empower adolescents to make informed choices about their sleep schedules
- Remind families of the utility of a relaxing presleep ritual.

ACKNOWLEDGMENTS

I thank the many colleagues, fellows, staff, and families who have contributed to the research from my group that is summarized in this paper. In addition, I acknowledge support from the National Institutes of Health, including MH45945, MH52415, MH58879, HL71120, MH076969, MH079179.

REFERENCES

1. Andrade M, Menna-Baretto L. Sleep patterns of high school students living in Sao Paula, Brazil. In: Carskadon MA, editor. Adolescent sleep patterns: biological, social, and psychological factors. New York: Cambridge University Press; 2002. p. 118–31.
2. Arakawa M, Taira K, Tanaka H, et al. A survey of junior high school students' sleep habit and lifestyle in Okinawa. Psychiatry Clin Neurosci 2001;55(3):211–2.
3. Bearpark HM, Michie PT. Prevalence of sleep/wake disturbances in Sidney adolescents. Sleep Res 1987;16:304.
4. Carskadon MA. Patterns of sleep and sleepiness in adolescents. Pediatrician 1990;17(1):5–12.
5. Dorofaeff TF, Denny S. Sleep and adolescence. Do New Zealand teenagers get enough? J Paediatr Child Health 2006;42(9):515–20.
6. Gau SF, Soong WT. The transition of sleep–wake patterns in early adolescence. Sleep 2003;26(4):449–54.
7. Gibson ES, Powles AC, Thabane L, et al. Sleepiness is serious in adolescence: two surveys of 3235 Canadian students. BMC Public Health 2006;6:116.
8. Laberge L, Petit D, Simard C, et al. Development of sleep patterns in early adolescence. J Sleep Res 2001;10(1):59–67.
9. Park YM, Matsumoto K, Seo YJ, et al. Changes of sleep or waking habits by age and sex in Japanese. Percept Mot Skills 2002;94:1199–213.
10. Reid A, Maldonado CC, Baker FC. Sleep behavior of South African adolescents. Sleep 2002;25(4):423–7.
11. Saarenpaa-Heikkila OA, Rintahaka PJ, Laippala PJ, et al. Sleep habits and disorders in Finnish schoolchildren. J Sleep Res 1995;4(3):173–82.
12. Strauch I, Meier B. Sleep need in adolescents: a longitudinal approach. Sleep 1988;11(4):378–86.
13. Thorleifsdottir B, Bjornsson JK, Benediktsdottir B, et al. Sleep and sleep habits from childhood to young adulthood over a 10-year period. J Psychosom Res 2002;53(1):529–37.
14. Wolfson AR, Carskadon MA. Sleep schedules and daytime functioning in adolescents. Child Dev 1998;69(4):875–87.
15. Yang CK, Kim JK, Patel SR, et al. Age-related changes in sleep/wake patterns among Korean teenagers. Pediatrics 2005;115(Suppl 1):250–6.
16. National Sleep Foundation. 2006 Sleep in America Poll summary findings. Available at: http://www.sleepfoundation.org/site/c.hulXKjM0IxF/b.2419037/k.1466/2006_Sleep_in_America_Poll.htm. Accessed February 14, 2007.
17. Iglowstein I, Jenni OG, Molinari L, et al. Sleep duration from infancy to adolescence: reference values and generational trends. Pediatrics 2003;111(2):302–7.
18. Carskadon MA, Orav EJ, Dement WC. Evolution of sleep and daytime sleepiness in adolescents. In: Guilleminault C, Lugaresi E, editors. Sleep/wake disorders: natural history, epidemiology, and long-term evolution. New York: Raven Press; 1983. p. 201–16.
19. Carskadon MA, Harvey K, Duke P, et al. Pubertal changes in daytime sleepiness. Sleep 1980;2:453–60.

20. Carskadon MA, Acebo C, Seifer R. Extended nights, sleep loss, and recovery sleep in adolescents. Arch Ital Biol 2001;139(3):301–12.
21. Borbély AA. A two-process model of sleep regulation. Hum Neurobiol 1982;1(3): 195–204.
22. Czeisler CA, Allan JS, Kronauer RE. A method for assaying the effects of therapeutic agents on the period of the endogenous circadian pacemaker in man. In: Montplaisir J, Godbout R, editors. Sleep and biological rhythms: basic mechanisms and applications to psychiatry. New York: Oxford University Press; 1990. p. 87–98.
23. Andrade MM, Benedito-Silva AA, Domenice S, et al. Sleep characteristics of adolescents: a longitudinal study. J Adolesc Health 1993;14:401–6.
24. Tanner JM. Growth at adolescence. 2nd edition. Oxford (UK): Blackwell; 1962.
25. Carskadon MA, Vieira C, Acebo C. Association between puberty and delayed phase preference. Sleep 1993;16(3):258–62.
26. Hagenauer MH, Perryman JI, Lee TM, et al. Adolescent changes in the homeostatic and circadian regulation of sleep. Dev Neurosci 2009;31(4):276–84.
27. McGinnis MY, Lumia AR, Tetel MJ, et al. Effects of anabolic androgenic steroids on the development and expression of running wheel activity and circadian rhythms in male rats. Physiol Behav 2007;92:1010–8.
28. Carskadon MA, Labyak SE, Acebo C, et al. Intrinsic circadian period of adolescent humans measured in conditions of forced desynchrony. Neurosci Lett 1999; 260(2):129–32.
29. Weinert D, Eimert H, Erkert HG, et al. Resynchronizatin of the circadian corticosterone rhythm after a light/dark shift in juvenile and adult mice. Chronobiol Int 1994;11:222–31.
30. Carskadon MA, Acebo C, Arnedt JT, et al. Melatonin sensitivity to light in adolescents: preliminary results. Sleep 2001;24:A190–1.
31. Borbély AA, Achermann P. Sleep homeostasis and models of sleep regulation. In: Kryger MH, Roth T, Dement WC, editors. Principles and practice of sleep medicine. 3rd edition. Philadelphia: W.B. Saunders Company; 2000. p. 377–90.
32. Jenni OG, Carskadon MA. Spectral analysis of the sleep electroencephalogram during adolescence. Sleep 2004;27(4):774–83.
33. Campell IG, Darchia N, Higgins LM, et al. Adolescent changes in homeostatic regulation of EEG activity in the delta and theta frequency bands during NREM sleep. Sleep 2011;34(1):83–91.
34. Tarokh L, Carskadon MA, Rusterholz T, et al. Homeostatic sleep regulation in adolescents: longitudinal perspectives. Sleep, in press.
35. Jenni OG, Achermann P, Carskadon MA. Homeostatic sleep regulation in adolescents. Sleep 2005;28(11):1446–54.
36. Taylor DJ, Jenni OG, Acebo C, et al. Sleep tendency during extended wakefulness: insights into adolescent sleep regulation and behavior. J Sleep Res 2005;14(3):239–44.
37. Carskadon MA. The second decade. In: Guilleminault C, editor. Sleep and waking disorders: indications and techniques. Menlo Park (CA): Addison Wesley; 1982. p. 99–125.
38. Gangwisch JE, Babiss LA, Malaspina D, et al. Earlier parental set bedtimes as a protective factor against depression and suicidal ideation. Sleep 2010;33(1): 97–106.
39. Short MA, Gradisar M, Wright H, et al. Time for bed: parent-set bedtimes associated with improved sleep and daytime functioning in adolescents. Sleep, in press.

40. Cain N, Gradisar M. Electronic media use and sleep in school-aged children and adolescents. Sleep Med 2010;11(8):735–42.
41. Brainard GC, Hanifin JP, Greeson JM, et al. Action spectrum for melatonin regulation in humans: evidence for a novel circadian photoreceptor. J Neurosci 2001; 21(16):6405–12.
42. Thapan K, Arendt J, Skene DJ. An action spectrum for melatonin suppression: evidence for a novel nonrod, noncone photoreceptor system in humans. J Physiol 2001;535:261–7.
43. Khalsa SB, Jewett ME, Cajochen C, et al. A phase response curve to single bright light pulses in human subjects. J Physiol 2003;549:945–52.
44. Carskadon MA, Wolfson AR, Acebo C, et al. Adolescent sleep patterns, circadian timing, and sleepiness at a transition to early school days. Sleep 1998;21(8): 871–81.

Cognitive, Behavioral, and Functional Consequences of Inadequate Sleep in Children and Adolescents

Dean W. Beebe, PhD

KEYWORDS

- Sleep deprivation • Sleep quality • Pediatrics • Cognition
- Psychological • School functioning

The premise that inadequate sleep can cause problems with cognition, behavior, or other aspects of daytime functioning has been long discussed in Western culture. Relevant writings date back to antiquity,[1] and once technological advances allowed for a popular press, it disseminated definitively worded advice on proper sleep patterns for children.[2] Physicians and the lay public could not be blamed, however, for a healthy dose of skepticism. After all, the advice seemed to change among investigators, and it did not take much digging to see that it was based on thinly veiled personal observations and opinions. Over the past several decades, however, scientific data have largely replaced subjective observations and personal speculation and have confirmed that at least some of early observers' impressions were correct. This article reviews the available data, and then outlines why that evidence is particularly concerning from a developmental perspective.

METHODOLOGICAL CONSIDERATIONS

This review focuses on data collected in children and adolescents. There is a large and well-developed literature on sleep deprivation in adults that can provide initial

This work was supported by grant No. R01 HL092149 from the National Institutes of Health.
Neuropsychology Program, Division of Behavioral Medicine and Clinical Psychology (ML3015), Cincinnati Children's Hospital Medical Center, University of Cincinnati College of Medicine, 3333 Burnet Avenue, Cincinnati, OH 45229, USA
E-mail address: dean.beebe@cchmc.org

guidance for pediatric research, but cannot be extrapolated to children without studying children, for several reasons. Whereas the large majority of adult experimental studies have examined the impact of 1 to 2 nights of complete sleep deprivation, it is reasonable to question how these findings generalize to children, whose overall sleep need is greater and who far more often experience chronic partial sleep restriction than total sleep deprivation. Moreover, circadian rhythms shift developmentally, and adolescence brings tremendous changes in sleep physiology, particularly within the lower slow-wave electroencephalographic (EEG) frequency ranges, that may alter the response to sleep restriction.[3–5] Finally, the contexts in which children must function differ substantially from adults. Adult research findings on how experimental sleep deprivation affects truck drivers, medical residents, or other professionals are important, but these findings provide only a rough guess as to the effect of chronic sleep restriction on classroom behaviors or learning, the development of new driving skills, or behavioral and social functioning in developing children.

Studying children and adolescents poses methodological challenges. The primary research design for adult sleep deprivation studies, in which participants stay in lab to allow for greater control of sleep and activity schedules, is less of an option for child researchers because parents are often reluctant to leave their children in the care of unfamiliar adults, participants may be resistant to a prolonged stay away from home, and children's sleep may be particularly subject to disruption in an unfamiliar environment.[6,7] Further, children are a vulnerable population, for whom additional protections against risk may be required. Although it seems that any health effects of short-term sleep restriction are reversible with 1 to 2 nights of recovery sleep, researchers must consider the risk of events that could occur during sleep restriction (eg, a poor school grade, auto accident for young drivers) and attempt to mitigate that risk. As a result, there have been few experimental studies.

High-quality studies using multiple research designs are needed because each has strengths and weaknesses. Correlational, case-control, and quasi-experimental studies lend themselves well to assessing the real-world associations between sleep and daytime function, often in impressively large samples that promote subgroup analyses and generalization of findings. However, the potential for uncontrolled confounding factors (eg, parent work schedules, parenting styles, family structure, child daytime activities/habits, teen employment) limits causal inferences, and measurements of both sleep and outcome variables are often imprecise. In contrast, experimental studies allow for more confident attribution of causality and more measurement precision, but the conclusions can be limited by small samples and by methods and measures that do not map cleanly onto real-world circumstances.

Like research designs, different cognitive and behavioral assessment techniques have complementary strengths and weaknesses.[8] Questionnaires have the advantages of easy administration, low cost, and ready assessment of real-world functioning, but are prone to reporter biases. Office-based standardized neuropsychological tests avoid such bias and can parse out specific cognitive skills. However, some domains of functioning, particularly attention and executive functioning (eg, planning, organization, mood, and behavior regulation), are difficult to assess in an office-based testing environment.[9,10] Direct systematic rating of child behaviors by trained observers can provide an objective perspective in applied settings but is logistically very difficult; the 2 studies that have used such techniques in the sleep-behavior literature used simulated classrooms rather than embedding raters in subjects' schools.[11,12]

In the end, there is no single best way to study the effect of sleep on the daytime functioning of children and adolescents. The best conclusions tend to be drawn from an accumulation of studies with complementary strengths and weaknesses.

CORRELATIONAL AND CASE-CONTROL STUDIES

The largest research base that links sleep in children to daytime functioning comes from correlational studies in epidemiologic samples. As summarized in recent major reviews,[13–16] children's quantity and/or quality of sleep repeatedly has been shown to correlate with their levels of daytime sleepiness and performance at school. The strength of that association may vary by student age and sex; one recent meta-analysis of sleep and school functioning reported that studies of younger children, particularly those that enrolled more boys, tended to show the largest effects.[16] To some degree, research in this area could be criticized for an overreliance on parent- or self-report of sleep and academic performance. However, such reports correlate well with objective measures,[15,17] and importantly, the association between sleep and academic functioning has been reported even when both constructs were measured objectively.[18]

Even so, findings have not been universal. Mayes and colleagues recently suggested that sleep is minimally associated with academic knowledge.[19] This study relied heavily on office-based tests of academic knowledge, which are only partial predictors of classroom performance. Classroom performance also depends on skills that are difficult to test in the office, including sustained attention, behavior regulation, planning, and organization.[20] Indeed, school-identified learning problems did significantly correlate with poor parent-reported sleep quality in the Mayes and colleagues' study. However, this effect disappeared after statistically covarying for symptoms of attention-deficit/hyperactivity disorder (ADHD), which led to the speculation that any apparent link between sleep and learning problems could be because of the confounding effects of ADHD. Alternatively, however, symptoms of ADHD may not represent confounding factors but the mechanism by which poor sleep quality was linked to learning problems.

Indeed, inadequate sleep has been linked to difficulties with attention, impulse control, and behavior regulation,[21–24] with potential consequences that extend beyond the classroom. Poor sleep quality is associated with crash risk in teen drivers,[25] and short sleep has been linked to accidental injuries in young children[26–28] and adolescents,[27] as well as risk-taking behaviors in adolescents.[29] Because poor regulation of attention and behavior are the key features of ADHD, it has been concluded that a subgroup of children with primary sleep problems may be misdiagnosed with ADHD. However, the relationship between ADHD and sleep is complex, and the reader is referred to the relevant article elsewhere in this issue and several other recent reviews for detailed coverage.[30–32]

The links between sleep and other psychiatric diagnoses, including depression and anxiety disorders, are similarly complex and extend beyond the current discussion. Briefly, sleep problems are disproportionately present in many psychiatric conditions, and the direction of causation seems to be reciprocal rather than unidirectional.[33] There is also evidence that the presence or severity of sleep disturbance predicts psychiatric symptom severity and functional impairment.[34,35] However, it is difficult to know how to apply this information to the general population; although sleep disruption seems to be linked to mood, studies have yielded mixed associations between sleep duration and emotional functioning.[36–38] Indeed, within one study, parent-reported mood problems and behavior problems had variable associations with sleep duration, depending on the source of information on behavior/mood (parent- vs self-report) and sleep duration (parent vs actigraphy).[39]

Of greater interest are studies of daytime functioning of children and adolescents with obstructive sleep apnea (OSA), a largely treatable disorder in which the upper airway is chronically and/or repeatedly obstructed during sleep. As reviewed by

Beebe,[40] OSA has been linked to poor classroom grades, sleepiness, inattention, hyperactivity, oppositional behaviors, and mood dysregulation (but not ongoing mood disturbance) in the vast majority of relevant studies, most of which have targeted children aged 5 to 12 years. Beebe and colleagues[20] recently extended those findings through the adolescent years. Office-based tests of intelligence have yielded inconsistent results in children with OSA, with the most consistent evidence of IQ deficits during the preschool and early grade-school years.[40] Other tests of cognition have yielded mixed results, but there is some evidence of poor scores on tests of attention, executive functioning, and learning/memory in children with OSA.[40–42] OSA is of particular interest in this article not only because a large number of studies have examined behavioral outcomes of children with this condition but also because treatments focus on the airway and would not be expected to affect behavior in a manner independent of sleep. Nonrandomized studies have shown improved daytime functioning following surgical intervention for uncomplicated OSA,[40,43] bolstering the suggestion that OSA is causally related to daytime dysfunction. However, the results of the childhood adenotonsillectomy (CHAT) study are awaited, an ongoing large randomized adenotonsillectomy trial for OSA with blinded outcome measures.

There have been studies that have linked other treatable sleep conditions, most notably restless legs syndrome (RLS) and periodic limb movement disorder, to daytime dysfunction, particularly to hyperactivity/impulsivity and inattention.[44,45] However, compared with OSA, studies have been few, causal implications are unclear, and intervention data are difficult to interpret because the relevant sleep treatments can also directly affect daytime functioning. For more information on RLS, see the article by Durmer and colleagues elsewhere in this issue.

Outside OSA, only a handful of correlational and case-controlled studies of pediatric sleep have used objective measures of cognitive functioning. In 2 studies, poor quality sleep was significantly associated with poor attention, working memory, and/or impulse control.[22,23] A recent study linked objectively defined short sleep with lower IQ test scores.[46] However, other studies have reported either (1) no relationship between sleep duration and IQ[47] or (2) an association only for males and on selected aspects of intelligence.[48] Two studies of large sample size on young children have arrived at conflicting results with respect to overall cognitive functioning and sleep.[49,50]

In summary, correlational and case-control studies have yielded good evidence of the association between inadequate sleep and disturbances in children's behavior and attention regulation, daytime sleepiness, academic performance, and, to the extent that it has been explored, executive functioning. However, the possibility of uncontrolled confounding factors limits the degree to which causal inferences can be drawn from these studies.

QUASI-EXPERIMENTAL STUDIES

As summarized in **Table 1**, there have been several quasi-experimental studies in which scientists have carefully observed that in middle- and high-school students, sleep duration was systematically influenced by school start times. In an impressive illustration of how public policy can affect health, starting school later in the morning is associated with students getting more sleep, regardless of whether comparing across schools (between groups),[51–54] within a group of students over time,[55,56] or within individuals over time.[57] The link between more sleep and later school start time is primarily when students awaken; bedtimes are relatively unchanged. Not surprisingly, later start times are also associated with less subjective and physiologic sleepiness.[51–54,57] Finally, later start times seem to be associated with improved enrollment stability,[53,54] better attendance among the least stable students,[53,54] less tardiness,[53,54] fewer teen driving accidents,[55] and slightly fewer sick days and depressive symptoms.[53,54]

Limitations of many of these studies include an unknown risk for uncontrolled confounding factors (eg, school management, historical events, child development), reliance on self-report of daytime functioning, and samples consisting of superhealthy individuals who may not reflect the general population. Importantly, evidence of academic gains or improvements on standardized test scores is sparse, and none of these studies has yet demonstrated that students learn more with later school start times.

EXPERIMENTAL STUDIES

Since 1896, hundreds of publications have documented the impact of experimental sleep deprivation or restriction on adults' sleep-wake regulation, affect regulation, cognitive performance, real-world functioning (eg, driving), and neuronal activity.[58] In contrast, as of late 2010, there had been only 7 analogous published studies of pediatric populations, all in print since 1980 (**Table 2**). These studies so far allow for 5 broad conclusions.

First, compared with when they are well-rested, sleep-deprived children fall asleep more easily during the day, self-report sleepiness, and look sleepier.[7,11,59–62] Second, children are less attentive when sleep deprived. It has been difficult to demonstrate this conclusion on formal attention tests, but shortened sleep results in visibly more inattentive behaviors, whether reported by individuals who are not blind to sleep condition,[7,11] teachers who were likely blind to sleep condition,[62] or observers whose blind state was rigorously maintained.[17] Third, no experimental study has yet shown that sleep restriction induces hyperactivity, impulsivity, or other externalizing behaviors in children, despite the correlational and case-control evidence that these changes should occur. Fourth, there is some evidence that depriving children of sleep affects their higher-level cognitive skills. One study documented diminished creativity and reasoning skills following a single night of shortened sleep, but overall study results were mixed.[63] Another study reported that sleep-deprived adolescents showed diminished higher-level executive functioning skills according to parent- and self-report forms.[7] Fifth, there is evidence that the impact of sleep deprivation is substantial enough to result in real-world impairment. Sleepiness and inattention in real-world settings have been reported by teachers, parents, and subjects.[7,61,62] One study also found deficits in executive functioning as applied to daily life,[7] and 2 studies reported learning difficulties in a simulated or real classroom.[12,62]

These findings are important because they infer that inadequate sleep causes daytime deficits. However, to date, there simply have been too few studies to answer many important questions. In children, there is little to no knowledge (1) of how circadian rhythms interact with sleep restriction to affect functioning, (2) of the response to sleep restriction as it accumulates over time, and (3) on whether and why some individuals are more vulnerable to sleep restriction. Moreover, the existing studies have generally had limited statistical power because of small sample sizes and/or the use of between-subjects research designs. The samples also have been largely composed of superhealthy individuals, with limited ethnic and socioeconomic diversity. Young children have been overlooked entirely in published work, although this age range may show unique symptoms (eg, greater impulsivity). In addition, although it is clear that sleep restriction results in impairments that extend beyond simple

Table 1
Quasi-experimental studies involving differences in school start times

Authors	Grade Level	Analytic Design	Comparison	Findings
Dexter et al[51]	10th–11th	Between groups	2 nearby schools serving students with similar demographics, one starting at 7:50 AM and the other at 8:35 AM	Students at the school that started at 7:50 AM reported significantly less sleep and a trend toward more sleepiness. Sleepiness ratings at both schools approached the pathologically sleepy range
Wolfson et al[52]	7th–8th	Between groups	2 nearby schools serving students with similar demographics, one starting at 7:15 AM and the other at 8:37 AM	Students at the school that started at 7:15 AM reported significantly less sleep on school nights and greater sleepiness and had more school-documented tardiness. Reported class grades differed across schools for 8th graders, but not 7th graders
Hansen et al[56]	Incoming 9th grade honors students	Within group	Student sleep diaries the month before school started were compared with those completed at the first 2 wk of high school and again several months later	Weeknight sleep duration dropped dramatically from summer into the school year. It then lengthened a bit across the school year, but remained well less than summertime levels
Carskadon[57]	Students shifting from 9th to 10th grades	Within subjects	Students wore actigraphs in the spring of 9th grade at a school that started at 8:25 AM and again in the fall of 10th grade after transitioning to a school that started at 7:20 AM. Sleepiness was also assessed during each period	School night bedtimes did not change over time, but rise time became significantly earlier with the transition to the 7:20 AM start time, resulting in less sleep. Students' physiologic sleepiness was higher during the second time point as well

Study	Grades	Design	Description	Results
Wahlstrom[53,54]	9th–12th	Mixed within group and between groups	7 schools in one district (district A) changed start time from 7:15–8:40 AM. Letter grades and enrollment data were compared before and after the schedule change. Also, after the school start time change, student-reported sleep and affect ratings were compared against analogous ratings in a nearby, demographically similar district that had a 7:30 AM start time (district B)	After start time change, students in district A changed schools less, and those who changed schools had higher attendance rates. There were no differences in overall student grades from before to after the start time change, but methodological issues complicated analyses. Focusing on the post–change period, compared with district B, students in district A had only slightly later bedtimes, but markedly later rise times, resulting in almost an hour more sleep per night. Also students in district A reported less daytime sleepiness, less tardiness due to oversleeping, and marginally fewer sick days and symptoms of depression
Danner & Phillips[55]	9th–12th	Mixed within group and between groups	Students reported on sleep before and after start times were shifted from 7:30–8:30 AM in a countywide district. Motor vehicle crash data for 17–18-year-old adolescents in the county were contrasted with trends for other counties in the state	Compared with before the change in start times, after the start time had been changed, students' school night sleep time increased significantly, weekend night sleep time decreased significantly, and motor vehicle crashes by teens in the county decreased. During the same period, teen crashes were stable or increased slightly elsewhere in the same state

Table 2
Experimental studies of cognitive and behavioral effects of sleep restriction in children and adolescents

Authors	Sample	Analytic Design	Comparison	Findings
Carskadon et al[59]	9 subjects aged 11–13 y	Within subject, no crossover	Objective sleepiness and cognitive testing after a baseline night (10 h in bed), 1 night of 4 h in bed, and a recovery night (10 h in bed)	Objective sleepiness increased after sleep restriction. No significant changes across nights were noted on the cognitive tests, which included measures of complex addition, word learning/ memory, and sustained auditory attention
Carskadon et al[60]	12 subjects aged 11–14 y	Within subject, no crossover	Objective and subjective sleepiness and cognitive testing after baseline night (10 h in bed), 1 night of no sleep at all, and 2 recovery nights (10 h each)	After sleep deprivation, objective and subjective sleepiness increased and performance on all cognitive tests diminished, reaching significance on complex addition and word learning/memory, and showing trends on sustained attention tests
Randazzo et al[63]	16 subjects aged 10–14 y	Between subject	Cognitive test scores after random assignment to 11 h in bed or 5 h in bed for a single night	Significant effects on 3 indexes of creativity and a measure of concept formation/reasoning. No such effects were evident on a second measure of concept formation/reasoning, a test of verbal learning, or 7 other indexes of creativity
Sadeh et al[61]	77 subjects aged 9–12 y	Mixed within & between subject	Cognitive tests after 2 nights of normal sleep and 3 nights of a randomly assigned sleep condition (normal sleep duration ±1 h)	There were cross-condition effects for sleepiness and session-by-group interactions for reaction time and attention span, favoring the lengthened sleep condition. No such interactions were evident on tests of finger tapping speed, sustained attention, impulse control, working memory, or learning/memory

Study	Subjects	Design	Protocol	Findings
Fallone et al[11]	82 subjects aged 8–15 y	Between subjects	Cognitive testing, sleepiness, and behaviors in a simulated academic setting after one in an optimized sleep condition (10 h in bed) or restricted sleep condition (4 h in bed)	Observers rated those with restricted sleep as less attentive but not more hyper/impulsive. In the academic setting, subjects who had restricted sleep were sleepy but not hyper/impulsive. Self-report and objective sleepiness were higher in the restricted sleep condition. There were few cross-group effects on attention tests
Fallone et al[62]	74 subjects aged 6–12 y	Within subject, with crossover	Teacher behavior ratings while subjects underwent 3-wk protocol: baseline week (self-selected sleep duration), followed in counterbalanced order by optimized sleep (10+ h/night) vs sleep restriction (6.5–8 h/night)	Cross-condition effects were seen on teacher ratings of academic problems, sleepiness, and inattention; the worst ratings occurred during the restricted sleep condition, although otherwise the pattern of scores varied. There were no significant cross-condition effects on teacher ratings of hyperactivity/impulsivity, internalizing/mood issues, or oppositional/aggressive behaviors
Beebe et al[7,12,64]	19 subjects aged 13–16 y	Within subject, with crossover	Parent and subject ratings of behavior, simulated classroom performance, and EEG and fMRI assessments during a 3-wk protocol: baseline (self-selected sleep duration), followed in counterbalanced order by extended (10 h/night) vs restricted sleep (6.5 h/night)	Parents rated their teenage children as sleepier and having more problems with attention, oppositionality, behavior regulation, and metacognition; similar effects were also self-reported. Effects on reported hyperactivity/impulsivity were minimal. In the simulated classroom, learning was poorer and there was behavioral and EEG evidence of sleepiness/low arousal during sleep restriction. fMRI suggested compensatory neural mechanisms

Abbreviation: fMRI, functional magnetic resonance imaging.

sleepiness, some constructs remain underexplored (eg, problem solving, memory) and others are unexplored but theoretically at risk (eg, affect regulation). Finally, only 1 pilot study so far has examined how pediatric sleep restriction affects waking neural activity.[12,64]

ADDING A DEVELOPMENTAL CONTEXT

The findings presented so far are important, but few address developmental issues that are particularly salient during childhood, such as the parallel development of the brain and its cognitive and behavioral functions, as well as unique contexts involving children.

Developmental changes are evident in the brain throughout the life span, but the most dramatic neurodevelopment occurs during childhood, guided by an interaction between genetic programming and environmental factors.[65,66] Chronic or extreme exposure to stress or toxins during development can lead to aberrant neural connections, resulting in disruption of cognitive, behavioral, or emotional functioning.[66] Inadequate sleep may be one such exposure; animal models have demonstrated that even short-term sleep deprivation can alter neural plasticity.[67–73] Further, a rodent model of OSA suggests a developmental gradient, with particularly marked effects on the brain and learning during the period equivalent to early childhood.[74,75] These findings are notable in light of human data that suggest that OSA has the greatest effect on behavioral functioning in boys younger than 8 years[76] and on intelligence in preschool children.[40] Inadequate sleep state can be prolonged in humans, so even low levels of inadequacy might result in changed neurodevelopmental patterns and trajectories over time. Notably, the anterior brain regions that show the most protracted development across childhood are also those that are thought to experience the greatest functional impact of sleep deprivation.[77–79]

There have been few publications on the neural response to sleep deprivation in children, but noninvasive technologies hold promise for providing additional data. Four relevant studies have been published. Magnetic resonance spectroscopy of school-aged children with severe OSA found region-specific chemical abnormalities suggestive of neuronal injury.[80] Also, in young children with subclinical sleep-disordered breathing, altered neuronal processing of speech sounds has been detected via evoked response potentials, leading to the speculation that the brain may be attempting to compensate for sleep disturbance.[81] A similar explanation was evoked to explain altered activation-deactivation patterns in attention-related brain regions of adolescents during sleep restriction.[64] These adolescents also showed EEG slowing in a simulated classroom while sleep deprived.[12] All these findings are preliminary, and at present, it is impossible to draw coherent conclusions because of the differences in sample size, research designs, and measures. However, these studies support the suggestion that inadequate sleep can substantively alter neural processing.

Paralleling neurodevelopment, key functional skills develop across childhood. While academic skills are most easily appreciated as requiring learning, it is no exaggeration to state that every foundation skill necessary for adult functioning matures substantially during childhood and adolescence. To the degree that sleep deprivation affects a young child's ability to engage with and learn from the environment—and the evidence reviewed earlier suggests that it does—maturation may be delayed or disrupted. Older children and adolescents may be vulnerable in other ways because their behaviors can have costly irreversible consequences.[78] For example, there is a spike in accidental injuries during adolescence,[78] and adolescent school underperformance increases the odds of school dropout, failure to enroll in or complete college, adult mental illness or substance abuse, and low occupational attainment.[82–86] If sleep quality or quantity affects injury risk or school success, as described previously, then the long-term legacy of pediatric sleep problems may be considerable.

In humans, it is neither feasible nor ethical to experimentally expose children to prolonged sleep restriction. However, longitudinal studies can examine the natural associations between inadequate sleep and later functioning. Over a dozen relevant studies have been published, and a well-replicated finding is that childhood sleep problems (variously defined) predict the development of anxiety and depressive symptoms over time, even after controlling for baseline mood difficulties and other potential confounds. This finding has been reported across time frames spanning preschool to midchildhood,[87,88] preschool to midadolescence,[89,90] midchildhood to late childhood,[39,91] midchildhood to young adulthood,[92] and adolescence to young adulthood.[93] Longitudinal associations between sleep problems and externalizing behaviors, such as hyperactivity, aggression, or conduct, have tended to be weaker or less consistent, but also have been reported.[39,87,88,92] Consistent with such associations, the presence of loud snoring, a hallmark symptom of OSA, in young children has been shown to predict later hyperactivity and poor school performance.[94,95] Finally, sleep problems at the ages of 3 to 8 years have also been found to predict the early onset of substance use in adolescents.[90]

However, such longitudinal relationships have not always been straightforward. One group has suggested that inadequate sleep has the greatest effects in children from homes of lower socioeconomic status.[39,47] In several other studies, the initial presence of sleep problems was less important in predicting later functioning than whether these problems persisted or worsened over time.[38,96,97] Such complexity has also been evident in studies of cognitive and learning outcomes. Especially among children from low-income homes, the presence of sleep problems in third grade predicts intellectual stagnation, whereas longer sleep predicts better reading development, over the following 2 years.[47] Persistent or worsening sleep problems during childhood also predict poorer scores later on tests of executive functioning, but not on memory, nonverbal reasoning, vocabulary, or fine motor skills.[97–99]

These longitudinal findings cannot prove causation but are consistent with a developmental model in which inadequate sleep is viewed as a noxious exposure that results, over time, in increased risk for adverse functional outcomes.

SUMMARY

Findings from studies that used complementary research methods have converged to strongly suggest that inadequate sleep quality and quantity are causally linked to sleepiness, inattention, and probably other cognitive and behavioral deficits that affect daytime functioning, with potential implications for long-term development. Important research questions remain, but the available data not only support the integration of sleep screening and interventions into routine clinical care (see related article elsewhere in this issue) but also support advocacy for public policy changes to improve the sleep of children and adolescents, with the goal of preventing long-term functional deficits.[53,54]

As the pediatric sleep discipline moves forward, it is worth reflecting on other domains of public health that focus on prevention. When causes of adult conditions are earlier in development, treatments performed in adulthood are usually inefficient and not entirely efficacious; for example, skin cancer can be treated in adulthood but with mixed success and sometimes at great personal and societal cost. In contrast, better understanding of the early effects of sun exposure during childhood has led to more effective primary prevention.[100] Effective prevention has also emerged when childhood exposure to a suspected pathogen is studied to determine its deleterious mechanisms and lifetime effects. This was the case with inorganic lead exposure that, until studied in children, was tolerated at levels later shown to cause long-term adaptive deficits.[101] In both of these examples, it is noteworthy that causal conclusions, and the effective preventive strategies that followed, were derived from a combination of translational, experimental, correlational, and longitudinal data. If similarly diverse data continue to bear out the developmental model described earlier, chronic sleep problems or sleep restriction might not be considered any more tolerable during childhood or adolescence than noxious serum lead levels or unregulated artificial tanning facilities.

REFERENCES

1. Thorpy MJ. History of sleep and man. In: Thorpy MJ, Yager J, editors. The encyclopedia of sleep and sleep disorders. New York: Facts on File, Inc; 1991. p. ix–xxx.
2. Stearns PN, Rowlands P, Giarnella L. Children's sleep: sketching historical change. J Soc Hist 1996;30:345–66.
3. Carskadon MA, Acebo C. Regulation of sleepiness in adolescents: update, insights, and speculation. Sleep 2002;25:606–14.
4. Jenni OG, Achermann P, Carskadon MA. Homeostatic sleep regulation in adolescents. Sleep 2005;28:1446–54.
5. Campbell IG, Higgins LM, Trinidad JM, et al. The increase in longitudinally measured sleepiness across adolescence is related to the maturational decline in low-frequency EEG power. Sleep 2007;30:1677–87.
6. Fallone G, Seifer R, Acebo C, et al. How well do school-aged children comply with imposed sleep schedules at home? Sleep 2002;25:739–45.
7. Beebe DW, Fallone G, Godiwala N, et al. Feasibility and behavioral effects of an at-home multi-night sleep restriction protocol for adolescents. J Child Psychol Psychiatry 2008;49:915–23.
8. Beebe DW. Assessing neurobehavioral outcomes in childhood sleep disordered breathing: a primer for non-neuropsychologists. In: Marcus C, Carroll J, Loughlin G, et al, editors. Sleep in children: developmental changes in sleep patterns. 2nd edition. New York: Informa Healthcare; 2008. p. 345–65.
9. Gioia GA, Isquith PK, Guy SC, et al. BRIEF – Behavior Rating Inventory of Executive Function. Odessa (FL): Psychological Assessment Resources; 2000.
10. Baron IS. Neuropsychological evaluation of the child. New York: Oxford University Press; 2004.
11. Fallone G, Acebo C, Arnedt JT, et al. Effects of acute sleep restriction on behavior, sustained attention, and response inhibition in children. Percept Mot Skills 2001;93:213–29.
12. Beebe DW, Rose D, Amin R. Attention, learning, and arousal of experimentally sleep-restricted adolescents in a simulated classroom. J Adolesc Health 2010; 47:523–5.
13. Drake C, Nickel C, Burduvali E, et al. The pediatric daytime sleepiness scale (PDSS): sleep habits and school outcomes in middle-school children. Sleep 2003;26:455–8.
14. Fallone G, Owens JA, Deane J. Sleepiness in children and adolescents: clinical implications. Sleep Med Rev 2002;6:287–306.
15. Wolfson AR, Carskadon MA. Understanding adolescents' sleep patterns and school performance: a critical appraisal. Sleep Med Rev 2003;7:491–506.

16. Dewald JF, Meijer AM, Oort FJ, et al. The influence of sleep quality, sleep duration and sleepiness on school performance in children and adolescents: a meta-analytic review. Sleep Med Rev 2010;14:179–89.

17. Wolfson AR, Carskadon MA, Acebo C, et al. Evidence for the validity of a sleep habits survey for adolescents. Sleep 2003;26:213–6.

18. Keller PS, El-Sheikh M, Buckhalt JA. Children's attachment to parents and their academic functioning: sleep disruptions as moderators of effects. J Dev Behav Pediatr 2008;29:441–9.

19. Mayes SD, Calhoun SL, Bixler EO, et al. Nonsignificance of sleep relative to IQ and neuropsychological scores in predicting academic achievement. J Dev Behav Pediatr 2008;29:206–12.

20. Beebe DW, Ris MD, Kramer ME, et al. The association between sleep-disordered breathing, academic grades, and cognitive and behavioral functioning among overweight subjects during middle to late childhood. Sleep 2010;33:1447–56.

21. Paavonen EJ, Raikkonen K, Lahti J, et al. Short sleep duration and behavioral symptoms of attention-deficit/hyperactivity disorder in healthy 7- to 8-year-old children. Pediatrics 2009;123:e857–64.

22. Sadeh A, Gruber R, Raviv A. Sleep, neurobehavioral functioning, and behavior problems in school-age children. Child Dev 2002;73:405–17.

23. Steenari MR, Vuontela V, Paavonen EJ, et al. Working memory and sleep in 6- to 13-year-old schoolchildren. J Am Acad Child Adolesc Psychiatry 2003;42:85–92.

24. Paavonen EJ, Porkka-Heiskanen T, Lahikainen AR. Sleep quality, duration and behavioral symptoms among 5–6-year-old children. Eur Child Adolesc Psychiatry 2009;18:747–54.

25. Pizza F, Contardi S, Antognini AB, et al. Sleep quality and motor vehicle crashes in adolescents. J Clin Sleep Med 2010;6:41–5.

26. Koulouglioti C, Cole R, Kitzman H. Inadequate sleep and unintentional injuries in young children. Public Health Nurs 2008;25:106–14.

27. Stallones L, Beseler C, Chen P. Sleep patterns and risk of injury among adolescent farm residents. Am J Prev Med 2006;30:300–4.

28. Owens JA, Fernando S, Mc Guinn M. Sleep disturbance and injury risk in young children. Behav Sleep Med 2005;3:18–31.

29. O'Brien EM, Mindell JA. Sleep and risk-taking behavior in adolescents. Behav Sleep Med 2005;3:113–33.

30. Gruber R. Sleep characteristics of children and adolescents with attention deficit-hyperactivity disorder. Child Adolesc Psychiatr Clin N Am 2009;18:863–76.

31. Owens JA. Sleep disorders and attention-deficit/hyperactivity disorder. Curr Psychiatry Rep 2008;10:439–44.

32. Cortese S, Faraone SV, Konofal E, et al. Sleep in children with attention-deficit/hyperactivity disorder: meta-analysis of subjective and objective studies. J Am Acad Child Adolesc Psychiatry 2009;48:894–908.

33. Ivanenko A, Crabtree VM, Gozal D. Sleep in children with psychiatric disorders. Pediatr Clin North Am 2004;51:51–68.

34. Liu X, Buysse DJ, Gentzler AL, et al. Insomnia and hypersomnia associated with depressive phenomenology and comorbidity in childhood depression. Sleep 2007;30:83–90.

35. Liu X, Hubbard JA, Fabes RA, et al. Sleep disturbances and correlates of children with autism spectrum disorders. Child Psychiatry Hum Dev 2006;37:179–91.

36. Moore M, Kirchner HL, Drotar D, et al. Relationships among sleepiness, sleep time, and psychological functioning in adolescents. J Pediatr Psychol 2009;34:1175–83.

37. Wolfson AR, Carskadon MA. Sleep schedules and daytime functioning in adolescents. Child Dev 1998;69:875–87.
38. Fredriksen K, Rhodes J, Reddy R, et al. Sleepless in Chicago: tracking the effects of adolescent sleep loss during the middle school years. Child Dev 2004;75:84–95.
39. El-Sheikh M, Kelly RJ, Buckhalt JA, et al. Children's sleep and adjustment over time: the role of socioeconomic context. Child Dev 2010;81:870–83.
40. Beebe DW. Neurobehavioral effects of childhood sleep-disordered breathing (SDB): a comprehensive review. Sleep 2006;29:1115–34.
41. Spruyt K, Capdevila OS, Kheirandish-Gozal L, et al. Inefficient or insufficient encoding as potential primary deficit in neurodevelopmental performance among children with OSA. Dev Neuropsychol 2009;34:601–14.
42. Kheirandish-Gozal L, De Jong MR, Spruyt K, et al. Obstructive sleep apnoea is associated with impaired pictorial memory task acquisition and retention in children. Eur Respir J 2010;36:164–9.
43. Garetz SL. Behavior, cognition, and quality of life after adenotonsillectomy for pediatric sleep-disordered breathing: summary of the literature. Otolaryngol Head Neck Surg 2008;138:S19–26.
44. Cortese S, Konofal E, Lecendreux M, et al. Restless legs syndrome and attention-deficit/hyperactivity disorder: a review of the literature. Sleep 2005;28:1007–13.
45. O'Brien LM. The neurocognitive effects of sleep disruption in children and adolescents. Child Adolesc Psychiatr Clin N Am 2009;18:813–23.
46. Gruber R, Laviolette R, Deluca P, et al. Short sleep duration is associated with poor performance on IQ measures in healthy school-age children. Sleep Med 2010;11:289–94.
47. Buckhalt JA, El-Sheikh M, Keller PS, et al. Concurrent and longitudinal relations between children's sleep and cognitive functioning: the moderating role of parent education. Child Dev 2009;80:875–92.
48. Ortega FB, Ruiz JR, Castillo R, et al. Sleep duration and cognitive performance in adolescence. The AVENA study. Acta Paediatr 2010;99:454–6.
49. Touchette E, Petit D, Seguin JR, et al. Associations between sleep duration patterns and behavioral/cognitive functioning at school entry. Sleep 2007;30:1213–9.
50. Nixon GM, Thompson JM, Han DY, et al. Short sleep duration in middle childhood: risk factors and consequences. Sleep 2008;31:71–8.
51. Dexter D, Bijwadia J, Schilling D, et al. Sleep, sleepiness and school start times: a preliminary study. WMJ 2003;102:44–6.
52. Wolfson AR, Spaulding NL, Dandrow C, et al. Middle school start times: the importance of a good night's sleep for young adolescents. Behav Sleep Med 2007;5:194–209.
53. Wahlstrom KL. Accommodating the sleep patterns of adolescents within current educational structures: an uncharted path. In: Carskadon MA, editor. Adolescent sleep patterns: biological, social, and psychological influences. Cambridge (United Kingdom): Cambridge University Press; 2002. p. 172–97.
54. Wahlstrom KL. Changing times: findings from the first longitudinal study of later high school start times. NAASP Bulletin 2002;96:3–21.
55. Danner F, Phillips B. Adolescent sleep, school start times, and teen motor vehicle crashes. J Clin Sleep Med 2008;4:533–5.
56. Hansen M, Janssen I, Schiff A, et al. The impact of school daily schedule on adolescent sleep. Pediatrics 2005;115:1555–61.
57. Carskadon MA. Adolescent sleep patterns: biological, social, and psychological influences. Cambridge (United Kingdom): Cambridge University Press; 2002.

58. Goel N, Rao H, Durmer JS, et al. Neurocognitive consequences of sleep deprivation. Semin Neurol 2009;29:320–39.
59. Carskadon MA, Harvey K, Dement WC. Acute restriction of nocturnal sleep in children. Percept Mot Skills 1981;53:103–12.
60. Carskadon MA, Harvey K, Dement WC. Sleep loss in young adolescents. Sleep 1981;4:299–312.
61. Sadeh A, Gruber R, Raviv A. The effects of sleep restriction and extension on school-age children: what a difference an hour makes. Child Dev 2003;74: 444–55.
62. Fallone G, Acebo C, Seifer R, et al. Experimental restriction of sleep opportunity in children: effects on teacher ratings. Sleep 2005;28:1561–7.
63. Randazzo AC, Muehlback MJ, Schweitzer PK, et al. Cognitive function following acute sleep restriction in children ages 10–14. Sleep 1998;21:861–8.
64. Beebe DW, Difrancesco MW, Tlustos SJ, et al. Preliminary fMRI findings in experimentally sleep-restricted adolescents engaged in a working memory task. Behav Brain Funct 2009;5:9.
65. Beebe DW. Sleep and behavior in children: a multi-system, developmental heuristic model. In: Ivanenko A, editor. Sleep and psychiatric disorders in children and adolescents. New York: Informa; 2008. p. 1–10.
66. Michel GF. A developmental-psychobiological approach to developmental neuropsychology. Dev Neuropsychol 2001;19:11–32.
67. Mirmiran M, Ariagno RL. Role of REM sleep in brain development and plasticity. In: Maquet P, Smith C, Stickgold R, editors. Sleep and brain plasticity. New York: Oxford University Press; 2003. p. 181–7.
68. Frank MG, Stryker MP. The role of sleep in the development of central visual pathways. In: Maquet P, Smith C, Stickgold R, editors. Sleep and brain plasticity. New York: Oxford University Press; 2003. p. 190–206.
69. Dang-Vu TT, Desseilles M, Peigneux P, et al. A role for sleep in brain plasticity. Pediatr Rehabil 2006;9:98–118.
70. Frank MG. The mystery of sleep function: current perspectives and future directions. Rev Neurosci 2006;17:375–92.
71. Guzman-Marin R, Ying Z, Suntsova N, et al. Suppression of hippocampal plasticity-related gene expression by sleep deprivation in rats. J Physiol 2006; 575:807–19.
72. Lopez J, Roffwarg HP, Dreher A, et al. Rapid eye movement sleep deprivation decreases long-term potentiation stability and affects some glutamatergic signaling proteins during hippocampal development. Neuroscience 2008;153: 44–53.
73. Tartar JL, Ward CP, McKenna JT, et al. Hippocampal synaptic plasticity and spatial learning are impaired in a rat model of sleep fragmentation. Eur J Neurosci 2006;23:2739–48.
74. Gozal E, Row BW, Schurr A, et al. Developmental differences in cortical and hippocampal vulnerability to intermittent hypoxia in the rat. Neurosci Lett 2001;305:197–201.
75. Row BW, Kheirandish L, Neville JJ, et al. Impaired spatial learning and hyperactivity in developing rats exposed to intermittent hypoxia. Pediatr Res 2002;52: 449–53.
76. Chervin RD, Archbold KH, Dillon JE, et al. Inattention, hyperactivity, and symptoms of sleep-disordered breathing. Pediatrics 2002;109:449–56.
77. Harrison Y, Horne JA. The impact of sleep deprivation on decision making: a review. J Exp Psychol Appl 2000;6:236–49.

78. Dahl RE. Adolescent brain development: a period of vulnerabilities and opportunities. Keynote address. Ann N Y Acad Sci 2004;1021:1–22.
79. Dahl RE, Lewin DS. Pathways to adolescent health sleep regulation and behavior. J Adolesc Health 2002;31:175–84.
80. Halbower AC, Degaonkar M, Barker PB, et al. Childhood obstructive sleep apnea associates with neuropsychological deficits and neuronal brain injury. PLoS Med 2006;3:e301.
81. Key AP, Molfese DL, O'Brien L, et al. Sleep-disordered breathing affects auditory processing in 5–7-year-old children: evidence from brain recordings. Dev Neuropsychol 2009;34:615–28.
82. Iramaneerat C. Predicting academic achievement in the medical school with high school grades. J Med Assoc Thai 2006;89:1497–505.
83. Dubow EF, Huesmann LR, Boxer P, et al. Middle childhood and adolescent contextual and personal predictors of adult educational and occupational outcomes: a mediational model in two countries. Dev Psychol 2006;42:937–49.
84. Crum RM, Juon HS, Green KM, et al. Educational achievement and early school behavior as predictors of alcohol-use disorders: 35-year follow-up of the Woodlawn Study. J Stud Alcohol 2006;67:75–85.
85. Locke TF, Newcomb MD. Adolescent predictors of young adult and adult alcohol involvement and dysphoria in a prospective community sample of women. Prev Sci 2004;5:151–68.
86. Rosenbaum JE. Beyond college for all. New York: Sage; 2001.
87. Jaspers M, de Winter AF, de Meer G, et al. Early findings of preventive child healthcare professionals predict psychosocial problems in preadolescence: the TRAILS study. J Pediatr 2010;157:316–321.e2.
88. Gregory AM, Eley TC, O'Connor TG, et al. Etiologies of associations between childhood sleep and behavioral problems in a large twin sample. J Am Acad Child Adolesc Psychiatry 2004;43:744–51.
89. Gregory AM, O'Connor TG. Sleep problems in childhood: a longitudinal study of developmental change and association with behavioral problems. J Am Acad Child Adolesc Psychiatry 2002;41:964–71.
90. Wong MM, Brower KJ, Zucker RA. Childhood sleep problems, early onset of substance use and behavioral problems in adolescence. Sleep Med 2009;10:787–96.
91. Gregory AM, Rijsdijk FV, Lau JY, et al. The direction of longitudinal associations between sleep problems and depression symptoms: a study of twins aged 8 and 10 years. Sleep 2009;32:189–99.
92. Gregory AM, Van der Ende J, Willis TA, et al. Parent-reported sleep problems during development and self-reported anxiety/depression, attention problems, and aggressive behavior later in life. Arch Pediatr Adolesc Med 2008;162:330–5.
93. Roane BM, Taylor DJ. Adolescent insomnia as a risk factor for early adult depression and substance abuse. Sleep 2008;31:1351–6.
94. Chervin RD, Ruzincka DL, Archbold KH, et al. Snoring predicts hyperactivity four years later. Sleep 2005;28:885–90.
95. Gozal D, Pope D. Snoring during early childhood and academic performance at ages thirteen to fourteen years. Pediatrics 2001;107:1394–9.
96. Gregory AM, Caspi A, Eley TC, et al. Prospective longitudinal associations between persistent sleep problems in childhood and anxiety and depression disorders in adulthood. J Abnorm Child Psychol 2005;33:157–63.

97. Quach J, Hiscock H, Canterford L, et al. Outcomes of child sleep problems over the school-transition period: Australian population longitudinal study. Pediatrics 2009;123:1287–92.

98. Friedman NP, Corley RP, Hewitt JK, et al. Individual differences in childhood sleep problems predict later cognitive executive control. Sleep 2009;32:323–33.

99. Gregory AM, Caspi A, Moffitt TE, et al. Sleep problems in childhood predict neuropsychological functioning in adolescence. Pediatrics 2009;123:1171–6.

100. MacNeal RJ, Dinulos JG. Update on sun protection and tanning in children. Curr Opin Pediatr 2007;19:425–9.

101. Dietrich KN. Environmental toxicants and psychological development. In: Yeates KO, Ris MD, Taylor HG, et al, editors. Pediatric neuropsychology: research, theory, and practice. 2nd edition. New York: Guilford; 2010. p. 211–64.

A Framework for the Assessment and Treatment of Sleep Problems in Children with Attention-Deficit/Hyperactivity Disorder

Penny Corkum, PhD[a],*, Fiona Davidson, BSc[a],
Marilyn MacPherson, MD, FRCPC[b]

KEYWORDS

- Attention-deficit/hyperactivity disorder • Sleep • Assessment
- Intervention

There are several published guidelines describing the assessment and treatment of attention-deficit/hyperactivity disorder (ADHD), including practice parameters developed by the American Academy of Pediatrics (AAP),[1,2] the American Academy of Child and Adolescent Psychiatry (AACAP),[3] the Canadian Attention Deficit Hyperactivity Disorder Resource Alliance (CADDRA),[4] and the National Institute for Health and Clinical Excellence (NICE).[5] Recent research has indicated that primary care clinicians are aware of these guidelines and generally follow the clinical practice recommendations provided.[6] However, while available ADHD practice parameters are fairly comprehensive, it is notable that the important role of sleep in the assessment and treatment of ADHD is either not mentioned at all (eg, AAP) or receives little focus. Therefore, the goal of this review is to provide pediatricians involved in the assessment and treatment of ADHD in school-aged children with a framework for evaluating and managing sleep-related concerns in the clinical setting.

This work was supported by Grant No. MOP-81191 from Canadian Institute of Health Research.
The authors have nothing to disclose.
[a] Department of Psychology, Dalhousie University, 1355 Oxford Street, Halifax, Nova Scotia, B3H 4J1, Canada
[b] Pediatrics, Colchester East Hants Health Authority, 207 Willow Street, Truro, Nova Scotia, B2N 5A1, Canada
* Corresponding author.
E-mail address: penny.corkum@dal.ca

Pediatr Clin N Am 58 (2011) 667–683
doi:10.1016/j.pcl.2011.03.004
0031-3955/11/$ – see front matter © 2011 Elsevier Inc. All rights reserved.

pediatric.theclinics.com

ATTENTION-DEFICIT/HYPERACTIVITY DISORDER

ADHD is the most common childhood mental health disorder, affecting approximately 5% of school-aged children worldwide.[7] Children are typically diagnosed with ADHD during the elementary school years, with boys being diagnosed more often than girls (sex ratio ranges from 3:1 to 8:1). ADHD is often chronic in nature with symptoms persisting into adolescence and adulthood in approximately two-thirds of children.[8] Children with ADHD typically display a heterogeneous combination of disruptive behavior, academic underachievement, and difficulty with social and familial relations, as well as high rates of comorbidity with other clinical disorders.[7] In fact, research has found that the vast majority (up to 87%) of children with ADHD meet criteria for one other mental health disorder and approximately half of all children diagnosed with ADHD have 2 or more comorbid disorders, with the most common being disruptive behavior disorders (ie, oppositional defiant disorder and conduct disorder), anxiety and mood disorders, and learning disabilities.[7]

ADHD is conceptualized as a neurobiological disorder in which the primary cause is thought to result from a complex set of genetic factors, although nongenetic factors (eg, perinatal stress, prematurity, traumatic brain injury, maternal substance abuse during pregnancy) have also been postulated to play a role in the etiology of this disorder.[7,8] These genetic and nongenetic factors are thought to influence brain structure (ie, the integrity of the prefrontal cortical-striatal network) and function (ie, neurotransmitter systems such as the catecholamine system), and ultimately affect behavior.[7] In terms of theoretical models, the cognitive-energetic model is one that provides a particularly comprehensive framework for understanding the neurocognitive deficits associated with ADHD.[9] This model indicates that problems associated with ADHD occur at 3 levels: (1) cognitive mechanisms (eg, response outputs such as motor organization), (2) energetic pools (eg, arousal, activation, and effort), and (3) executive functioning (eg, inhibition, working memory, planning). It is assumed that these problems are related to differences in the underlying neural architecture and modulator systems in individuals with ADHD.

ADHD increases the risk for numerous adverse health outcomes later in development, including substance abuse, motor vehicle accidents, and involvement with the justice system.[7,10,11] As such, ADHD represents a significant burden to individuals, their families, and society. Given the heterogeneity of the disorder in its 3 recognized subtypes (namely Predominately Inattentive, Predominately Hyperactive-Impulsive, Combined),[12] and its pervasive impact on children, it is often recommended that treatment involve multiple modalities, including behavioral, psychoeducational, and pharmacological interventions.[11] Long-term prospective studies, however, such as the Multimodal Treatment Study of Children with ADHD (MTA), have suggested that an optimal level of pharmacological medication is the single most effective treatment for ADHD in most children, at least for the first year of treatment.[13] Moreover, stimulant medication alone remains the most common treatment for ADHD.[14]

ADHD and Sleep

ADHD has one of the highest rates of sleep problems of all child mental health disorders.[15] There have been numerous systematic reviews of the literature on the sleep characteristics of children with ADHD,[16–23] as well as articles written about this relationship for clinical audiences.[24–27] All reviews concur that parents of children with ADHD report more sleep problems than do parents of typically developing children. Prevalence estimates of sleep problems based on parent reporting have varied widely, but have been consistently high (ie, 50%–80%), depending on the operational definition of sleep problem used.[17,28] The sleep problems most commonly reported by parents of children with ADHD are difficulties initiating or maintaining sleep, both of which typically shorten sleep duration and can cause problems for the family and child. Although sleep problems are common in children with ADHD, these are often overlooked and rarely included in research examining the comorbidity of ADHD. For example, the largest treatment trial of ADHD, the MTA study, examined comorbidities associated with ADHD but did not include sleep disorders.[29]

Sleep problems have also been shown to be related to ADHD subtype. Most research has indicated that children with the Combined subtype of ADHD have more sleep problems compared with children with the Inattentive or Hyperactive/Impulsive subtypes of ADHD.[30,31] However, there is also some evidence that children with the Inattentive subtype of ADHD may be sleepier during the day than their typically developing peers, despite their nocturnal sleep being similar.[32] A recent study also found that hypersomnia was more prevalent in the Inattentive subtype, whereas circadian rhythm problems were more prevalent in the Combined subtype.[33] When interpreting these results, it is important to consider the potential confound of ADHD symptom severity across the subtypes and the possible impact of this on research findings.

The high rates of sleep problems reported by parents of children with ADHD are not often verified by research using objective measures of sleep (eg, actigraphy and polysomnography [PSG]).[17,34] Although several individual research studies have found a higher rate of a specific sleep disorders (eg, sleep apnea) or a specific sleep architecture variation (eg, differences in rapid eye movement [REM] sleep), a meta-analysis by Sadeh and colleagues[21] found that the only consistent finding across studies was a higher rate of periodic limb movement disorder (PLMD) in children with ADHD when compared with typically developing children. All other sleep disorders (eg, sleep apnea) and differences in sleep architecture were associated with ADHD through mediating factors including age, gender, and comorbidity. This finding is in contrast to results of the meta-analysis by Cortese and colleagues[19] of PSG studies, which found that children with ADHD had higher scores on the index indicating sleep apnea. Unfortunately, periodic limb movements were not included in the analyses. The investigators of both of these meta-analyses highlight that there is wide variability across studies in terms of definitions and measurement of these sleep disorders, and that this variability may result in inconsistent findings across studies.

STIMULANT MEDICATION AND SLEEP

Current estimates are that 2% to 9% of North American children receive stimulant medications for the treatment of ADHD,[35,36] and standard practice has changed from twice-a-day regimes (ie, medication given morning and noon to provide coverage during school hours) to sustained-release formulations that treat symptoms inside and outside of school hours.[37,38] Current treatment with stimulant medication has been reported to affect sleep,[30,39–42] with stimulant treated children sleeping approximately 1 hour less per night during an acute medication trial.[43] In particular, the trend toward the use of controlled-release preparations may have a significant impact on sleep in these children. In addition, there is preliminary evidence that stimulant medication may change the strength and timing of the circadian rhythm.[44] Moreover, research has demonstrated that performance on a measure of sustained attention was most improved by medication in children with ADHD who had poor sleep quality as compared with children with ADHD with good sleep quality.[45] This finding implies that sleep quality during pharmacological treatment of ADHD may moderate the effectiveness of stimulant medication in enhancing attention.

ADHD ASSESSMENT

ADHD and sleep disorders can present similarly, therefore it is difficult to know which disorder is causing the child's inattention and/or impulsivity/hyperactivity. There are 3 possible relationships: (1) ADHD may cause sleep problems (eg, a child with ADHD develops insomnia as he or she is not able to slow down his or her thoughts to settle for sleep), (2) a primary sleep disorder may cause ADHD-like symptoms (eg, sleep apnea results in daytime sleepiness and as such the child displays difficulties with attention and increased motor activity), or (3) a third variable may cause both ADHD and sleep disorders or problems (eg, dysregulation of arousal resulting in ADHD and insomnia). It is important to take these 3 possible relationships between ADHD and sleep into consideration when conducting an ADHD assessment.

Differential Diagnosis

The goal of the ADHD assessment process is twofold; first, to "rule in" ADHD symptoms to confirm that the clinical presentation meets diagnostic criteria, and second, to "rule out" other possible diagnoses that would account for the ADHD symptoms. In other words, pediatricians should consider a differential diagnosis, which is a process of weighing the probability of one disorder versus another to best explain a patient's symptoms. This step is often overlooked in the assessment and diagnosis of ADHD, yet is critical for understanding prognosis and for treatment planning.

Sleep disorders are an important consideration in the differential diagnosis of ADHD.[46] The most comprehensive classification system of sleep disorders, the International Classification of Sleep Disorders (ICSD-2),[47] organizes sleep disorders into 8 categories: (1) Insomnia, (2) Sleep-related breathing disorders, (3) Hypersomnias of central origin, (4) Circadian rhythm sleep disorders, (5) Parasomnias, (6) Sleep-related movement disorders, (7) Isolated symptoms and normal variants, and (8) Other sleep disorders. Although pediatric sleep disorders are well represented in the ICDS-2, it continues to be a challenge to identify sleep disorders within the context of the wide range of typical sleep behaviors in children.[48]

Sleep problems are not specific to ADHD, but rather are a common symptom of many mental health disorders. For example, general sleep disturbances can be a symptom of major depression; decreased need for sleep can be a symptom of mania; refusal to sleep alone and persistent nightmares of separation are symptoms of separation anxiety, whereas the following are possible symptoms of generalized anxiety: becoming easily tired/appearing tired, difficulties falling or staying asleep, and restless unsatisfying sleep. Moreover, there is no sleep problem or sleep disorder that is associated specifically with ADHD. Therefore, screening for a range of potential sleep disorders and sleep problems should be undertaken as part of the ADHD assessment.

The first step in an ADHD assessment typically involves gathering information to better understand the concerns about the child and to conduct a screening for ADHD symptoms. This step should also include a screening for other possible explanations for the child's presenting ADHD symptoms, including sleep disorders. During this initial meeting, the pediatrician should ask the parent about the child's sleep. Therefore, the inclusion of a brief sleep screen is recommended as an integral component of this step in the ADHD diagnostic process. An example is the 5-item sleep-screening instrument called the BEARS (B = Bedtime issues, E = Excessive daytime sleepiness, A = night Awakenings, R = Regularity and duration of sleep, S = Snoring), which has been found to be user-friendly in a primary care setting[49] (http://www.kidzzzsleep.org).

Often parent and teacher questionnaires are used as part of this assessment process; however, these questionnaires rarely screen for sleep problems/disorders. Therefore, it is recommended that pediatricians include a questionnaire that will screen for sleep disorders and sleep problems. One such example is the Children's Sleep Habits Questionnaire[50] (http://www.kidzzzsleep.org), which is a parent-report survey that may be useful in identifying sleep problems. The questionnaire includes 45 items comprising 8 scales: (1) Bedtime resistance, (2) Sleep onset delay, (3) Sleep duration, (4) Sleep anxiety, (5) Night awakenings, (6) Parasomnias, (7) Sleep disordered breathing and (8) Daytime sleepiness. Elevated scores on any of these 8 scales or an overall score of more than 41 may indicate sleep problems that require further investigation. (See Spruyt and Gozal[51] for a listing and critique of the most common pediatric sleep questionnaires.)

If sleep concerns are raised either during the interview or on the sleep questionnaire, then additional information about the child's sleep is required. The pediatrician should consider asking the parent and/or youth (depending on the child's age and ability level) to complete a sleep diary for 2 weeks. A graphic sleep diary that collects information about sleep quantity and quality is best, as patterns related to sleep problems (eg, late bedtime, short sleep, multiple night awakenings) are more obvious than when the information is collected in written format. Child-friendly sleep diaries can be ordered from the National Sleep Foundation at http://www.sleepfoundation.org/ or can be downloaded from www.kidzzzsleep.com. For a review of the various sleep measures, including sleep diaries and polysomnography, the reader is referred to Sheldon,[52] Weiss[27] , and Luginbuehl and Kohler.[53]

When collecting information about the child's sleep, the pediatrician must consider several primary sleep disorders (eg, sleep apnea, PLMD/restless legs syndrome, circadian sleep disorders), as these can all result in increased inattention, impulsivity, and hyperactivity, and as such have the potential to be misdiagnosed as ADHD.[25,27,46,54,55] A referral for a sleep study (ie, PSG study) is only necessary if the initial sleep assessment indicates that there may be a primary sleep disorder for which a PSG study is useful for diagnostic purposes (eg, sleep apnea, PLMD). For example, if the parent reports that the child snores loudly, at times has been heard to snort and gasp while sleeping, and tends to fall asleep in the car while being driven relatively short distances, then it would be appropriate for the child to have a PSG study to examine the possibility of sleep apnea.

Comorbid Diagnosis

Comorbidity refers to the presence of one (or more) disorders in addition to the primary disorder. As already noted, comorbidity is very common in children with ADHD, and has important implications for understanding prognosis and for developing treatment plans. A disorder is considered comorbid with ADHD if there is evidence for both disorders and if one disorder does not fully account for the symptoms of the other disorder. For example, a child who presents with ADHD and separation anxiety symptoms might receive a diagnosis of both disorders, and as such both of these disorders need to be considered in treatment planning. The most common comorbid sleep disorder seen in the context of an ADHD assessment is behavioral insomnia. Based on the ICSD-2, there are three types of behavioral insomnia of childhood (BIC): (1) Sleep onset association type (difficulties with initiating sleep as sleep onset is paired with an external cue such as a parent's presence); (2) Limit setting type (parents are not consistent with limit setting at bedtime and/or reinforce behaviors incompatible with sleep); and (3) Combined type. Behavioral insomnias of childhood present clinically with bedtime resistance, difficulty falling asleep, and/or problems staying asleep.[56] Given that BIC is the most common sleep problem in school-aged children with ADHD, it is this comorbid sleep disorder that we will focus on in the Treatment Considerations section below.

Assessment of Sleep Problems in Children Previously Diagnosed with ADHD

As previously described, sleep problems should be evaluated in the initial ADHD assessment; however, reassessment of sleep problems may be required at a later date if new sleep problems arise or if past sleep problems are exacerbated. The assessment approach will depend on whether the child is on medication, and the type and dose of the medication. If the child is not on medication then the sleep assessment should proceed as outlined earlier. However, if the child is on stimulant medication, the impact of the medication on sleep must be determined. The most common impact of stimulant medication is delayed sleep onset, which often reduces sleep duration. If the parent reports that the sleep problem either started or worsened during the course of treatment with stimulants, consideration should be given to changing the timing and/ or dose of the medication. There are many stimulant medications used in the treatment of ADHD, and all have different durations of effects and release properties. If changing the dose and/or timing of the stimulant medication is ineffective, a different stimulant or a nonstimulant medication could be considered for the treatment of ADHD.[57] For a review of ADHD medications and their properties, see Kratochvil and colleagues[58] or the following Web sites: http://www.addwarehouse.com/shopsite_sc/store/html/article3.htm; http://www.caddra.ca/cms4/pdfs/medication-adhd-canada_April2010.pdf.

Some pediatricians recommend an additional dose of stimulant medication in the evening, as it is believed that difficulties falling asleep are the result of "rebound effects" (ie, increased irritability, agitation, and emotional liability) as the child's daytime medication wanes. Although an additional dose is commonly used, there is no empirical evidence for this practice. In fact, of the few studies conducted, most have found that sleep onset is further delayed with an additional dose of medication.[59,60] Other considerations in medication use include the presence of comorbid conditions. For example, treatment of ADHD symptoms with atomoxetine has been found to improve nocturnal enuresis associated with ADHD,[61,62] and therefore could be considered when both ADHD and enuresis are diagnosed and in need of treatment.

TREATMENT CONSIDERATIONS

The primary focus of this section is the treatment of behavioral insomnias of childhood (particularly sleep-onset association disorder), as this is the most common sleep disorder in both unmedicated and medicated children with ADHD. Additional information on behavioral insomnias of childhood can be found in an article elsewhere in this issue. Unfortunately, there is very little research on the effectiveness of interventions for insomnia specific to children with ADHD, which has resulted in this area being identified as a top research priority by a consensus group on insomnia in children.[63] The evidence-based interventions for typically developing children[56,64] are reviewed and, when possible, research focused on children with ADHD is highlighted; how these interventions could be modified for children with ADHD is also discussed. The treatment overview includes relevant behavioral, pharmacological, and complementary treatments for insomnia in school-aged children. This section ends with a brief overview of research that has evaluated specific interventions in children with ADHD for sleep disorders other than insomnia (eg, restless leg syndrome, PLMD, circadian disorders, and obstructive sleep apnea).

Behavioral Interventions

Given that pediatric sleep problems occur in the context of the parent-child relationship, many of the psychosocial treatments are behaviorally based parent management strategies. Mindell and colleagues[65] conducted a systematic literature review of 52 behavioral intervention studies and reported that 94% of these interventions were efficacious in treating behavioral insomnia, and significantly improved sleep in 80% of children. Despite the strong efficacy data, caution needs to be exercised in generalizing these results to school-aged populations, as these studies were primarily focused on infants and young children. It is unfortunate that so little research has been conducted in school-aged children, as this age group accounts for the highest percentage of visits to primary pediatricians regarding sleep concerns.[66] The most commonly used behavioral interventions for school-aged children are sleep hygiene, positive routines, faded bedtime with response cost, and cognitive strategies. These approaches are described in more detail below. Based on the findings of pediatric sleep research and knowing that children with ADHD have difficulty with cognitive processes and executive functions, it may be necessary to make some adaptations to behavioral interventions for treating insomnia in children with ADHD.

Sleep hygiene

Educating parents on the importance and implementation of good sleep hygiene for their children has received empirical support.[67] Good sleep hygiene is achieved by several factors, some of which occur during the day and others at night. Diet is one daytime factor that plays an important role in promoting healthy sleep. For example, high levels of caffeine consumption during the day (eg, cola and chocolate), especially in the late afternoon and evening, can lead to delayed sleep onset.[68] Another dietary issue that should be considered is the types of food children are consuming during the day. One study demonstrated that when children with ADHD were put on a diet consisting mainly of fruit, vegetables, rice, and meat, they complained less of physical problems and sleep problems than did children in a control group.[69]

Another daytime factor that plays a role in sleep hygiene is physical activity (eg, exercise, outdoor activity). Studies with adults suggest that moderate physical activity is associated with sleep-promoting benefits.[70] However, active play should be limited as bedtime approaches (eg, within 3 hours), as children should be engaging in quieter, relaxing activities to help them wind down, rather than being overstimulated before sleep.[67] Activities involving electronics (eg, television and computer) should also be limited before bed, as these can also stimulate the child rather than have a calming effect. For example, Owens and colleagues[71] found that increased duration of television watching, and television watching at bedtime, were both associated with increased sleep difficulties, especially when the television was in the child's bedroom. It is recommended that all electronic devices (including cell phones, computers, and television) are turned off at least one hour before bedtime. The above recommendations are particularly important for children with ADHD, as these children tend to have more sedentary lifestyles, watch more television, and play more videogames than their typically developing peers.[72,73]

The sleep environment is also important to consider as part of healthy sleep hygiene. A child should have a comfortable bed, with a quiet, dark (or lowly lit) room, and a comfortable room temperature. Children will not sleep as well if the environment is either too hot or too cold.[67] If possible, children should not be punished by being confined to their room during the day,[68] as they should learn to associate their bed/bedroom as a place for relaxation and sleep rather than play or worry.

A study by Weiss and colleagues[74] examined the efficacy of sleep hygiene and melatonin treatment for stimulant-treated children and adolescents with ADHD who were experiencing insomnia (sleep-onset latency >60 minutes). In this study, children and adolescents were given a sleep hygiene intervention during which time parents were provided information on consistency in bedtime routines, as well as being instructed to avoid caffeine and naps. Findings indicated that less than 20% of the children were effectively treated with sleep hygiene alone. Based on this one study, it seems that for many children with ADHD (on stimulant medication), sleep hygiene strategies may be necessary but not sufficient to treat their symptoms of insomnia.

Positive bedtime routines

Establishing consistent bedtime routines for children can help them learn appropriate behaviors for bedtime and reduce the stress of going to bed. Positive bedtime routines involve a consistent bedtime each night and a consistent bedtime routine (ie, a set of activities to help the child get ready and wind down before bed).[65,75] Bedtime routines work best if they occur in the same way each night, so the child knows exactly what will happen and when it will happen. Having the same activities occurring each night can help children calm down before bed, as novel or unexpected events can increase stimulation.[76] Typical bedtime routines may include a reminder from parents that it will soon be time to get ready for bed, a snack, brushing teeth, washing up, getting pajamas on, a story/time with parents, and lights out. Parents should ensure that there is an appropriate amount of time for the bedtime routine, as it should not be a rushed process. The bedtime routine can also provide some positive one-on-one interaction between children and their parents.[68] It is also important to have a wake time that is similar across weekends and weekdays, and the rule of thumb is no more than a 30 minutes difference between these two wake times.

One area where children with ADHD may have more difficulty than typically developing children is with the bedtime routine. Children with ADHD may benefit from more warnings before being called to bed so that they know that bedtime is coming. These children may also require an increased number of prompts during the bedtime routine to keep them on track and to help them transition from one activity to the next in a timely manner. The routine should be structured in a way to allow for sufficient time to complete each activity (eg, brushing teeth), but not so much time that the child has opportunities to become distracted. Because children with ADHD may have difficulty following through with multi-step instructions, parents should give their child instructions one step at a time. It may also be helpful to have the bedtime routine posted (with pictorial representations of the activities for younger children) in a location where the child can see it, and can check off each activity as it is completed. This method may be particularly beneficial to children with ADHD, as it gives them a visual reminder of the bedtime routine in a step-by-step fashion. These modifications may help parents of children with ADHD, and the children themselves, follow the bedtime routine with more success.

Faded bedtime with response cost

A faded bedtime with response cost is a process whereby the child is put to bed at a specific time and if he or she is not able to fall asleep within a predetermined time (eg, 20 minutes), he or she has to leave his or her bed and engage in a quiet activity for a pre-set length of time without being permitted to fall asleep (ie, response cost).[65] The point is to make associations for the child so that he or she falls asleep when in bed (ie, stimulus control). Once the child is falling asleep within the first 20 minutes of being placed in bed for a few consecutive nights, the bedtime is moved earlier by 15- to 30-minute increments until the goal bedtime is reached.[65,77] A consistent wake time needs to be put in place as well. This technique focuses on increasing appropriate bedtime behaviors instead of reducing less appropriate bedtime behaviors, and also results in sleep restriction so the child is tired when going to bed.[65]

Sleep interventions for children with ADHD

There is only one published study examining behaviorally based sleep interventions for children with ADHD. Mullane and Corkum[78] examined the effect of a 5-week behavioral intervention for 3 unmedicated children with ADHD and difficulties initiating and/or maintaining sleep. Parents were provided with a manual and received weekly telephone sessions with a paraprofessional facilitator to review material covered in the manual. The topics covered in the treatment manual included the following: (1) basic sleep physiology and the different types of sleep problems/disorders, their impact, and treatments, (2) sleep hygiene and bedtime routines, (3) faded bedtime strategy with a response cost and positive reinforcement, (4) implementing a faded bedtime strategy and reward program, and (5) fine tuning and fading the program. Results indicated that children's sleep improved and that these gains were generally maintained at the 3-month follow-up.[78] These findings provided a foundation for a larger randomized controlled trial completed by Corkum and colleagues.[79] This trial evaluated the efficacy of their sleep intervention method in typically developing children and children with ADHD (who comprised ~30% of the total sample of 54 children aged 6–12 years). Preliminary analyses indicate that the treatment group had significantly improved sleep compared to the wait-list control group, and that children with ADHD were as responsive to the treatment as typically developing children (Penny Corkum, PhD, Fiona Davidson, BSc, Lingley-Pottie, et al, unpublished data, 2009).

In older children and adolescents, the inclusion of cognitive strategies such as relaxation and guided imagery may be helpful in reducing anxiety and psychological arousal at bedtime. Although there is a strong research base for these strategies with adults who suffer from insomnia, there is no research on the effectiveness in school-aged children.[80]

Pharmacological Interventions

Sleep disorders are one of the primary reasons for the use of medication in children.[81] A survey of community-based pediatricians in the United States showed that the use of prescription and over-the-counter medications in treating sleep problems in children is relatively common, with approximately one-fourth of children with sleep problems being prescribed a medication.[82] The results from a recent survey of child psychiatrists also indicated that there is a wide range of variability in the medications and approaches used to treat insomnia in children.[81] In this study, α-agonists were most commonly used for treating children with ADHD or other neurodevelopmental delays; however, our knowledge of the efficacy and safety of these medications for children is limited because of a lack of clinical medication trials for children with sleep disorders and sleep problems.[65] There are currently no medications approved for use in children with insomnia in the United States, and furthermore, recent clinical guidelines emphasize that pharmacologic treatment is rarely the first-line approach and should instead be combined with sleep hygiene and behavioral interventions.[63,81]

The general classes on medications used for the treatment of insomnia in children with ADHD in clinical practice settings include sedative-hypnotic medicines, benzodiazepines, nonbenzodiazepines, ramelteon, and melatonin. The discussion of pharmacological interventions here is limited to only those medications for which some empirical data exist regarding use in children with ADHD and insomnia. A nonbenzodiazepine hypnotic agent, zolpidem, has been researched for its effectiveness in treating pediatric sleep-onset insomnia in children with ADHD. In a controlled clinical trial, a dose of 0.25 mg/kg per day (to a maximum of 10 mg/d) of zolpidem was not effective in reducing sleep-onset insomnia in youths between the ages of 6 and 17 years based on actigraphy and PSG.[83] Reported side effects of zolpidem included dizziness, headaches, and hallucinations.

A commonly prescribed medication for children with ADHD and insomnia is clonidine, an α-agonist. Clonidine has been found to be helpful in treating children with ADHD and sleep problems, due to its sedating effects for insomnia.[84] Clonidine has a duration of action between 3 and 5 hours and a half life of 12 to 16 hours. It is typically given orally at bedtime, and its effects last for approximately 4 hours in children.[85] Although there is evidence that clonidine may be effective for managing sleep problems in children with ADHD, case study reports show that some children have experienced adverse responses to clonidine, including low blood pressure and weight loss.[86] Case study reports have also identified withdrawal effects including shortness of breath, high blood pressure, and tachycardia, and there are concerns with the interactions with stimulant medications.[87,88] Sleep and clonidine research on adults has also shown that medium to high doses of clonidine may decrease REM sleep.[89] These reports indicate that pediatricians should exercise caution when prescribing clonidine, and monitor the child for side effects and withdrawal effects as well as appropriate dosage.

The most common medication used to treat sleep problems in children with ADHD is the supplement melatonin. Giving children with ADHD synthetic melatonin has been found to be effective in decreasing sleep-onset latency.[74] In unmedicated children with ADHD, melatonin in large doses (ie, 5 mg) before bedtime was found to decrease sleep onset and increase sleep duration; however, the supplement was not effective in improving daytime problem behaviors or cognitive performance.[90] Although melatonin appears to be effective at improving sleep problems in children in the short term, there is limited research on its efficacy in the long term, although one study did find that children taking melatonin for an average of 3.7 years continued to benefit.[91] No adverse effects have been noted in some studies,[91] whereas other studies have found that melatonin use has been associated with a lowered seizure threshold and exacerbation of asthma symptoms, and may contribute to delayed onset of puberty in children.[92] In addition, there is no consensus on the best therapeutic dose of melatonin,[93] and the formulation is not well regulated so varying responses can occur.

There is a small body of literature examining the use of other complementary and alternative medicine and strategies (see Larzelere and colleagues[94] for a review). Most of this work has been done in infants and adults, with next to no research on school-aged children. Although some parents report anecdotally that these treatments are effective at improving their children's sleep problems, such reports have not be verified by research.

Treatment of Other Common Comorbid Primary Sleep Disorders in Children with ADHD

Movement disorders: periodic limb movement disorder, restless leg syndrome

PLMD is characterized by periodic episodes of repetitive and involuntary rhythmic movements of the legs during sleep. The core symptoms of restless legs syndrome (RLS) include the urge to move the legs that worsens when resting, such as in the evening or at bedtime. Research has shown that lower serum ferritin levels have been associated with PLMD and RLS in children with ADHD,[95,96] and children with lower levels of serum ferritin had higher scores on objective measures of problems sleep and symptoms of ADHD.[95] Treatment with supplemental iron has been anecdotally reported to alleviate RLS symptoms in children,[97] although no randomized trials have been conducted.

Circadian rhythm disorders

Melatonin is used to treat circadian rhythm disorders, specifically delayed sleep phase disorder, which is characterized by a delayed sleep episode relative to the desired clock time. This delay can result in daytime sleepiness, symptoms of sleep-onset insomnia, and difficulty awakening at the desired time. Adult data suggest that optimal timing and dose may be different for melatonin used as a chronobiotic. Chronotherapy (ie, successively delaying sleep-onset times around the clock until the actual sleep-onset time is realigned with a desired earlier bedtime) and bright light therapy (ie, use of light boxes to emit full-spectrum fluorescent light and filter out ultraviolet wavelengths) have been suggested in the literature as potential treatments for sleep problems in children with ADHD.[55] To date there has been very little research on these interventions. There is one case study,[98] which found that a combination of chronotherapy and a behavioral intervention was successful in a young girl with ADHD and delayed sleep phase insomnia. Positive benefits from morning bright light therapy was reported in one study of adults with ADHD[99] and in a single case study of a child with ADHD.[100]

Obstructive sleep apnea

Although there is compelling evidence that treatment of obstructive sleep apnea can improve neurocognitive functioning, including attention, in typically developing children,[25] there are few studies that have examined the outcome of treatments for sleep apnea specifically in children diagnosed with ADHD. One recent study[101] examined treatment outcomes for children with ADHD and mild sleep apnea that were self-selected into 3 groups: methylphenidate treatment, surgical treatment (adenotonsillectomy), and no treatment. The surgical group demonstrated the greatest improvement in ADHD symptoms.[101] Several other studies have also demonstrated the benefits that children with ADHD and obstructive sleep apnea can experience after surgical treatment.[102,103] These results underscore the importance of treating obstructive sleep apnea in the context of ADHD, and potentially speak to the need for differential diagnosis between ADHD and sleep.

SUMMARY

Although there are many unanswered questions, it is clear that ADHD and sleep are intimately linked and that sleep needs to be considered in the assessment and treatment of ADHD. Sleep disorders can mimic ADHD symptoms, therefore an assessment that includes sleep in the differential diagnosis is critical. Sleep disorders can also coexist with ADHD, and can modify prognosis and treatment responses. Given the lack of efficacy and safety data for the pharmacological treatment of sleep problems in children, it is critical that pediatricians use behavioral intervention strategies, such as sleep hygiene and positive bedtime routines, as a first line of treatment.

REFERENCES

1. Clinical practice guideline: diagnosis and evaluation of the child with attention-deficit/hyperactivity disorder. American Academy of Pediatrics. Pediatrics 2000; 105(5):1158–70.
2. American Academy of Pediatrics. Clinical practice guideline: treatment of the school-aged child with attention-deficit/hyperactivity disorder. Pediatrics 2001; 108:1033–44.
3. American Academy of Child and Adolescent Psychiatry. Practice parameter for the assessment and treatment of children and adolescents with attention-deficit/hyperactivity disorder. J Am Acad Child Psychiatry 2007;46:894–921.

4. Canadian ADHD Practice Guidelines (CADDRA). 2008. Available at: http://www. caddra.ca/cms4/index.php?option=com_content&view=article&id=26&Itemid= 70&lang=en. Accessed October, 2010.
5. NICE guideline no. 72. Attention deficit hyperactivity disorder. In: The NICE guidelines on diagnosis and management of ADHD in children, young people and adults. British Psychological Society & Royal College of Psychiatrists Publications; 2009. Available at: http://guidance.nice.org.uk/CG72/Guidance/pdf/ English. Accessed October, 2010.
6. Rushton JL, Fant KE, Clark SJ. Use of practice guidelines in the primary care of children with attention-deficit/hyperactivity disorder. Pediatrics 2004;114(1): e23–8.
7. Schachar R. Attention deficit hyperactivity disorder in children, adolescents, and adults. Continuum Lifelong Learning Neurology 2009;15(6):78–97.
8. Remschmidt H. Global consensus on ADHD/HKD. Eur Child Adolesc Psychiatry 2005;14(3):127–37.
9. Sergeant JA, Geurts H, Huijbregts S, et al. The top and the bottom of ADHD: A neuropsychological perspective. Neurosci Biobehav Rev 2003;27(7): 583–92.
10. Root RW, Resnick RJ. An update on the diagnosis and treatment of attention-deficit/hyperactivity disorder in children. Prof Psychol Res Pr 2003;34(1):34–41.
11. Waschbusch DA, Hill GP. Empirically supported, promising, and unsupported treatments for children with attention-deficit/hyperactivity disorder. In: Lohr JM, editor. Science and pseudoscience in clinical psychology. New York: Guilford Press; 2003. p. 333–62.
12. Diagnostic and statistical manual of mental disorders, revised. 4th edition. Washington, DC: American Psychiatric Association; 2000.
13. Swanson J, Arnold L, Wigal T, et al. Evidence, interpretation, and qualification from multiple reports of long-term outcomes in the multimodal treatment study of children with ADHD (MTA): part I: executive summary. J Atten Disord 2008; 12(1):4–14.
14. Pelham WE Jr, Fabiano GA. Evidence-based psychosocial treatments for attention-deficit/hyperactivity disorder. J Clin Child Adolesc Psychol 2008; 37(1):184–214.
15. Meltzer LJ, Mindell JA. Sleep and sleep disorders in children and adolescents. Psychiatr Clin North Am 2006;29(4):1059–76.
16. Bullock GL, Schall U. Dyssomnia in children diagnosed with attention deficit hyperactivity disorder: a critical review. Aust N Z J Psychiatry 2005;39(5):373–7.
17. Corkum P, Tannock R, Moldofsky H. Sleep disturbances in children with attention-deficit/ hyperactivity disorder. J Am Acad Child Psychiatry 1998; 37(6):637–46.
18. Cortese S, Konofal E, Yateman N, et al. Sleep and alertness in children with attention-deficit/hyperactivity disorder: a systematic review of the literature. Sleep 2006;29(4):504–11.
19. Cortese S, Faraone SV, Konofal E, et al. Sleep in children with attention-deficit/ hyperactivity disorder: meta-analysis of subjective and objective studies. J Am Acad Child Psy 2009;48(9):894–908.
20. Hoban TF. Sleep disturbances and attention deficit hyperactivity disorder. Sleep Medicine Clinics 2008;3:469–78.
21. Sadeh A, Pergamin L, Bar-Haim Y. Sleep in children with attention-deficit hyperactivity disorder: a meta-analysis of polysomnographic studies. Sleep Med Rev 2006;10(6):381–98.

22. Owens JA. The ADHD and sleep conundrum: a review. J Dev Behav Pediatr 2005;26(4):312–22.
23. Van der Heijden KB, Smits MG, Gunning WB. Sleep-related disorders in ADHD: a review. Clin Pediatr 2005;44(3):201–10.
24. Gruber R. Sleep characteristics of children and adolescents with attention deficit-hyperactivity disorder. Child Adolesc Psychiatr Clin N Am 2009;18(4):863–76.
25. Konofal E, Lecendreux M, Cortese S. Sleep and ADHD. Sleep Med 2010;11(7): 652–8.
26. Owens JA. A clinical overview of sleep and attention-deficit/hyperactivity disorder in children and adolescents. J Can Acad Child Adolesc Psychiatry 2009;18(2):92–102.
27. Weiss MD. The unique aspects of assessment of ADHD. Primary Psychiatry 2010;17(5):21–5.
28. Ivanenko A, Barnes ME, Crabtree VM, et al. Psychiatric symptoms in children with insomnia referred to a pediatric sleep medicine center. Sleep Med 2004; 5(3):253–9.
29. Jensen PS, Hinshaw SP, Kraemer HC, et al. ADHD comorbidity findings from the MTA study: comparing comorbid subgroups. J Am Acad Child Psy 2001;40(2): 147–58.
30. Corkum P, Moldofsky H, Hogg-Johnson S, et al. Sleep problems in children with attention-deficit/hyperactivity disorder: impact of subtype, comorbidity, and stimulant medication. J Am Acad Child Psy 1999;38(10):1285–93.
31. Mayes SD, Calhoun SL, Bixler EO, et al. ADHD subtypes and comorbid anxiety, depression, and oppositional-defiant disorder: differences in sleep problems. J Pediatr Psychol 2009;34(3):328–37.
32. Lecendreux M, Konofal E, Bouvard M, et al. Sleep and alertness in children with ADHD. J Child Psychol Psychiatry 2000;41(6):803–12.
33. Chiang HL, Gau SSF, Ni HC, et al. Association between symptoms and subtypes of attention-deficit hyperactivity disorder and sleep problems/disorders. J Sleep Res 2010;19(4):535–45.
34. Corkum P, Tannock R, Moldofsky H, et al. Actigraphy and parental ratings of sleep in children with attention-deficit/hyperactivity disorder (ADHD). Sleep 2001;24(3):303–12.
35. Rowland AS, Umbach DM, Catoe KE, et al. Studying the epidemiology of attention-deficit hyperactivity disorder. Can J Psychiatry 2001;46(10):931–40.
36. Habel LA, Schaefer CA, Levine P, et al. Treatment with stimulants among youths in a large California health plan. J Child Adolesc Psychopharmacol 2005;15(1):62–7.
37. Buitelaar J, Medori R. Treating attention-deficit/hyperactivity disorder beyond symptom control alone in children and adolescents: a review of the potential benefits of long-acting stimulants. Eur Child Adolesc Psychiatry 2010;19(4): 325–40.
38. Kutcher S, Aman M, Brooks SJ, et al. International consensus statement on attention-deficit/hyperactivity disorder (ADHD) and disruptive behavior disorders (DBDs): clinical implications and treatment practice suggestions. Eur Neuropsychopharmacol 2004;14(1):11–28.
39. Galland BC, Tripp EG, Taylor BJ. The sleep of children with attention deficit hyperactivity disorder on and off methylphenidate: a matched case-control study. J Sleep Res 2009;19(2):366–73.
40. Mick E, Biederman J, Jetton J, et al. Sleep disturbances associated with attention deficit hyperactivity disorder: The impact of psychiatric comorbidity and pharmacotherapy. J Child Adolesc Psychopharmacol 2000;10(3):223–31.

41. Sangal RB, Owens J, Allen AJ, et al. Effects of atomoxetine and methylphenidate on sleep in children with ADHD. Sleep 2006;29(12):1573–85.

42. Stein MA. Unravelling sleep problems in treated and untreated children with ADHD. J Child Adolesc Psychopharmacol 1999;9(3):157–68.

43. Corkum P, Panton R, Ironside S, et al. Acute impact of immediate release methylphenidate administered three times a day on sleep in children with attention-deficit/hyperactivity disorder. J Pediatr Psychol 2008;33(4):368–79.

44. Ironside S, Davidson F, Corkum P. Circadian motor activity affected by stimulant medication in children with attention-deficit/hyperactivity disorder. J Sleep Res 2010;19:546–51.

45. Gruber R, Grizenko N, Schwartz G, et al. Performance on the continuous performance test in children with ADHD is associated with sleep efficiency. Sleep 2007;30(8):1003–9.

46. Archbold KH. Sleep disorders and attention-deficit hyperactivity disorder in children: a missing differential diagnosis. J Am Psychiatr Nurses Association 2006; 12(4):216–24.

47. American Academy of Sleep Medicine. The international classification of sleep disorders: diagnostic and coding manual, ICSD-2. 2nd edition. Westchester (IL): American Academy of Sleep Medicine; 2005.

48. Owens J. Classification and epidemiology of childhood sleep disorders. Sleep Medicine Clinics 2007;2:353–61.

49. Owens JA, Dalzell V. Use of the 'BEARS' sleep screening tool in a pediatric residents' continuity clinic: a pilot study. Sleep Med 2005;6(1):63–9.

50. Owens JA, Spirito A, McGuinn M. The Children's sleep habits questionnaire (CSHQ): Psychometric properties of a survey instrument for school-aged children. Sleep 2000;23(8):1–9.

51. Spruyt K, Gozal D. Pediatric sleep questionnaires as diagnostic or epidemiological tools: a review of currently available instruments. Sleep Med Rev 2011; 15(1):19–32.

52. Sheldon SH. Diagnostic methods in pediatric sleep medicine. Sleep Medicine Clinics 2007;2:343–51.

53. Luginbuehl M, Kohler WC. Screening and evaluation of sleep disorders in children and adolescents. Child Adolesc Psychiatr Clin N Am 2009;18(4):825–38.

54. Prihodova I, Paclt I, Kemlink D, et al. Sleep disorders and daytime sleepiness in children with attention-deficit/hyperactivity disorder: a two-night polysomnographic study with a multiple sleep latency test. Sleep Med 2010;11(9): 922–8.

55. Walters AS, Silvestri R, Zucconi M, et al. Review of the possible relationship and hypothetical links between ADHD and the simple sleep related movement disorders, parasomnias, hypersomnias, and circadian rhythm disorders. J Clin Sleep Med 2008;4(6):591–600.

56. Reid GJ, Huntley ED, Lewin DS. Insomnias of childhood and adolescence. Child Adolesc Psychiatr Clin N Am 2009;18(4):979–1000.

57. Kratochvil CJ, Lake M, Pliszka SR, et al. Pharmacological management of treatment-induced insomnia in ADHD. J Am Acad Child Psy 2005;44(5): 499–501.

58. Kratochvil CJ, Vaughan BS, Barker A, et al. Review of pediatric attention deficit/hyperactivity disorder for the general psychiatrist. Psychiatr Clin North Am 2009; 32(1):39–56.

59. Ahmann PA, Waltonen SJ, Olson KA, et al. Placebo-controlled evaluation of ritalin side effects. Pediatrics 1993;91(6):1101–6.

60. Stein MA, Blondis TA, Schnitzler ER, et al. Methylphenidate dosing: twice daily versus three times daily. Pediatrics 1996;98(4):748–56.
61. Shreeram S, He J, Kalaydjian A, et al. Prevalence of enuresis and its association with attention-deficit/hyperactivity disorder among U.S. children: results from a nationally representative study. J Am Acad Child Psy 2009;48(1):35–41.
62. Sumner CR, Schuh KJ, Sutton VK, et al. Placebo-controlled study of the effects of atomoxetine on bladder control in children with nocturnal enuresis. J Child Adolesc Psychopharmacol 2006;16(6):699–711.
63. Mindell JA, Emslie G, Blumer J, et al. Pharmacologic management of insomnia in children and adolescents: consensus statement. Pediatrics 2006;117(6): e1223–32.
64. Owens JA, Moturi S. Pharmacologic treatment of pediatric insomnia. Child Adolesc Psychiatr Clin N Am 2009;18(4):1001–16.
65. Mindell JA, Kuhn B, Lewin DS, et al. Behavioral treatment of bedtime problems and night wakings in infants and young children. Sleep 2006;29(10): 1263–76.
66. Stojanovski SD, Rasu RS, Balkrishnan R, et al. Trends in medication prescribing for pediatric sleep difficulties in US outpatient settings. Sleep 2007;30(8): 1013–7.
67. Galland BC, Mitchell EA. Helping children sleep. Arch Dis Child 2010;95:850–3.
68. Davis KF, Parker KP, Montgomery GL. Sleep in infants and young children. Part one: normal sleep. J Pediatr Health Care 2004;18(2):65–71.
69. Pelsser L, Frankena K, Buitelaar J, et al. Effects of food on physical and sleep complaints in children with ADHD: a randomised controlled pilot study. Eur J Pediatr 2010;169(9):1129–38.
70. Driver HS, Taylor SR. Exercise and sleep. Sleep Med Rev 2000;4(4):387–402.
71. Owens J, Maxim R, McGuinn M, et al. Television-viewing habits and sleep disturbance in school children. Pediatrics 1999;104(3):e27.
72. Acevedo-Polakovich I, Lorch EP, Milich R. Comparing television use and reading in children with ADHD and non-referred children across two age groups. Media Psychology 2007;9(2):447–72.
73. Chan PA, Rabinowitz T. A cross-sectional analysis of video games and attention deficit hyperactivity disorder symptoms in adolescents. Ann Gen Psychiatry 2006;5.
74. Weiss MD, Wasdell MB, Bomben MM, et al. Sleep hygiene and melatonin treatment for children and adolescents with ADHD and initial insomnia. J Am Acad Child Psy 2006;45(5):512–9.
75. Ramchandani P, Wiggs L, Webb V, et al. A systematic review of treatments for settling problems and night waking in young children. BMJ 2000;320:209–13.
76. Jan J, Owens J, Weiss M, et al. Sleep hygiene for children with neurodevelopmental disabilities. Pediatrics 2008;122(6):1343–50.
77. Kuhn BR, Elliott AJ. Treatment efficacy in behavioral pediatric sleep medicine. J Psychosom Res 2003;54(6):587–97.
78. Mullane J, Corkum P. Case series: evaluation of a behavioural sleep intervention for three children with attention-deficit/hyperactivity disorder and dyssomnia. J Atten Disord 2006;10(2):217–27.
79. Corkum P, Davidson F, Lingley-Pottie P, et al. Behavioral treatment for diagnosed pediatric insomnia in school-aged children. Fifth Annual Conference on Pediatric Sleep Medicine. (Symposium). Denver (CO), October 3, 2009.
80. Tikotzky L, Sadeh A. The role of cognitive-behavioral therapy in behavioral childhood insomnia. Sleep Med 2010;11(7):686–91.

81. Owens JA, Rosen CL, Mindell JA, et al. Use of pharmacotherapy for insomnia in child psychiatry practice: a national survey. Sleep Med 2010;11(7):692–700.

82. Owens JA, Rosen CL, Mindell JA. Medication use in the treatment of pediatric insomnia: results of a survey of community-based pediatricians. Pediatrics 2003;111(5):e628–35.

83. Blumer JL, Findling RL, Shih WJ, et al. Controlled clinical trial of zolpidem for the treatment of insomnia associated with attention-deficit/ hyperactivity disorder in children 6 to 17 years of age. Pediatrics 2009;123(5):e770–6.

84. Palumbo DR, Sallee FR, Pelham WE Jr, et al. Clonidine for attention-deficit/ hyperactivity disorder: I. efficacy and tolerability outcomes. J Am Acad Child Psy 2008;47(2):180–8.

85. Rains A, Scahill L. Nonstimulant medications for the treatment of ADHD. J Child Adolesc Psychiatr Nurs 2006;19(1):44–7.

86. McCracken JT, Martin W. Clonidine side effect. J Am Acad Child Psy 1997;36(2): 160–1.

87. Cantwell DP, Swanson J, Connor DF. Case study: adverse response to clonidine. J Am Acad Child Psy 1997;36(4):539–44.

88. Mcdonald CA, Guttinger R, Joyce D. Case report: clonidine withdrawal after atypically high-dose maintenance treatment. J Paediatr Child Health 2005; 41(11):609–10.

89. Miyazaki S, Uchida S, Mukai J, et al. Clonidine effects on all-night human sleep: opposite action of low-and medium-dose clonidine on human NREM-REM sleep proportion. Psychiatry Clin Neurosci 2004;58(2):138–44.

90. Van der Heijden KB, Smits MG, van Someren EJ, et al. Effect of melatonin on sleep, behavior, and cognition in ADHD and chronic sleep-onset insomnia. J Am Acad Child Psy 2007;46(2):233–41.

91. Hoebert M, Van der heijden KB, Van Geijlswijk IM, et al. Long-term follow-up of melatonin treatment in children with ADHD and chronic sleep onset insomnia. J Pineal Res 2009;47(1):1–7.

92. Armour D, Paton C. Melatonin in the treatment of insomnia in children and adolescents. Psychiatric Bulletin 2004;28(6):222–4.

93. Famuyiwa O, Adewuya A. Reflections on melatonin: focus on child mental health. Psychiatric Bulletin 2008;32(12):444–8.

94. Larzelere MM, Campbell JS, Robertson M. Complementary and alternative medicine usage for behavioral health indications. Primary Care 2010;37(2): 213–36.

95. Cortese S, Konofal E, Bernardina BD, et al. Sleep disturbances and serum ferritin levels in children with attention-deficit/hyperactivity disorder. Eur Child Adolesc Psychiatry 2009;18(7):393–9.

96. Konofal E, Cortese S, Marchand M, et al. Impact of restless legs syndrome and iron deficiency on attention-deficit/hyperactivity disorder in children. Sleep Med 2007;8(7):711–5.

97. Konofal E, Lecendreux M, Deron J, et al. Effects of iron supplementation on attention deficit hyperactivity disorder in children. Pediatr Neurol 2008;38(1):20–6.

98. Dahl RE, Pelham WE, Wierson M. The role of sleep disturbances in attention deficit disorder symptoms: a case study. J Pediatr Psychol 1991;16(2):229–39.

99. Rybak YE, McNeely HE, Mackenzie BE, et al. An open trial of light therapy in adult attention-deficit/hyperactivity disorder. J Clin Psychiatry 2006;67(10): 1527–35.

100. Gruber R, Grizenko N, Joober R. Delayed sleep phase syndrome, ADHD, and bright light therapy. J Clin Psychiatry 2007;68(2):337–8.

101. Huang Y, Guilleminault C, Li H, et al. Attention-deficit/hyperactivity disorder with obstructive sleep apnea: a treatment outcome study. Sleep Med 2007;8(1): 18–30.
102. Dillon JE, Blunden S, Ruzicka DL, et al. DSM-IV diagnoses and obstructive sleep apnea in children before and 1 year after adenotonsillectomy. J Am Acad Child Psy 2007;46(11):1425–36.
103. Chervin RD, Ruzicka DL, Giordani BJ, et al. Sleep-disordered breathing, behavior, and cognition in children before and after adenotonsillectomy. Pediatrics 2006;117(4):e769–78.

Sleep and Autism Spectrum Disorders

Ann M. Reynolds, MD[a],*, Beth A. Malow, MD, MS[b]

KEYWORDS

- Autism spectrum disorders • Sleep • Neurodevelopment
- Quality of life

Autism spectrum disorders (ASD) are neurodevelopmental disorders characterized by dysfunction in social interaction and communication, as well as the presence of restricted interests or repetitive behaviors. ASD include autistic disorder, Asperger syndrome, and pervasive developmental disorder, not otherwise specified. Sleep problems are common in children with ASD and have a significant effect on the quality of life of children with ASD and their families.

NEUROBIOLOGY OF SLEEP AND WAKEFULNESS IN CHILDREN WITH ASD

Although a detailed examination of neurobiological alterations in the regulation of the sleep-wake cycle in children with ASD compared with that in typically developing children is beyond the scope of this review, some discussion of potential factors that may be related to abnormal sleep patterns in these children is warranted. Several neurotransmitters involved in these systems have also been implicated in the cause of ASD and include γ-aminobutyric acid (GABA), serotonin, and melatonin. In autism, GABAergic interneurons seem to be disrupted[1] and a genetic susceptibility region has been identified on chromosome 15q that contains GABA-related genes.[2] Abnormal expression of GABA may interfere with its inhibitory function, which may in turn interfere with sleep. Melatonin, a sleep-promoting substance that is inhibited by light and released by the pineal gland,[3] is synthesized from serotonin.[4] There are reports of abnormal platelet serotonin levels in children with autism.[5] The relationship between hyperserotonemia and sleep requires further study[6]; however, melatonin secretion has also been noted to be low in individuals with ASD,[7–10] and in one study, the level of the major metabolite of melatonin (6-sulfoxymelatonin) was directly related to the level of deep sleep in children with ASD.[11] Jonsson and colleagues[12] found mutations in regulatory regions in 3 genes in the melatonin pathway: acetylserotonin-O-methyltransferase (ASMT), melatonin receptor 1A, and melatonin receptor

[a] Department of Pediatrics, The Children's Hospital, University of Colorado Denver School of Medicine, 13123 East 16th Avenue, B-140, Aurora, CO 80045, USA
[b] Department of Neurology, Vanderbilt University Medical Center, 1161 21st Avenue South, Room A-0106 MCN, Nashville, TN 37232-2551, USA
* Corresponding author.
E-mail address: reynolds.ann@tchden.org

Pediatr Clin N Am 58 (2011) 685–698
doi:10.1016/j.pcl.2011.03.009
0031-3955/11/$ – see front matter © 2011 Elsevier Inc. All rights reserved.

1B in children with ASD, whereas Cai and colleagues[13] found a higher rate of abnormalities in ASMT in children with ASD compared with controls. Melke and colleagues[8] also found ASMT polymorphisms and lower levels of ASMT activity in children with ASD. In contrast, Toma and colleagues[14] examined ASMT variants in Finnish, Italian, and multiplex European families and found no differences from controls. Nonetheless, these findings are provocative and suggest that ASMT variability contributes to abnormalities in the synthesis of serotonin to melatonin. Treatment with melatonin has also been found to be helpful in treating insomnia in children with ASD (see later discussion). Other genes worthy of study in children with autism and insomnia include clock genes that regulate sleep phase (eg, Per 3 is associated with delayed sleep phase) or sleep duration (eg, BMAL and CRY are associated with short sleep duration); however, the function of these genes on sleep is still being explored.[15] It is expected that a better understanding of these genetic variations and their effects on sleep will lead to better treatments in the future.

PREVALENCE OF SLEEP PROBLEMS IN ASD

Sleep problems are common in children with ASD, with prevalence rates of approximately 50% to 80% compared with 9% to 50% in children with typical development.[16–19] Children with ASDs are also reported to have sleep problems more frequently than children with other developmental disabilities.[20,21] Although children with developmental disorders in general have a high rate of sleep problems, children with autism differ within that group. Although lower cognitive level and younger age are associated with the presence of higher rates of sleep problems in other developmental disorders, these associations are not necessarily seen in ASD.[17,22,23] Cognitive level and age do not always predict severity of sleep problems in ASD because children with high-functioning autism and Asperger syndrome have a high rate of sleep disturbance as well.[24] In one series, parents of younger children (<8 years) reported more severe sleep concerns than parents of older children.[25] However, a larger series comparing children younger and older than 8 years found no age differences, with the exception that behavioral sleep problems, including limit-setting sleep disorder and sleep-onset association disorder, were more common in the younger group. These discrepancies may reflect differences in methodology and the heterogeneity in this population.

EFFECTS OF SLEEP PROBLEMS IN CHILDREN WITH ASD

Sleep disturbances may contribute to stress in families of children with ASD and developmental disabilities. Parents of children with ASD who report sleep problems in their children also report more frequent daily stress and more intense hassles.[26] Quine[27] found a correlation between sleep problems in children with developmental disorders and maternal stress and parental sleep disruption. Sleep problems may worsen daytime behavior in individuals with developmental disabilities[28] and in children with epilepsy.[29] Behavioral issues such as inattention and hyperactivity may be worsened by the presence of sleep disorders such as sleep disordered breathing.[30,31] In ASD, short sleep duration has been associated with higher rates of stereotypic behavior, as well as higher overall autism severity scores and social skills deficits.[32] Sleep problems have been associated with increased repetitive behaviors and need for sameness on the Repetitive Behavior Scale[33]; however, the relationship may also have been moderated by level of cognitive ability in that particular study. It is critical to identify and address sleep problems in children with ASD because of the effect on health and quality of life in both the children and their parents.

TYPES OF SLEEP DISORDERS IN CHILDREN WITH ASD
Insomnia

Symptoms of insomnia, defined as difficulty initiating or maintaining sleep, are the major sleep concerns reported by parents of children with ASD. Questionnaires and sleep diaries completed by parents have shown that children with ASD are more likely to exhibit insomnia with prolonged sleep latency (time to fall asleep), bedtime resistance, decreased sleep efficiency (decreased time asleep in relation to time in bed), decreased sleep duration and continuity, and increased awakenings.[16,17,22,34] Overall, sleep-onset insomnia (difficulty falling asleep) is more prevalent, compared with sleep maintenance insomnia (difficulty staying asleep),[17,34] although children with ASD frequently experience aspects of both.

Insomnia is a symptom with many causes, and the causes of insomnia in ASD are multifactorial. They include neurobiological factors such as aberrations in neurotransmitter systems that promote sleep and establish a regular sleep-wake cycle (eg, melatonin) and medical disorders that disrupt sleep continuity (eg, neurologic conditions such as epilepsy, gastrointestinal disorders such as reflux, and primary sleep disorders such as sleep apnea). Psychiatric comorbidities, including anxiety/depression, attention-deficit/hyperactivity disorder (ADHD), and obsessive/repetitive behavior, can also contribute to insomnia and may also be exacerbated by insomnia. Medications used to treat seizures and psychiatric conditions can also disrupt sleep. The core behavioral deficits associated with ASD may also impede the establishment of sound bedtime behaviors and routines. For example, children with ASD may have difficulty with emotional regulation (eg, ability to calm self) or transitioning from preferred or stimulating activities to sleep. Children with ASD can also perseverate on an activity or thought that can interfere with settling for sleep. Because of deficits in communication skills, children with ASD may not readily understand the expectations of parents related to going to bed and falling asleep. Sorting out the cause of insomnia in children with ASD can be challenging, especially because multiple issues may be contributing to the sleep problems simultaneously.

Sleep Disordered Breathing

Sleep disordered breathing encompasses disorders related to airway obstruction and includes obstructive sleep apnea (OSA). Although not necessarily more common in autism, sleep disordered breathing is common in the general pediatric population and can adversely affect daytime behavior, contributing to sleepiness or ADHD symptoms, with improvement after adenotonsillectomy.[31,35,36] Hypotonia, which can be seen in children with ASD and other developmental disorders, can also contribute to sleep disordered breathing. Therefore, it is important to recognize sleep disordered breathing in this population. In one report, treatment of OSA in a child with ASD improved daytime behaviors.[37]

Parasomnias

Non–rapid eye movement arousal disorders
The non–rapid eye movement (NREM) arousal disorders, such as night terrors, sleep walking, and confusional arousals, usually occur in the first half of the night and during deeper levels of NREM (ie, deep, slow wave, or δ) sleep. Although they have not been extensively studied in children with ASD, some (but not all) studies report more parasomnias in individuals with ASD than in comparison groups.[20,24,25,38]

Rapid eye movement–associated sleep abnormalities
In one study that performed 1 night of polysomnography (PSG), rapid eye movement (REM) sleep percentage was noted to be lower in children with ASD compared with children with typical development and children with developmental disorders, 14.5% versus 22.6% and 25% respectively (P<.001).[39] Another group of investigators found that REM sleep percentage was lower on night 1 but not night 2 of PSG, with the difference between nights attributable to a first-night effect (sleep is more disrupted on the first night in the sleep laboratory than on subsequent nights).[8] The significance of these potential differences in REM percentage is not fully understood, but may reflect underlying central nervous system dysregulation in these children.

REM sleep behavior disorder (RBD), in which individuals act out their dreams because of the absence of the normal physiologic generalized muscle paralysis during REM sleep, has been reported in one case series of children with ASD who were studied with PSG.[40] However, a larger polysomnographic study that excluded children on psychotropic medication did not document REM sleep without atonia or RBD.[23] REM sleep behavior disorder can occur in association with psychotropic medications that affect REM sleep, such as the selective serotonin reuptake inhibitors,[41] which are frequently used in children with ASD.

Sleep-related Movement Disorders

Rhythmical movement disorder
Rhythmical movement disorder is characterized by repetitive motion of the head (including head banging), trunk, or limbs, usually during the transition from wakefulness to sleep.[42] It may also arise during sustained sleep. Although the condition most often affects infants and toddlers with typical development in a transient and self-limited fashion, it may be more persistent and increased in intensity in children with autism and other developmental disabilities. Padding the sleeping environment can be helpful.

Restless legs syndrome/periodic limb movements in sleep/periodic limb movement disorder Restless legs syndrome (RLS) is a sensorimotor disorder that involves an urge to move the legs and that typically occurs at bedtime, is worse at rest, and is relieved by movement. An accompanying uncomfortable sensory component or dysthesias in the lower extremities is common and may be expressed as growing pains. Periodic limb movements in sleep (PLMS) are defined by repetitive stereotypic movements of the limbs during sleep. Periodic limb movement disorder (PLMD) includes both repetitive stereotypic movements but also is associated with insomnia or daytime sleepiness. Although most patients with PLMD do not report symptoms of RLS, approximately 63% to 74% of pediatric patients with RLS have PLMS.[43]

Diagnosing RLS is difficult even in typically developing children less than 5 years of age, because of their inability to fully communicate symptoms.[43] Because difficulty communicating is a core feature of ASD, the diagnosis of RLS is even more challenging in children with ASD. Also, because PLMS on PSG may be helpful in corroborating the diagnosis of RLS in children who are nonverbal or who do not meet classic criteria,[43] making a diagnosis in children with ASD is further complicated because they are often unable to tolerate PSG because of tactile sensitivities or anxiety in novel situations.

ADDITIONAL CONSIDERATIONS
Medical and Psychiatric Issues

Insomnia may result from coexisting medical conditions that disrupt sleep. Addressing medical issues that have an effect on sleep is paramount to successful treatment of sleep disorders. Co-occurring disorders that cause pain or discomfort must be addressed; these include, but are not limit to, reflux esophagitis, constipation, dental issues, reactive airway disease, eczema, or oversensitivity to the environment (discomfort caused by diaper or pajamas). For example, if a child has severe eczema accompanied by pruritus and is uncomfortable at night, then sleep hygiene is unlikely to be successful until the eczema is addressed. Identifying these issues may be particularly challenging in children with ASD who often have difficulty communicating pain or discomfort.

Potential causes of sleep-onset and maintenance insomnia in children with ASD include primary sleep disorders such as sleep disordered breathing and restless leg syndrome. One potential risk factor for sleep disorders is nutritional deficiency, which is common in children with ASD and often related to issues such as severely restricted diets, food neophobia, and mealtime rituals[32,44]; as many as 70% to 90% of children with ASD have atypical feeding behaviors.[45–48] In particular, both RLS and PLMD are associated with iron deficiency; specifically, a serum ferritin level of less than 50 ng/ml.[43,49] There is 1 small study that reported a high rate of iron deficiency in children with ASD,[50] and another small study that reported low ferritin, a marker of iron deficiency, in children with ASD who also had restless sleep.[49] Both the ferritin levels and restless sleep responded to iron treatment in that small, open-label study.[49]

Psychiatric conditions such as ADHD, anxiety, or depression can interfere with sleep, as can the psychotropic medications often used to treat these conditions. Depression may be manifested by early morning waking, and bipolar disorder by decreased need for sleep. Anxiety, which is particularly common in children with Asperger syndrome, may lead to difficulty falling asleep alone, obsessive-compulsive disorder may result in prolonged sleep latency caused by excessive bedtime rituals, and sensory hypersensitivities (eg, to extraneous noises) may be an unrecognized cause of difficulty falling asleep. Coexisting epilepsy or its treatment may also disrupt sleep and, if there is a concern for sleep-related seizures, referral for PSG with electroencephalogram may be appropriate.[51]

EVALUATION AND TREATMENT OF SLEEP DISORDERS IN ASD

As with any child, it is important to take a comprehensive sleep history and refer for appropriate work-up as indicated. Sleep problems in children with ASD may be overlooked because daytime behavioral issues often take precedence. The sleep history should include bedtime, waking time, napping during the day, and any waking during the night, with estimated durations and associated behaviors. Daytime functioning should be assessed, including hyperactivity as well as sleepiness, because daytime sleepiness may manifest as hyperactivity in children. Parents should be encouraged to keep a sleep diary to assess sleep latency, total sleep time, night waking, and response to treatment. A sleep questionnaire, such as the Children's Sleep Habits Questionnaire,[52] is a useful adjunctive tool to assess multiple domains of sleep problems including sleep-related breathing disorders, sleep anxiety, bedtime resistance, and daytime sleepiness. The Family Inventory of Sleep Habits (FISH) is a parentally completed instrument that provides a quantitative measure of sleep habits, including bedtime routine, sleep environment, and parental interactions.[53] A behavioral rating scale such as the Child Behavior Checklist[54] can screen other behavioral domains including anxiety, aggression, and hyperactivity that may affect sleep. When appropriate, a psychiatric evaluation to assess for bipolar disorder, depression, or anxiety disorder should be obtained, because all of these conditions can affect sleep.

The presence of symptoms of and risk factors for treatable primary sleep disorders such as sleep-related breathing disorders, RLS, seizures, or narcolepsy should be assessed. Although PSG is the gold standard for measuring sleep in children with autism, including the detection of sleep apnea, seizures, interictal epileptiform discharges, parasomnias, and periodic limb movements, it does have limitations in terms of child tolerance, timely availability, and expense. However, desensitization therapy before PSG can work well for many children with ASD. Actigraphy, a methodology that measures sleep and wake patterns based on limb movement, represents an alternative to PSG for documenting sleep patterns in children with autism. It is especially helpful in insomnia. Actigraphy is performed in the child's home environment, and may be especially helpful in those with tactile sensitivities or anxiety in novel environments such as a hospital sleep laboratory.

Addressing sleep issues in children with ASD is a priority of the Autism Treatment Network (ATN), which is a group of 17 sites across the United States and Canada that have been funded by Autism Speaks to address medical conditions in children with ASD. The ATN is currently developing an algorithm and a behavioral sleep medicine toolkit for the evaluation and treatment of insomnia in children with ASD. The algorithm emphasizes screening for sleep problems in children with ASD, followed by identification and treatment of associated medical comorbidities that may affect sleep (**Box 1** and **Fig. 1**). Implementation of sleep education and behavioral strategies are then considered the first-line treatment.

TREATMENT OF INSOMNIA IN ASD

Once treatable medical and psychiatric disorders are addressed, the treatment of insomnia in children with ASD should include an approach that includes attention to the sleep environment, good sleep hygiene, establishment of a bedtime routine, and other educational and behavioral interventions. When a family is unable to implement these educational and behavioral interventions, or these interventions are not successful, consultation with a sleep specialist may be warranted. In these cases,

---

Box 1
Causes of sleep disturbance in autism

Poor sleep habits

Hypersensitivity to environmental stimuli

Hyperarousal/difficulty with self regulation

Medical concerns that may cause pain, discomfort, or sleep disruption (eg, constipation, gastroesophageal reflux, eczema, tooth pain, coughing/asthma)

Repetitive thoughts or behaviors that interfere with settling

Inability to benefit from communication/social cues regarding sleep

Co-occurring psychiatric conditions (eg, anxiety, depression)

Psychotropic medications

Coexisting epilepsy

OSA

RLS/periodic limb movements of sleep

Circadian rhythm abnormalities

Screening Checklist for Medical Comorbidities Associated with Sleep Problems
©Reynolds and Malow

Gastrointestinal

1. Does your child have a history of reflux?	☐ Yes	☐ No
If yes, when did it resolve? _____		
2. Are there any ongoing symptoms?	☐ Yes	☐ No
If yes, list: _____		
3. Does your child have constipation?	☐ Yes	☐ No
If yes, is it controlled?	☐ Yes	☐ No
What medication(s) is used for control? _____		
4. Does your child have abdominal pain?	☐ Yes	☐ No
5. Does abdominal pain occur at night?	☐ Yes	☐ No
How often does this occur? _____		

Seizures and Other Nighttime Events

1. Does your child have seizures?	☐ Yes	☐ No
If yes, does your child have seizures that happen multiple times a night?	☐ Yes	☐ No
2. Does our child have unusual events (behaviors or movements) during the night?	☐ Yes	☐ No
If yes, is the event similar every time (suggests seizure)?	☐ Yes	☐ No

Sleep Disordered Breathing

1. Does your child snore/breathe loudly?	☐ Yes	☐ No
2. Does your child gasp for breath or stop breathing (if no, child may still have sleep disordered breathing)	☐ Yes	☐ No
3. Does your child have allergies/nasal congestion?	☐ Yes	☐ No

Asthma/Sinusitis

1. Does your child cough at night?	☐ Yes	☐ No

Pain/Itching/Discomfort

1. Does your child see a dentist regularly?	☐ Yes	☐ No
2. Could your child have any tooth pain?	☐ Yes	☐ No
3. Does your child have eczema?	☐ Yes	☐ No
If yes, is it currently well controlled?		
What medication is used for this? _____		
When is this medication used (i.e. daily, as needed?)_____		
Do you think that the eczema causes your child to be itchy or have pain?	☐ Yes	☐ No
4. Could your child be hungry at night?	☐ Yes	☐ No
5. Is your child overly sensitive to light, sounds, or textures of clothing?		
6. Can you think of anything that may be causing your child pain or discomfort?	☐ Yes	☐ No
If yes, explain: _____		

Nutrition

1. Does your child eat at least 1 – 2 ounces of meat per day?	☐ Yes	☐ No
2. If not, does your child take a multivitamin with iron?	☐ Yes	☐ No
How often? _____		

Restless Sleep

	☐ Yes	☐ No
1. Does your child have restless sleep?		
2. Does your child have leg pains/"growing pains"?	☐ Yes	☐ No
3. Does your child experience frequent leg movements during sleep or complain of unusual feelings involving the legs when in bed?)		

Medication

1. Is your child on medication?	☐ Yes	☐ No
What is the name of the medication? _____		

Physical Exam

1. Does child have large tonsils?	☐ Yes	☐ No
2. Is child hypotonic?	☐ Yes	☐ No
3. Does child have nasal congestion or signs of allergic rhinitis?	☐ Yes	☐ No
4. Dental issues?	☐ Yes	☐ No
5. Wheezing?	☐ Yes	☐ No
6. Significant eczema/dry itchy skin?	☐ Yes	☐ No

Fig. 1. Screening checklist for medical comorbidities associated with sleep problems. This checklist was developed by the Autism Treatment Network to screen for medical issues that might have a negative effect on sleep. Intended for use by clinicians when interviewing families. (*Courtesy of* Ann M. Reynolds, MD and Beth A. Malow, MD.)

melatonin or other medications may be effective in promoting sleep and may sometimes allow for the successful implementation of educational/behavioral interventions.

Good Sleep Practices and Sleep Education

Despite parents of children with ASD facing many stressors and multiple priorities, a sleep education program is considered an important component for treatment of insomnia in children with ASD. Healthy sleep practices (sleep hygiene) can be divided into the following categories: daytime habits, evening habits, sleep environment, and bedtime routines. Daytime habits should include adequate exercise and exposure to light, limiting caffeine, and limiting naps. Evening habits should include decreasing stimulation, decreasing light, decreasing exposure to electronics, and a good bedtime routine. The sleep environment should be cool with minimal light and sound. Children with ASD may be hypersensitive to stimuli in their environment such as light and sound. A continual noise machine may be helpful for some children. Textures can also present a challenge, such as pajamas, sheets, or diapers. Children with ASD may respond more favorably to deep pressure than a light touch. A study of use of a weighted blanket is underway in England (Lucy Wiggs, personal communication, November 2010). A bedtime routine should include a series of bedtime tasks or activities that occur at the same time and place every night. The routine should be simple enough to occur nightly. Clinicians and families may benefit from completing a sleep habits checklist that identifies potential areas of concern that can be targeted for improvement.[55] For a more in-depth review of sleep hygiene in children with neurodevelopmental disabilities please see Jan and colleagues.[56]

Behavioral Treatment

Behavioral treatment of sleep problems in children with intellectual disabilities reduces parental stress, increases parents' satisfaction with their own sleep and their child's sleep, and heightens their sense of control and ability to cope with their child's sleep.[57] Behavioral sleep interventions must be tailored to meet the needs of the child and family but generally adhere to strategies that are successful for children with typical development. Until recently, case studies[58,59] have mainly been reported regarding the effectiveness of behavioral interventions for sleep in children with ASD. Reed and colleagues[53] showed subjective and objective (actigraphy) improvements in insomnia as well as aspects of daytime behavior and parental stress[53] after a group intervention program for parents of children with ASD that included both parental education and behavioral strategies. Moon and colleagues[60] reported improvement in sleep with a controlled trial of behavioral intervention. Studies determining the most effective methods for delivering sleep behavioral interventions are underway at several sites in the United States, Canada, and United Kingdom.

Children with ASD typically respond well to visual cues and routines once established. A visual schedule can be helpful for children with ASD. It should include pictures of each step of the bedtime routine (**Fig. 2**).The child should be trained to follow the visual schedule after a cue from parents, which may be accomplished using physical prompts. Back-to-bed reminders on the door also communicate parental expectations to the child. Stories that describe other children going to sleep and their struggles can also be helpful for communicating expectations for sleep to a child with adequate language to understand the story. Sleep restriction (decreasing total hours expected to sleep) and fading (move bedtime to a later time, often the time that the child usually falls asleep, and then gradually moving the bedtime to an earlier time once the child is in the habit of falling asleep more quickly) may also be helpful, especially for children who do not seem sleepy at bedtime.

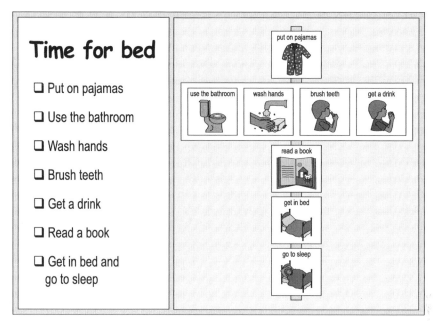

Fig. 2. Picture schedule. Picture schedules can be particularly helpful for children with ASD who respond better to visual stimuli than to auditory stimuli.

It is important for children to learn to fall asleep on their own. Fears and/or unhelpful rituals must also be addressed. If the child has anxiety about falling asleep alone, parents may temporarily set up a bed or rocking chair next to the child's bed. No physical contact or eye contact should be made during this phase of treatment. The rocking chair can be gradually moved closer to the door on successive nights until it is through the door. This transition may need to be done slowly.

The Bedtime Pass developed by Friman,[61] which limits nighttime waking, can also be helpful for children, especially those with comorbid anxiety, who can understand actions and consequences. The child may use the pass for 1 curtain call or opportunity to check in. If the child has not used the pass during the night, then the child can turn in the pass for a reinforcer in the morning. If the pass is the picture of a favorite toy or character, then keeping the pass may be its own reinforcer.

Melatonin for Insomnia and Circadian Rhythm Sleep Disorders

Whether the sleep problem primarily involves sleep initiation or a circadian phase shift, a combination of sleep hygiene and melatonin may be useful before considering other medications. Synthetic melatonin is available as a dietary supplement. Although studies have not been shown to support the use of melatonin to treat sleep disorders in children with typical development, a meta-analysis that included studies of children with ASD[62] found that melatonin seems to be safe and effective in the short term in individuals with an intellectual disability. There have also been some studies that evaluated the use of melatonin specifically in children with ASD. A retrospective open-label study of 107 children with ASD that included long-term follow-up[63] and several small open-label or randomized trials found improvement in sleep latency with melatonin and minimal adverse effects.[64–67] Although there is the need for larger placebo controlled trials, there seems to be enough evidence to consider use of melatonin in children with ASD who have significant issues with sleep-onset latency.

In the studies referenced earlier, and in practice, melatonin is generally used as a hypnotic with doses of 1 mg or higher given 30 minutes before bedtime. Doses may be rapidly titrated up to 3 mg if needed; rarely, 6 mg or more is needed. Melatonin may also be used as a chronobiotic, to shift or advance timing of sleep onset. In this latter case, melatonin is usually given in lower doses (300 μg), 3 to 5 hours before bedtime. Once a sleep cycle is established for 6 weeks or more, the melatonin may be discontinued, although long-term use is often necessary to maintain sleep patterns.[66] The use of melatonin for sleep maintenance is less well studied and less likely to be efficacious given that the half-life of melatonin is less than 1 hour. Extended-release preparations may be helpful in those circumstances.[66,68] Although generally regarded as a low-risk alternative, melatonin has not been rigorously tested for safety or efficacy in either adults or children; however, no serious long-term adverse effects have been reported with this widely used supplement.

Other Pharmacologic Treatments

When behavioral therapies and melatonin are ineffective, pharmacologic treatment can be considered. Although many different medications have been used in clinical practice, including clonidine, trazodone and other sedating antidepressants, and atypical antipsychotics,[69] there are few data to guide the use of psychotropic medications in children with ASD. One open-label, retrospective case series of clonidine use in children with ASD found that all children with difficulty with sleep initiation had a reduction in sleep-onset time by parent report, and 16 of 17 with night waking had improvement in the frequency of night waking.[70]

A helpful principle for prescribing sleep medications in children with coexisting neurologic or psychiatric disorders is to consider the overlapping neurologic systems that are affected. Wherever possible, prescribe a medication for the coexisting condition that also assists with sleep, and avoid those that cause insomnia. For example, in children with coexisting epilepsy or bipolar disorder, mood stabilizers with sedating properties, such as atypical antipsychotics or anticonvulsants, may be a reasonable choice. The antiepileptic regimen can be adjusted to administer a bedtime dose of medication that provides sedation and promotes sleep. Children with comorbid bipolar disorder, extreme mood irritability, aggression, or self-injurious behavior may benefit from treatment with the sedating atypical neuroleptics (eg, risperidol, olanzapine). The dosages of these medications can be adjusted to give the higher dose at bedtime. In children with anxiety or depression, antidepressants that promote sleep, such as mirtazepine, may be considered.

For a review of pharmacologic treatment of pediatric insomnia see Owens and Moturi.[71]

SUMMARY

Sleep disorders are common in children with ASD and have a significant effect on daytime function and parental stress. The cornerstone of treatment is to establish the cause of the sleep concern, which is often multifactorial. Identifying and treating sleep disorders may result not only in more consolidated sleep, more rapid time to fall asleep, and avoidance of night waking but also favorably affect daytime behavior and parental stress. Targeting effective treatment strategies is dependent on understanding the underlying cause/causes of sleep problems in children with ASD, therefore further research is paramount.

REFERENCES

1. Levitt P, Eagleson KL, Powell EM. Regulation of neocortical interneuron development and the implications for neurodevelopmental disorders. Trends Neurosci 2004;27(7):400–6.
2. McCauley JL, Olson LM, Delahanty R, et al. A linkage disequilibrium map of the 1-Mb 15q12 GABA(A) receptor subunit cluster and association to autism. Am J Med Genet B Neuropsychiatr Genet 2004;131(1):51–9.
3. Gooley JJ, Saper CB. Anatomy of the mammalian circadian system. In: Kryger MH, Roth T, Dement WC, editors. Principles and practice of sleep medicine. Philadelphia: Elsevier Saunders; 2011. p. 376–89.
4. Lin-Dyken DC, Dyken ME. Use of melatonin in young children for sleep disorders. Inf Young Children 2002;15(2):20–37.
5. Rapin I, Katzman R. Neurobiology of autism. Ann Neurol 1998;43(1):7–14.
6. Portas CM, Bjorvatn B, Ursin R. Serotonin and the sleep/wake cycle: special emphasis on microdialysis studies. Prog Neurobiol 2000;60(1):13–35.
7. Kulman G, Lissoni P, Rovelli F, et al. Evidence of pineal endocrine hypofunction in autistic children. Neuro Endocrinol Lett 2000;21(1):31–4.
8. Melke J, Goubran Botros H, Chaste P, et al. Abnormal melatonin synthesis in autism spectrum disorders. Mol Psychiatry 2008;13(1):90–8.
9. Nir I, Meir D, Zilber N, et al. Brief report: circadian melatonin, thyroid-stimulating hormone, prolactin, and cortisol levels in serum of young adults with autism. J Autism Dev Disord 1995;25(6):641–54.
10. Tordjman S, Anderson GM, Pichard N, et al. Nocturnal excretion of 6-sulphatoxymelatonin in children and adolescents with autistic disorder. Biol Psychiatry 2005;57(2):134–8.
11. Leu RM, Beyderman L, Botzolakis EJ, et al. Relation of melatonin to sleep architecture in children with autism. J Autism Dev Disord 2011;41(4):427–33.
12. Jonsson L, Ljunggren E, Bremer A, et al. Mutation screening of melatonin-related genes in patients with autism spectrum disorders. BMC Med Genomics 2010;3:10.
13. Cai G, Edelmann L, Goldsmith JE, et al. Multiplex ligation-dependent probe amplification for genetic screening in autism spectrum disorders: efficient identification of known microduplications and identification of a novel microduplication in ASMT. BMC Med Genomics 2008;1:50.
14. Toma C, Rossi M, Sousa I, et al. Is ASMT a susceptibility gene for autism spectrum disorders? A replication study in European populations. Mol Psychiatry 2007;12(11):977–9.
15. Crocker A, Sehgal A. Genetic analysis of sleep. Genes Dev 2010;24(12): 1220–35.
16. Couturier JL, Speechley KN, Steele M, et al. Parental perception of sleep problems in children of normal intelligence with pervasive developmental disorders: prevalence, severity, and pattern. J Am Acad Child Adolesc Psychiatry 2005; 44(8):815–22.
17. Krakowiak P, Goodlin-Jones B, Hertz-Picciotto I, et al. Sleep problems in children with autism spectrum disorders, developmental delays, and typical development: a population-based study. J Sleep Res 2008;17(2):197–206.
18. Richdale AL, Schreck KA. Sleep problems in autism spectrum disorders: prevalence, nature, possible biopsychosocial aetiologies. Sleep Med Rev 2009;13(6): 403–11.
19. Souders MC, Mason TB, Valladares O, et al. Sleep behaviors and sleep quality in children with autism spectrum disorders. Sleep 2009;32(12):1566–78.

20. Schreck KA, Mulick JA. Parental report of sleep problems in children with autism. J Autism Dev Disord 2000;30(2):127–35.
21. Wiggs L, Stores G. Severe sleep disturbance and daytime challenging behaviour in children with severe learning disabilities. J Intellect Disabil Res 1996;40(Pt 6): 518–28.
22. Richdale AL. Sleep problems in autism: prevalence, cause, and intervention. Dev Med Child Neurol 1999;41(1):60–6.
23. Malow BA, Marzec ML, McGrew SG, et al. Characterizing sleep in children with autism spectrum disorders: a multidimensional approach. Sleep 2006;29(12): 1563–71.
24. Patzold LM, Richdale AL, Tonge BJ. An investigation into sleep characteristics of children with autism and Asperger's disorder. J Paediatr Child Health 1998;34(6): 528–33.
25. Richdale AL, Prior MR. The sleep/wake rhythm in children with autism. Eur Child Adolesc Psychiatry 1995;4(3):175–86.
26. Honomichl RD, Goodlin-Jones BL, Burnham M, et al. Sleep patterns of children with pervasive developmental disorders. J Autism Dev Disord 2002;32(6): 553–61.
27. Quine L. Sleep problems in children with mental handicap. J Ment Defic Res 1991;35(Pt 4):269–90.
28. Didde R, Sigafoos J. A review of the nature and treatment of sleep disorders in individuals with developmental disabilities. Res Dev Disabil 2001;22(4):255–72.
29. Stores G, Wiggs L, Campling G. Sleep disorders and their relationship to psychological disturbance in children with epilepsy. Child Care Health Dev 1998;24(1):5–19.
30. Chervin RD, Archbold KH. Hyperactivity and polysomnographic findings in children evaluated for sleep-disordered breathing. Sleep 2001;24(3):313–20.
31. Chervin RD, Archbold KH, Dillon JE, et al. Inattention, hyperactivity, and symptoms of sleep-disordered breathing. Pediatrics 2002;109(3):449–56.
32. Schreck KA, Mulick JA, Smith AF. Sleep problems as possible predictors of intensified symptoms of autism. Res Dev Disabil 2004;25(1):57–66.
33. Gabriels RL, Cuccaro ML, Hill DE, et al. Repetitive behaviors in autism: relationships with associated clinical features. Res Dev Disabil 2005;26(2):169–81.
34. Williams PG, Sears LL, Allard A. Sleep problems in children with autism. J Sleep Res 2004;13:265–8.
35. Gottlieb DJ, Vezina RM, Chase C, et al. Symptoms of sleep-disordered breathing in 5-year-old children are associated with sleepiness and problem behaviors. Pediatrics 2003;112(4):870–7.
36. Goldstein NA, Fatima M, Campbell TF, et al. Child behavior and quality of life before and after tonsillectomy and adenoidectomy. Arch Otolaryngol Head Neck Surg 2002;128(7):770–5.
37. Malow BA, McGrew SG, Harvey M, et al. Impact of treating sleep apnea in a child with autism spectrum disorder. Pediatr Neurol 2006;34(4):325–8.
38. Honomichl RD, Goodlin-Jones BL, Burnham MM, et al. Secretin and sleep in children with autism. Child Psychiatry Hum Dev 2002;33(2):107–23.
39. Buckley AW, Rodriguez AJ, Jennison K, et al. Rapid eye movement sleep percentage in children with autism compared with children with developmental delay and typical development. Arch Pediatr Adolesc Med 2010; 164(11):1032–7.
40. Thirumalai SS, Shubin RA, Robinson R. Rapid eye movement sleep behavior disorder in children with autism. J Child Neurol 2002;17(3):173–8.

41. Mahowald MW. REM sleep parasomnias. In: Kryger MH, Roth T, Dement WC, editors. Principles and practice of sleep medicine. Philadelphia: Elsevier Saunders; 2011. p. 1083–97.
42. Hoban TF. Rhythmic movement disorder in children. CNS Spectr 2003;8(2):135–8.
43. Simakajornboon N, Kheirandish-Gozal L, Gozal D. Diagnosis and management of restless legs syndrome in children. Sleep Med Rev 2009;13(2):149–56.
44. Valicenti-McDermott M, McVicar K, Rapin I, et al. Frequency of gastrointestinal symptoms in children with autistic spectrum disorders and association with family history of autoimmune disease. J Dev Behav Pediatr 2006;27(2 Suppl):S128–36.
45. Ahearn WH, Castine T, Nault K, et al. An assessment of food acceptance in children with autism or pervasive developmental disorder-not otherwise specified. J Autism Dev Disord 2001;31(5):505–11.
46. Schreck KA, Williams K, Smith AF. A comparison of eating behaviors between children with and without autism. J Autism Dev Disord 2004;34(4):433–8.
47. Nieminen-von Wendt T, Paavonen JE, Ylisaukko-Oja T, et al. Subjective face recognition difficulties, aberrant sensibility, sleeping disturbances and aberrant eating habits in families with Asperger syndrome. BMC Psychiatry 2005;5:20 1–8.
48. Schreck KA, Williams K. Food preferences and factors influencing food selectivity for children with autism spectrum disorders. Res Dev Disabil 2006;27: 353–63.
49. Dosman CF, Brian JA, Drmic IE, et al. Children with autism: effect of iron supplementation on sleep and ferritin. Pediatr Neurol 2007;36(3):152–8.
50. Latif A, Heinz P, Cook R. Iron deficiency in autism and Asperger syndrome. Autism 2002;6(1):103–14.
51. Malow BA. Sleep disorders, epilepsy, and autism. Ment Retard Dev Disabil Res Rev 2004;10(2):122–5.
52. Owens JA, Spirito A, McGuinn M. The Children's Sleep Habits Questionnaire (CSHQ): psychometric properties of a survey instrument for school-aged children. Sleep 2000;23(8):1043–51.
53. Reed HE, McGrew SG, Artibee K, et al. Parent-based sleep education workshops in autism. J Child Neurol 2009;24(8):936–45.
54. Achenbach TM, Rescorla LA. Manual for the ASEBA preschool forms and profiles. Burlington (VT): University of Vermont, Research Center for Children, Youth, and Families; 2001.
55. Malow BA, Crowe C, Henderson L, et al. A sleep habits questionnaire for children with autism spectrum disorders. J Child Neurol 2009;24(1):19–24.
56. Jan JE, Owens JA, Weiss MD, et al. Sleep hygiene for children with neurodevelopmental disabilities. Pediatrics 2008;122(6):1343–50.
57. Wiggs L, Stores G. Sleep patterns and sleep disorders in children with autistic spectrum disorders: insights using parent report and actigraphy. Dev Med Child Neurol 2004;46(6):372–80.
58. Christodulu KV, Durand VM. Reducing bedtime disturbance and night waking using positive bedtime routines and sleep restriction. Focus Autism Other Dev Disabl 2004;19(3):130–9.
59. Weiskop S, Richdale A, Matthews J. Behavioural treatment to reduce sleep problems in children with autism or fragile X syndrome. Dev Med Child Neurol 2005; 47:94–104.
60. Moon EC, Corkum P, Smith IM. Case study: a case-series evaluation of a behavioral sleep intervention for three children with autism and primary insomnia. J Pediatr Psychol 2011;36:47–54.

61. Moore BA, Friman PC, Fruzzetti AE, et al. Brief report: evaluating the Bedtime Pass Program for child resistance to bedtime–a randomized, controlled trial. J Pediatr Psychol 2007;32(3):283–7.
62. Braam W, Smits MG, Didden R, et al. Exogenous melatonin for sleep problems in individuals with intellectual disability: a meta-analysis. Dev Med Child Neurol 2009;51(5):340–9.
63. Andersen IM, Kaczmarska J, McGrew SG, et al. Melatonin for insomnia in children with autism spectrum disorders. J Child Neurol 2008;23(5):482–5.
64. Paavonen EJ, Nieminen-von Wendt T, Vanhala R, et al. Effectiveness of melatonin in the treatment of sleep disturbances in children with Asperger disorder. J Child Adolesc Psychopharmacol 2003;13(1):83–95.
65. Garstang J, Wallis M. Randomized controlled trial of melatonin for children with autistic spectrum disorders and sleep problems. Child Care Health Dev 2006; 32(5):585–9.
66. Giannotti F, Cortesi F, Cerquiglini A, et al. An open-label study of controlled-release melatonin in treatment of sleep disorders in children with autism. J Autism Dev Disord 2006;36(6):741–52.
67. Wright B, Sims D, Smart S, et al. Melatonin versus placebo in children with autism spectrum conditions and severe sleep problems not amenable to behaviour management strategies: a randomised controlled crossover trial. J Autism Dev Disord 2011;41:175–84.
68. Wasdell MB, Jan JE, Bomben MM, et al. A randomized, placebo-controlled trial of controlled release melatonin treatment of delayed sleep phase syndrome and impaired sleep maintenance in children with neurodevelopmental disabilities. J Pineal Res 2008;44(1):57–64.
69. Owens JA, Rosen CL, Mindell JA, et al. Use of pharmacotherapy for insomnia in child psychiatry practice: a national survey. Sleep Med 2010;11(7):692–700.
70. Ming X, Gordon E, Kang N, et al. Use of clonidine in children with autism spectrum disorders. Brain Dev 2008;30(7):454–60.
71. Owens JA, Moturi S. Pharmacologic treatment of pediatric insomnia. Child Adolesc Psychiatr Clin N Am 2009;18(4):1001–16.

Sleep Problems in Children and Adolescents with Common Medical Conditions

Amy S. Lewandowski, PhD[a], Teresa M. Ward, RN, PhD[b],
Tonya M. Palermo, PhD[a,c],*

KEYWORDS

• Sleep • Pediatric • Chronic illness

Sleep is intricately connected to health and well-being. Over the past decade, research has increasingly recognized the importance of sleep and the adverse daytime consequences and health outcomes of untreated sleep disturbances and sleep disorders. Studies have shown associations among sleep problems and key physiologic health parameters, including immune system functioning and metabolic/endocrine regulation.[1] In children, specifically, short duration of nighttime sleep has been associated with increased risk of subsequent overweight or obesity.[2]

Sleep disturbances are especially prevalent in children with both acute and chronic disease states (eg, juvenile rheumatoid arthritis, asthma, cancer). Studies have shown that both acute and chronic medical conditions increase the risk of sleep disruptions,[3–6] and there is some evidence that sleep problems are more often chronic and persistent in youth with chronic conditions compared with those without chronic conditions.[7] The association between sleep problems and medical conditions may be related to underlying disease-related mechanisms (eg, airway restriction, inflammation), treatment regimens (including medications), or hospitalization. Some medical

This work was supported in part by Grants No. HD05343 and No. HD060068 from the National Institutes of Health (T.P.).
The authors have nothing to disclose.
[a] Department of Anesthesiology and Pain Medicine, University of Washington School of Medicine, PO Box 5371, Seattle, WA 98145-5005, USA
[b] Department of Family and Child Nursing, University of Washington School of Nursing, Box 357262, Seattle, WA 98195, USA
[c] Department of Pediatrics, University of Washington School of Medicine, PO Box 5371, Seattle, WA 98145-5005, USA
* Corresponding author. Department of Anesthesiology, Seattle Children's Hospital Research Institute, PO Box 5371, Seattle, WA 98145-5005.
E-mail address: tonya.palermo@seattlechildrens.org

Pediatr Clin N Am 58 (2011) 699–713
doi:10.1016/j.pcl.2011.03.012
0031-3955/11/$ – see front matter © 2011 Elsevier Inc. All rights reserved.

pediatric.theclinics.com

conditions are associated with particular sleep disorders (eg, sleep-disordered breathing [SDB] and atopic disease, restless legs syndrome, and iron deficiency anemia). Regardless of the cause, sleep disturbances typically manifest as poor sleep quality, difficulty falling asleep, disrupted or fragmented sleep with frequent awakenings, and inadequate amount of sleep. Unfortunately, sleep disturbances are too often undiagnosed and not routinely assessed by clinicians.

Poor sleep and untreated sleep disturbances pose significant adverse daytime consequences, including problems with social and emotional functioning, deficits in neurocognitive performance, poor quality of life, school absenteeism, and poor school performance.[8–12] Sleep disturbances are also associated with fatigue and daytime sleepiness.[13–16] The impact of poor sleep in children with chronic medical conditions may be of more concern given the bidirectional relations between sleep and health. Sleep problems may worsen the chronic medical condition, and in turn, disease-related symptoms may contribute to sleep disruptions.[17–19]

In this review, the authors summarize the data linking sleep disturbances and sleep disorders in children and adolescents with various medical conditions, and discuss the potential underlying mechanisms resulting in sleep problems. The potential impact of treatment-related medications on sleep is also described. Although it is beyond the scope of this article to provide a comprehensive review of sleep in all pediatric medical conditions, illustrative examples from common medical disorders and information on clinical evaluation and management are provided. The authors refer the reader to other relevant articles in this issue pertaining to the relationship between obesity and sleep (Hart) and sleep in autism spectrum disorders (Malow), and therefore do not cover these conditions.

MEDICAL CONDITIONS ASSOCIATED WITH SLEEP PROBLEMS
Allergic Rhinitis

One of the most common medical problems in children is allergic rhinitis, a chronic inflammatory disease of the upper airway affecting 10% to 30% of the population, with the greatest frequency found in children and adolescents.[20,21] Chronic allergies are associated with sleep problems and a known risk factor for SDB including habitual snoring, obstructive sleep apnea, and adenoid hypertrophy due to the chronic effects of inflammation.[22,23] Atopic symptoms can also affect sleep in children, for example, nocturnal pruritus associated with chronic eczema.[24]

Asthma

Childhood asthma, a condition defined by airway inflammation, is associated with sleep problems including decreased sleep time, less stage 4 sleep, more frequent nighttime arousals, and SDB.[25–28] Research has shown that asthma symptoms often worsen at night as a result of physiological changes (eg, airway inflammation and resistance, episodic coughing, wheezing, shortness of breath, mucociliary clearance, and lower lung volume) (see review by Suratwala and Brooks[29]). These nighttime exacerbations are related to circadian variations in lung function. Youth with asthma also show increased nocturnal awakenings compared with healthy youth. Asthma severity has been associated with both objective and subjective sleep reports,[26] and sleep disturbance has been shown to predict more severe asthma symptoms the following day.[17]

Cancer

Children and adolescents with cancer commonly report nocturnal sleep disturbances, but their causes are not well understood. Studies report frequent night awakenings, difficulty falling asleep, and increased wake time during hospitalization[30,31] and at home.[32–35] A recent study by Walker and colleagues[32] found that adolescents with cancer reported poor sleep quality, with more problems going to bed, falling asleep, maintaining sleep, and reinitiating sleep than healthy adolescents. Sleep disturbances for children and adolescents with cancer likely has many causes. Brain tumors or intracranial neoplasms are believed to affect sleep by their impact on brain structures. Brain tumors can affect sleep regulation, particularly if the mass impinges on brain structures affecting the circadian and homeostatic systems such as the hypothalamic-pituitary axis.[36] For example, craniopharyngiomas (tumors located in the basal forebrain near sleep-regulating structures) have been linked to a host of childhood sleep disturbances, including night awakenings, inability to maintain sleep, and secondary narcolepsy.[37] Tumors located near the pineal gland can result in irregular melatonin secretion, contributing to sleep-wake disturbances.[38] Central nervous system–mediated effects may also affect alertness. For example, neoplasms in the hypothalamus, thalamus, and brainstem have been linked to excessive daytime sleepiness as well as SDB.[39] Cranial radiation has also been linked to daytime sleepiness as well as sleep problems, particularly through injury to the optic nerve or retinohypothalamic track.[36]

Chronic Pain Conditions

Pain is common in youth with medical problems. Chronic pain may be a symptom or consequence of the medical problem (eg, sickle cell, arthritis, or cancer) or pain can be the problem itself (eg, headaches, chronic abdominal pain). Pain can make it difficult for children to settle and stay asleep. Youth with chronic pain report shorter sleep duration,[3,40] poorer sleep quality,[41,42] and more night wakings[43] than healthy youth. Insomnia symptoms are also common; estimates from several studies show that over half of children with different chronic pain conditions (eg, musculoskeletal pain, abdominal pain) report insomnia.[44,45] On actigraphy, youth with chronic pain demonstrate lower sleep efficiency than healthy youth.[42] Sleep disturbances are related to children's pain intensity as well as to their depressive symptoms.[46] A recent study of adolescents with mixed chronic pain conditions found that poor nighttime sleep was associated with a higher level of pain next day.[47]

In terms of specific pain conditions such as headache, frequency and duration of migraine headaches have been associated with sleep disturbances including parasomnias and bedtime resistance.[48] Furthermore, one study examining associations among sleep and headaches in youth found that tension headaches were associated with bruxism; SDB was frequent in youth with migraine and nonspecific headache; and that children with severe and chronic migraine headaches had disrupted sleep architecture (shortened sleep time, prolonged sleep latency, reduced slow-wave and rapid eye movement [REM] sleep[49]).

Craniofacial Abnormalities

Children diagnosed with genetic disorders such as Trisomy 21 and Crouzon syndrome, and children with muscular dystrophy and cerebral palsy are predisposed to craniofacial anomalies. Children with craniofacial structural overdevelopment or underdevelopment are at risk for and are often diagnosed with SDB.[22] Retrognathia, macroglossia, or mid-facial hypoplasia is commonly seen in children with underlying genetic disorders and/or hypotonia, which affect the airway and sleep. For example, cleft lip/palate is associated with several airway structural anomalies that restrict the pharyngeal airway, increasing the risk for SDB (see review by MacLean and colleagues[50]). In one study, 87% of children with cleft lip/palate had symptoms of SDB, with 28% demonstrating severe breathing problems during sleep.[51] Studies have shown that even after

undergoing surgical repair, children may continue to experience nighttime sleep disturbances. A recent study by Rustemeyer and colleagues[52] showed that 40% of children
who underwent surgery continued to have posterior airway narrowing, increasing the
risk for SDB.

Cystic Fibrosis

Sleep problems in children with cystic fibrosis have also been associated with airway
restriction.[53] Cystic fibrosis is a hereditary disease of the exocrine glands that usually
develops during early childhood. The disease affects the pancreas, respiratory system,
and sweat glands, and is characterized by the production of abnormally viscous mucus
resulting in chronic respiratory infections and impaired pancreatic function. Studies
have shown frequent sleep complaints, more nocturnal wakings, and alteration in sleep
architecture in this population.[18] Children and adolescents with cystic fibrosis also
demonstrate nocturnal hypoxemia, low sleep efficiency, prolonged REM latency,
and a reduced percentage of REM sleep on polysomnography.[53,54] Structural alterations in airways of children with cystic fibrosis can result in obstructive sleep apnea,[55]
although the frequency of sleep apnea in this population is currently unknown.[54]
Recent findings suggest that the relations between sleep and symptoms secondary
to cystic fibrosis are bidirectional.[18] Further longitudinal studies are needed on the
impact of disturbed sleep on symptoms.

Epilepsy

Children with epilepsy may manifest significant sleepiness as a result of disruptions in
sleep architecture, such as longer stage 1 sleep and latency to REM sleep.[56] Children
with epilepsy have also been reported to have SDB and parasomnias.[14] The associations between epileptic seizures and sleep are thought to be bidirectional. Patients
with epilepsy experience electroencephalographic (EEG) discharges at night that
may affect sleep, and sleep deprivation may subsequently influence EEG discharges
and seizures (see review by Parisi and colleagues[19]).

Gastroesophageal Reflux Disease

Gastroesophageal reflux disease (GERD) is a chronic condition in which the lower
esophageal sphincter allows gastric acids to reflux into the esophagus, causing heart-
burn, acid indigestion, and possible injury to the esophageal lining. During sleep
periods, the esophageal mucosa has more contact time with acid, and acid clearance
is reduced.[57] Often GERD is a common culprit of nighttime awakenings in infants.
Children with reflux have demonstrated a high number of apneas and hypopneas
(transient episode of shallow breathing or abnormally low respiratory rate) at night,
particularly during REM sleep, and GERD is considered a risk factor for obstructive
sleep apnea.[58]

Rheumatological Conditions

Rheumatological conditions including juvenile idiopathic arthritis (JIA) and juvenile
fibromyalgia (JF) are associated with significant sleep disruption in children and adolescents. Youth with JIA report poor sleep quality and daytime sleepiness,[3,12,15,59] with
children and their parents endorsing symptoms suggestive of sleep disorders, including
insomnia, parasomnias (sleep terrors, sleepwalking), SDB, and daytime sleepiness.[59,60]
Objective reports of sleep in youth with JIA including polysomnography and multiple
sleep latency tests (MSLT) show mild SDB, sleep fragmentation (eg, sleep stage shifts,
wake bouts), and daytime sleepiness.[12,16,61] For example, Passarelli and colleagues[3]
found that compared with healthy controls, children with JIA had reduced total sleep

time, more transient EEG arousals (brief shifts in the EEG to fast frequency without an awakening), and increased limb movements. Longer mean self-reported nap duration (~1 hour) and shorter mean sleep latencies[12,15] in MSLTs have been reported in children with JIA compared with mean sleep latencies from previous studies of healthy children.[3,62] Pain related to arthritis has been identified as a correlate of sleep disturbances[59] and is a potential mechanism.

Disruptions in sleep architectures in youth with JF are also common.[63,64] Compared with controls, children with JF have prolonged sleep latency, less total sleep time, decreased sleep efficiency, and more periodic limb movements,[63] and sleep anomalies are related to the intensity of pain experienced by children. Roizenblatt and colleagues[64] found decreased sleep efficiency, increased arousals, and disturbed EEG frequency during slow-wave sleep in children with JF. The mechanisms accounting for sleep alterations in JF are unclear, and additional research is warranted.

Sickle Cell Disease

The clinical manifestations of sickle cell disease (SCD) include episodes of severe pain (also called vaso-occlusive crises), infections (especially pneumococcal), cerebrovascular accidents, anemic episodes (aplastic crises or sequestration crises), and fragmented sleep. Excessive adenoidal and tonsillar growth occurs in children with SCD secondary to lymphoid tissue hyperplasia or recurrent tonsillitis.[65] Adenotonsillar hypertrophy is a risk factor for obstructive sleep apnea and vaso-occlusive crisis due to periods of hypoxemia.[66] Sleep patterns in children with SCD have not been well characterized, although studies report associations among nocturnal hypoxemia, SDB, and sleep disruption secondary to pain.[46,67–69] Compared with healthy children, parents of children with SCD report more symptoms of SDB, nocturnal enuresis, parasomnias, and night wakings.[70] In children with greater SCD severity, these parents reported more restless sleep in their children when compared with children with lower disease severity. A recent study using polysomnography reported prolonged sleep latency, decreased total sleep time, increased wake time, poor sleep efficiency, increased obstructive events, and periodic limb movements in children with SCD (HbSS, HbSC genotypes).[71] In their sample, obstructive sleep apnea was also common. Compared with children with the HbSC genotype, those with the HbSS genotype experienced more severe nocturnal oxygen desaturation.

OTHER CAUSES AND CONTRIBUTING FACTORS
Hospitalization and Treatment-Related Factors

The experience of being in hospital is associated with sleep disruptions for many children with medical conditions.[31,72,73] For example, 25% of hospitalized children with cancer reported poor sleep involving, for example, sleep fragmentation and night wakings.[72] Sleep disturbances may be due to disruptions in routine, fears and anxiety about separation from parents, loss of privacy, and frequent interruptions by medical staff. Children may also have to alter their sleeping position because of intravenous placement or location of surgical incisions. Sleep disruptions may also relate to specific treatment regimens. For example, children with chronic kidney disease experience sleep problems, and this has been linked to both the pathology of the disease and the dialysis process.[74] In a sample of pediatric dialysis patients, 86% reported sleep problems, including daytime sleepiness (60%), SDB (46%), and restless legs syndrome (29%).[74] Similarly, 49 nondialysis youths (19 had undergone a renal transplant) also reported sleep problems, particularly restless leg syndrome/periodic limb movement disorder, and 37% of these youths met diagnostic criteria for a sleep disorder.[75]

Behavioral, Emotional, and Psychological Factors

Children with chronic medical conditions are at increased risk for psychological problems[76,77]; therefore, it is important to consider the role of behavioral, emotional, and psychological factors that influence sleep. In youth with chronic conditions, behavioral and emotional problems were predictive of difficulties initiating and maintaining sleep.[6] Of importance, depression and anxiety symptoms have been associated with daytime sleepiness in female adolescents with chronic musculoskeletal pain.[43] In another study of adolescents with chronic pain, higher levels of depressive symptoms were related to more severe sleep disturbances (eg, irregular sleep habits, prolonged sleep latency, and difficulties getting up in the morning) even after controlling for adolescents' pain levels.[46] Among survivors of childhood cancer, greater symptoms of global distress predicted fatigue and continued sleep problems.[78] Symptoms of SDB have also been shown to predict behavior problems in children with asthma.[27] While depression, inattention, and oppositional behaviors were associated with sleep problems in children with epilepsy, the severity of epilepsy did not predict sleep disturbances.[79] Finally, it is important to consider the potential impact on sleep of psychotropic medications that may be used to treat comorbid psychiatric symptoms in these children.

EFFECTS OF MEDICATION ON SLEEP

Both over-the-counter and prescription medications used to treat chronic medical conditions affect sleep. Therefore it is important for the clinician to understand the effects on sleep of commonly used medications including antihistamines, antidepressants, anticonvulsants, corticosteroids, opioids, and benzodiazepines.

Anticonvulsants

Antiepileptic drugs (AEDs) are used for seizure control in youth with epilepsy. In addition, anticonvulsants such as gabapentin are commonly used agents for pain control in youth with chronic musculoskeletal pain. AEDs have mixed effects on sleep, and these effects appear independent of their anticonvulsant actions. AEDs also have the side effect of weight changes in children. A recent study by Kaleyias and colleagues[67] reports SDB, primary snoring, and periodic limb movement disorder in a cohort of 40 children with epilepsy. Children with poor control of epilepsy were more obese, had lower sleep efficiency, and higher arousal index in comparison with children with good seizure control or children free of seizures.[67]

Antidepressants

Antidepressant medications may be prescribed to treat comorbid conditions (eg, chronic pain, depression, anxiety) in children with medical conditions, and may also be prescribed specifically to treat sleep disturbance, particularly insomnia. Antidepressants have several effects on sleep and daytime wakefulness, most of which has been learned from studies in adults. These studies show prolonged sleep latency, reduced REM latency, decreased slow-wave sleep, and sleep fragmentation.[80–82] Studies in adolescents also have found prolonged sleep latency and reduced REM latency.[83–85] Most antidepressants suppress REM and increase latency to REM sleep, and abrupt withdrawal may lead to REM rebound.[86] Tricyclic antidepressants (TCAs; eg, imipramine) prolong REM latency and decrease REM sleep, and abrupt withdrawal can result in REM rebound.[87] TCAs have sedating side effects and therefore may be considered for the patient with insomnia. However, disruptions in sleep architecture are reported in children and adolescents treated with TCAs, including REM sleep suppression, decreases in slow-wave sleep, increases in stage 2 sleep, and sleep fragmentation.[88] Selective serotonin reuptake inhibitors (SSRIs) including fluoxetine (Prozac), sertraline HCl (Zoloft), and paroxetine (Paxil) have fewer sedating effects than TCAs. Little is known about the influence of SSRIs on sleep architecture in children and adolescents. Armitage and colleagues[89] examined fluoxetine use in depressed children and adolescents and found increases in stage 1 sleep, number of arousals, REM density, and oculomotor abnormalities.

Antihistamines

Antihistamines such as diphenhydramine, chlorpheniramine, and hydroxyzine are first-generation H1-histamine receptor blockers that have multiple effects on the central and peripheral nervous systems. These medications cross the blood-brain barrier and are rapidly absorbed through the gastrointestinal tract.[90] Many over-the-counter medications such as antiemetic, antiallergy, and antitussive agents contain diphenhydramine. Clinically antihistamines induce drowsiness and sleepiness, and are given to promote sleep. Sleep-onset latency is shortened and these agents have little effect on sleep architecture.[91] Some of the side effects include daytime drowsiness, lethargy, and dry mouth. Antihistamines can also intensify primary sleep disorders such as restless legs syndrome.[92]

Benzodiazepines

Benzodiazepines, such as clonazepam and diazepam, have both anticonvulsant and anxiolytic as well as hypnotic properties, and are thus used clinically for a variety of purposes. Randomized controlled studies of benzodiazepines for insomnia in children and adolescents are lacking, and it has been shown that benzodiazepines can disrupt sleep architecture (eg, suppressed delta sleep, prolonged REM latency, and increased stage 2 sleep), worsen SDB, and are associated with daytime sleepiness and cognitive effects.[93] Thus the use of these medications in the pediatric population is clinically limited.[94]

Corticosteroids

Corticosteroids are frequently used in children with chronic conditions including asthma, JIA, and cancer. These agents have a wide range of effects on multiple organs and also effect sleep.[34,95,96] Prolonged sleep-onset latency, increased wake time after sleep onset, and reduced REM sleep have been reported.[34,93,95,96] A recent study by Vallance and colleagues[95] reports that increased frequency and dosage of dexamethasone was associated with increased wake after sleep onset, poor sleep efficiency, decreased total sleep time, and increased night awakenings, as measured by actigraphy in children diagnosed with acute lymphoblastic leukemia. In pediatric cancer, studies have shown that daytime fatigue is highest during the first few days after the start of chemotherapy, and that corticosteroid use and hemoglobin values are associated with significant fatigue.[13,97] Often children receive intensive multiagent chemotherapy, and each agent can produce immediate or delayed effects on sleep.

Opioids

Opioid medications, such as oxycodone, commonly used for pain management, have also been linked to disruption of sleep architecture. There is a paucity of pediatric research on effects of opioids on sleep; however, adult studies have shown opioid use is associated with reductions in REM and slow-wave sleep, and that chronic use of opioids is associated with obstructive sleep apnea.[98,99] Timing of opioids may also affect daytime alertness; short-acting agents often induce sleep during the day.

EVALUATION OF SLEEP PROBLEMS

The clinical evaluation of sleep and its related disorders in children with medical conditions is challenging. Some sleep disorders or disturbances have a gradual onset and remain undetected for an extended period of time, in part because of the absence of adequate sleep assessment. Parents, children, and adolescents may not be familiar with the signs and symptoms (ie, altered mood, daytime sleepiness, inattention, and hyperactivity) or may attribute sleep disruptions to their underlying medical condition. Accurate assessment is critical for guiding identification and treatment of sleep problems in children with medical conditions. Differential diagnosis is key, as it can be difficult to differentiate medical, psychiatric, and sleep disorders that commonly co-occur. Thus the assessment of sleep disorders in children and adolescents with medical conditions requires a multidisciplinary team that may include advanced practice nurses, staff nurses, neurologists, pediatricians, psychologists, psychiatrists, pulmonologists, otolaryngologists, and dentists.

Similar to the assessment of sleep in the otherwise healthy child, evaluation should begin with a thorough sleep and medical history, psychiatric, developmental, and social health history, medication history, and physical examination. The physical examination should evaluate a child's physical appearance, focusing on craniofacial characteristics (midfacial hypoplasia), nasal obstruction, the oral cavity (eg, sizes of soft palate, tongue and tonsils, adenoidal tissue), a neurological evaluation for hypotonia, and an obesity assessment.[100] In the context of the medical condition, assessment of additional factors including the sleep environment and experience of nighttime symptoms will be important. For example, in children with allergies or asthma, assessment should include the child's exposure to environmental allergens including pets in the household, mattress, linens, and the living environment that might be associated with symptom exacerbations at night. Sleep assessment includes a thorough sleep history, addressing subjective and objective characteristics of sleep and sleep disturbances, related factors, and consequences (eg, mood, fatigue, excessive daytime sleepiness). Where indicated, depending on the sleep disorder, specialized sleep testing in a sleep laboratory setting may be recommended. The reader is referred to articles elsewhere in this issue for further details on evaluating sleep disorders (Babcock) and regarding sleep in the family (Meltzer).

In the general medical history evaluation, the clinician should pay particular attention to the child's underlying chronic condition (eg, pulmonary for a child diagnosed with asthma). Assessments should include cardiopulmonary (eg, heart disease, lung disease), neurological (eg, seizure disorder, restless legs syndrome), immune disorders (ie, rheumatoid arthritis), gastroenterology (eg, GERD), screening for psychiatric conditions (eg, anxiety, depression, bipolar), as well as other pain-related conditions (eg, JF, SCD). In the family history, information about sleep and psychiatric and medical conditions should be obtained; for example, history of family members or relatives who snore or are diagnosed with SDB, restless legs syndrome, narcolepsy, insomnia, or other problems such as fibromyalgia, depression, and anxiety.

In the medication review, in addition to consideration of the potential effects of medications on sleep and alertness outlined earlier, it is important to consider several other aspects of pharmacological treatment. These factors include timing (ie, direct versus withdrawal effects), dosage (ie, some sleep-disruptive effects are dose dependent), and use of combinations of medications (ie, synergistic effects of sedating drugs). During medication review, it is important to differentiate whether daytime sleepiness is secondary to symptom management (eg, pain exacerbation), in response to taking sedating medicines during the day, or to compensate for sleep loss at nighttime.

TREATMENT OF SLEEP PROBLEMS

The clinician's approach to management of sleep problems in children with common medical conditions is challenging and complex. The goal of treatment involves promotion of healthy sleep habits, prevention strategies, and treatment of diagnosed sleep disorders. Similar to otherwise healthy children, treatment of SDB in children and adolescents with medical conditions includes tonsillectomy and adenoidectomy, pharmacological interventions, and the use of noninvasive ventilation devices (eg, continuous positive airway pressure [CPAP], bilevel positive airway pressure [BiPAP]), as well as behavioral treatments and sleep education for any coexisting behaviorally based sleep issues. In children diagnosed with obstructive sleep apnea, an adenotonsillectomy is typically the first-line treatment, particularly when there is evidence of adenotonsillar hypertrophy.[101] However, children with medical conditions may require additional monitoring in the postoperative period following surgical intervention. It is important for the treating clinician to know that despite surgical intervention, some children with medical conditions continue to have obstructive sleep apnea due to underlying craniofacial anomalies or oropharyngeal features that affect the airway.[102] In these particular cases, noninvasive ventilation including CPAP or BiPAP is commonly used to treat obstructive sleep apnea. CPAP delivers a constant pressure of air to stent open the airway, and BiPAP delivers an inspiratory and expiratory pressure to children during sleep through a face mask. CPAP has been effectively used in medical populations including children with SCD[103] and young adults with cystic fibrosis.[104]

Pharmacological Treatment

Prescription and over-the-counter medications have been used to treat sleep disturbances in youth with medical conditions. For example, exogenous melatonin has been successfully used to treat circadian rhythm disturbances and sleep-onset insomnia in children with epilepsy[105] and neurodevelopmental disabilities,[106] and in children who are blind.[107] Despite the use of prescription and over-the-counter medications, there is a paucity of knowledge on the pharmacological management of sleep disturbances in children with medical conditions. In 2006, a consensus statement on the pharmacological management of pediatric insomnia was developed, which reported concerns on the lack of clinical trials and knowledge about safety and efficacy, particularly in children with chronic conditions.[108] Additional research is warranted on the pharmacological practices for the management of pediatric insomnia in children with medical conditions.

Behavioral and Psychological Treatments

There is also a paucity of research on behavioral and psychological treatments for sleep problems in children with medical conditions. Cognitive-behavioral therapy (CBT) is a psychological treatment that incorporates both cognitive strategies and behavioral techniques to promote more adaptive behaviors that facilitate sleep. CBT for insomnia (called CBT-I) has been well described for the treatment of adults and has received much empirical support in diverse populations of adults with medical conditions.[109] Only a few studies of behavioral treatments for sleep problems have been conducted in pediatric medical populations. The findings are promising, however, showing improvements in sleep quality and reductions in pain and fatigue in children and adolescents with fibromyalgia and cancer.[36,110]

Given the importance of sleep for health and well-being, strategies to heighten clinician and parental awareness and educate children, adolescents, and parents about the importance of sleep in health outcomes (eg, school and work function, quality of life, psychosocial functioning) is essential in the management of pediatric medical conditions.

SUMMARY AND RECOMMENDATIONS

Sleep is an important consideration in the management of common medical conditions in children and adolescents. Sleep loss carries specific health risks that may exacerbate a chronic condition and disease-related symptoms. Because of the adverse effects of inadequate sleep and untreated sleep disorders on health outcomes, routine screening for sleep disturbances and disorders as well as sleep assessments are needed to improve the clinical care of children and adolescents with medical conditions. Future research is needed on sleep disturbances using subjective and objective measures to better understand the relationships among sleep, disease-related symptoms, and health outcomes in children and adolescents with medical conditions. Such knowledge will enable optimal tailoring of sleep interventions to the unique needs of different medical populations.

REFERENCES

1. Bryant PA, Trinder J, Curtis N. Sick and tired: does sleep have a vital role in the immune system? Nat Rev Immunol 2004;4(6):457–67.
2. Bell JF, Zimmerman FJ. Shortened nighttime sleep duration in early life and subsequent childhood obesity. Arch Pediatr Adolesc Med 2010;164(9):840–5.
3. Passarelli CM, Roizenblatt S, Len CA, et al. A case-control sleep study in children with polyarticular juvenile rheumatoid arthritis. J Rheumatol 2006;33(4): 796–802.
4. Yuksel H, Sogut A, Yilmaz O, et al. Evaluation of sleep quality and anxiety-depression parameters in asthmatic children and their mothers. Respir Med 2007;101(12):2550–4.
5. Huntley ED, Campo JV, Dahl RE, et al. Sleep characteristics of youth with functional abdominal pain and a healthy comparison group. J Pediatr Psychol 2007; 32(8):938–49.
6. Hysing M, Sivertsen B, Stormark KM, et al. Sleep in children with chronic illness, and the relation to emotional and behavioral problems—a population-based study. J Pediatr Psychol 2009;34(6):665–70.
7. Sivertsen B, Hysing M, Elgen I, et al. Chronicity of sleep problems in children with chronic illness: a longitudinal population-based study. Child Adolesc Psychiatry Ment Health 2009;3(1):22.
8. Warren S. Sleep in medically compromised children. Med Health 2006;89(3): 100–1.
9. Long AC, Krishnamurthy V, Palermo TM. Sleep disturbances in school-age children with chronic pain. J Pediatr Psychol 2008;33(3):258–68.
10. Bartlet LB, Westbroek R, White JE. Sleep patterns in children with atopic eczema. Acta Derm Venereol 1997;77(6):446–8.
11. Wirrell E, Blackman M, Barlow K, et al. Sleep disturbances in children with epilepsy compared with their nearest-aged siblings. Dev Med Child Neurol 2005;47(11):754–9.

12. Ward TM, Archbold K, Lentz M, et al. Sleep disturbance, daytime sleepiness, and neurocognitive performance in children with juvenile idiopathic arthritis. Sleep 2010;33(2):252–9.
13. Zwerdling T, Konia T, Silverstein M. Congenital, single system, single site, Langerhans cell histiocytosis: a new case, observations from the literature, and management considerations. Pediatr Dermatol 2009;26(1):121–6.
14. Maganti R, Hausman N, Koehn M, et al. Excessive daytime sleepiness and sleep complaints among children with epilepsy. Epilepsy Behav 2006;8(1):272–7.
15. Zamir G, Press J, Tal A, et al. Sleep fragmentation in children with juvenile rheumatoid arthritis. J Rheumatol 1998;25(6):1191–7.
16. Ward TM, Brandt P, Archbold K, et al. Polysomnography and self-reported sleep, pain, fatigue, and anxiety in children with active and inactive juvenile rheumatoid arthritis. J Pediatr Psychol 2008;33(3):232–41.
17. Hanson MD, Chen E. The temporal relationships between sleep, cortisol, and lung functioning in youth with asthma. J Pediatr Psychol 2008;33(3):312–6.
18. Amin R, Bean J, Burklow K, et al. The relationship between sleep disturbance and pulmonary function in stable pediatric cystic fibrosis patients. Chest 2005;128(3):1357–63.
19. Parisi P, Bruni O, Pia Villa M, et al. The relationship between sleep and epilepsy: the effect on cognitive functioning in children. Dev Med Child Neurol 2010;52(9):805–10.
20. Dykewicz MS, Fineman S, Skoner DP. Joint Task Force summary statements on diagnosis and management of rhinitis. Ann Allergy Asthma Immunol 1998;81(5 Pt 2):474–7.
21. Wallace DV, Dykewicz MS, Bernstein DI, et al. The diagnosis and management of rhinitis: an updated practice parameter. J Allergy Clin Immunol 2008;122(Suppl 2):S1–84.
22. Bixler EO, Vgontzas AN, Lin HM, et al. Sleep disordered breathing in children in a general population sample: prevalence and risk factors. Sleep 2009;32(6):731–6.
23. Redline S, Tishler PV, Schluchter M, et al. Risk factors for sleep-disordered breathing in children. Associations with obesity, race, and respiratory problems. Am J Respir Crit Care Med 1999;159(5 Pt 1):1527–32.
24. Meltzer EO, Blaiss MS, Derebery MJ, et al. Burden of allergic rhinitis: results from the Pediatric Allergies in America survey. J Allergy Clin Immunol 2009;124(Suppl 3):S43–70.
25. Kales A, Kales JD, Sly RM, et al. Sleep patterns of asthmatic children: all-night electroencephalographic studies. J Allergy 1970;46(5):300–8.
26. Sadeh A, Horowitz I, Wolach-Benodis L, et al. Sleep and pulmonary function in children with well-controlled, stable asthma. Sleep 1998;21(4):379–84.
27. Fagnano M, van Wijngaarden E, Connolly HV, et al. Sleep-disordered breathing and behaviors of inner-city children with asthma. Pediatrics 2009;124(1):218–25.
28. Dean BB, Calimlim BC, Sacco P, et al. Uncontrolled asthma among children: impairment in social functioning and sleep. J Asthma 2010;47(5):539–44.
29. Suratwala D, Brooks LJ. Pulmonary disorders affecting sleep in children. In: Butkov N, Lee-Chiong T, editors. Fundamentals of sleep technology. Philadelphia: Lippincott Williams & Wilkins; 2007. p. 575–9.
30. Hockenberry MJ, Hooke MC, Gregurich M, et al. Symptom clusters in children and adolescents receiving cisplatin, doxorubicin, or ifosfamide. Oncol Nurs Forum 2010;37(1):E16–27.

31. Hinds PS, Hockenberry M, Rai SN, et al. Nocturnal awakenings, sleep environment interruptions, and fatigue in hospitalized children with cancer. Oncol Nurs Forum 2007;34(2):393–402.
32. Walker AJ, Johnson KP, Miaskowski C, et al. Sleep quality and sleep hygiene behaviors of adolescents during chemotherapy. J Clin Sleep Med 2010;6(5): 439–44.
33. Zupanec S, Jones H, Stremler R. Sleep habits and fatigue of children receiving maintenance chemotherapy for ALL and their parents. J Pediatr Oncol Nurs 2010;27(4):217–28.
34. Hinds PS, Hockenberry MJ, Gattuso JS, et al. Dexamethasone alters sleep and fatigue in pediatric patients with acute lymphoblastic leukemia. Cancer 2007; 110(10):2321–30.
35. Gedaly-Duff V, Lee KA, Nail L, et al. Pain, sleep disturbance, and fatigue in children with leukemia and their parents: a pilot study. Oncol Nurs Forum 2006; 33(3):641–6.
36. Rosen GM, Shor AC, Geller TJ. Sleep in children with cancer. Curr Opin Pediatr 2008;20(6):676–81.
37. Palm L, Nordin V, Elmqvist D, et al. Sleep and wakefulness after treatment for craniopharyngioma in childhood; influence on the quality and maturation of sleep. Neuropediatrics 1992;23(1):39–45.
38. Gapstur R, Gross CR, Ness K. Factors associated with sleep-wake disturbances in child and adult survivors of pediatric brain tumors: a review. Oncol Nurs Forum 2009;36(6):723–31.
39. Rosen G, Brand SR. Sleep in children with cancer: case review of 70 children evaluated in a comprehensive pediatric sleep center. Support Care Cancer 2010. [Epub ahead of print].
40. Tsai SY, Labyak SE, Richardson LP, et al. Actigraphic sleep and daytime naps in adolescent girls with chronic musculoskeletal pain. J Pediatr Psychol 2008; 33(3):307–11.
41. Haim A, Pillar G, Pecht A, et al. Sleep patterns in children and adolescents with functional recurrent abdominal pain: objective versus subjective assessment. Acta Paediatr 2004;93(5):677–80.
42. Palermo TM, Toliver-Sokol M, Fonareva I, et al. Objective and subjective assessment of sleep in adolescents with chronic pain compared to healthy adolescents. Clin J Pain 2007;23(9):812–20.
43. Meltzer LJ, Logan DE, Mindell JA. Sleep patterns in female adolescents with chronic musculoskeletal pain. Behav Sleep Med 2005;3(4):193–208.
44. LaPlant MM, Adams BS, Haftel HM, et al. Insomnia and quality of life in children referred for limb pain. J Rheumatol 2007;34(12):2486–90.
45. Palermo TM, Wilson AC, Lewandowski AS, et al. Behavioral and psychosocial factors associated with insomnia in adolescents with chronic pain. Pain 2011; 152(1):89–94.
46. Palermo TM, Kiska R. Subjective sleep disturbances in adolescents with chronic pain: relationship to daily functioning and quality of life. J Pain 2005;6(3):201–7.
47. Lewandowski AS, Palermo TM, De la Motte S, et al. Temporal daily associations between pain and sleep in adolescents with chronic pain versus healthy adolescents. Pain 2010;151(1):220–5.
48. Miller VA, Palermo TM, Powers SW, et al. Migraine headaches and sleep disturbances in children. Headache 2003;43(4):362–8.
49. Vendrame M, Kaleyias J, Valencia I, et al. Polysomnographic findings in children with headaches. Pediatr Neurol 2008;39(1):6–11.

50. MacLean JE, Hayward P, Fitzgerald DA, et al. Cleft lip and/or palate and breathing during sleep. Sleep Med Rev 2009;13(5):345–54.
51. MacLean JE, Fitzsimons D, Hayward P, et al. The identification of children with cleft palate and sleep disordered breathing using a referral system. Pediatr Pulmonol 2008;43(3):245–50.
52. Rustemeyer J, Thieme V, Bremerich A. Snoring in cleft patients with velopharyngoplasty. Int J Oral Maxillofac Surg 2008;37(1):17–20.
53. Naqvi SK, Sotelo C, Murry L, et al. Sleep architecture in children and adolescents with cystic fibrosis and the association with severity of lung disease. Sleep Breath 2008;12(1):77–83.
54. de Castro-Silva C, de Bruin VM, Cavalcante AG, et al. Nocturnal hypoxia and sleep disturbances in cystic fibrosis. Pediatr Pulmonol 2009;44(11):1143–50.
55. Ramos RT, Salles C, Gregorio PB, et al. Evaluation of the upper airway in children and adolescents with cystic fibrosis and obstructive sleep apnea syndrome. Int J Pediatr Otorhinolaryngol 2009;73(12):1780–5.
56. Maganti R, Sheth RD, Hermann BP, et al. Sleep architecture in children with idiopathic generalized epilepsy. Epilepsia 2005;46(1):104–9.
57. Orr WC. Sleep and gastroesophageal reflux: what are the risks? Am J Med 2003;115(Suppl 3A):109S–13S.
58. Halpern LM, Jolley SG, Tunell WP, et al. The mean duration of gastroesophageal reflux during sleep as an indicator of respiratory symptoms from gastroesophageal reflux in children. J Pediatr Surg 1991;26(6):686–90.
59. Bloom BJ, Owens JA, McGuinn M, et al. Sleep and its relationship to pain, dysfunction, and disease activity in juvenile rheumatoid arthritis. J Rheumatol 2002;29(1):169–73.
60. Labyak S, Stein L, Bloom B, et al. Sleep in children with juvenile rheumatoid arthritis. Sleep 2001;24(Suppl):A15.
61. Lopes MC, Guilleminault C, Rosa A, et al. Delta sleep instability in children with chronic arthritis. Braz J Med Biol Res 2008;41(10):938–43.
62. Palm L, Persson E, Elmqvist D, et al. Sleep and wakefulness in normal preadolescent children. Sleep 1989;12(4):299–308.
63. Tayag-Kier CE, Keenan GF, Scalzi LV, et al. Sleep and periodic limb movement in sleep in juvenile fibromyalgia. Pediatrics 2000;106(5):E70.
64. Roizenblatt S, Tufik S, Goldenberg J, et al. Juvenile fibromyalgia: clinical and polysomnographic aspects. J Rheumatol 1997;24(3):579–85.
65. Tripathi A, Jerrell JM, Stallworth JR. Cost-effectiveness of adenotonsillectomy in reducing obstructive sleep apnea, cerebrovascular ischemia, vaso-occlusive pain, and ACS episodes in pediatric sickle cell disease. Ann Hematol 2011; 90(2):145–50.
66. Wali YA, al Okbi H, al Abri R. A comparison of two transfusion regimens in the perioperative management of children with sickle cell disease undergoing adenotonsillectomy. Pediatr Hematol Oncol 2003;20(1):7–13.
67. Kaleyias J, Mostofi N, Grant M, et al. Severity of obstructive sleep apnea in children with sickle cell disease. J Pediatr Hematol Oncol 2008;30(9):659–65.
68. Jacob E, Miaskowski C, Savedra M, et al. Changes in sleep, food intake, and activity levels during acute painful episodes in children with sickle cell disease. J Pediatr Nurs 2006;21(1):23–34.
69. Hargrave DR, Wade A, Evans JP, et al. Nocturnal oxygen saturation and painful sickle cell crises in children. Blood 2003;101(3):846–8.
70. Daniel LC, Grant M, Kothare SV, et al. Sleep patterns in pediatric sickle cell disease. Pediatr Blood Cancer 2010;55(3):501–7.

71. Rogers VE, Lewin DS, Winnie GB, et al. Polysomnographic characteristics of a referred sample of children with sickle cell disease. J Clin Sleep Med 2010; 6(4):374–81.
72. Jacob E, Hesselgrave J, Sambuco G, et al. Variations in pain, sleep, and activity during hospitalization in children with cancer. J Pediatr Oncol Nurs 2007;24(4): 208–19.
73. Cureton-Lane RA, Fontaine DK. Sleep in the pediatric ICU: an empirical investigation. Am J Crit Care 1997;6(1):56–63.
74. Davis ID, Baron J, O'Riordan MA, et al. Sleep disturbances in pediatric dialysis patients. Pediatr Nephrol 2005;20(1):69–75.
75. Sinha R, Davis ID, Matsuda-Abedini M. Sleep disturbances in children and adolescents with non-dialysis-dependent chronic kidney disease. Arch Pediatr Adolesc Med 2009;163(9):850–5.
76. Bennett DS. Depression among children with chronic medical problems: a meta-analysis. J Pediatr Psychol 1994;19(2):149–69.
77. Lavigne JV, Faier-Routman J. Psychological adjustment to pediatric physical disorders: a meta-analytic review. J Pediatr Psychol 1992;17(2):133–57.
78. Zeltzer LK, Recklitis C, Buchbinder D, et al. Psychological status in childhood cancer survivors: a report from the Childhood Cancer Survivor Study. J Clin Oncol 2009;27(14):2396–404.
79. Becker DA, Fennell EB, Carney PR. Sleep disturbance in children with epilepsy. Epilepsy Behav 2003;4(6):651–8.
80. Oberndorfer S, Saletu-Zyhlarz G, Saletu B. Effects of selective serotonin reuptake inhibitors on objective and subjective sleep quality. Neuropsychobiology 2000;42(2):69–81.
81. Clark NA, Alexander B. Increased rate of trazodone prescribing with bupropion and selective serotonin-reuptake inhibitors versus tricyclic antidepressants. Ann Pharmacother 2000;34(9):1007–12.
82. Emslie GJ, Rush AJ, Weinberg WA, et al. Children with major depression show reduced rapid eye movement latencies. Arch Gen Psychiatry 1990;47(2):119–24.
83. Dahl RE, Ryan ND, Matty MK, et al. Sleep onset abnormalities in depressed adolescents. Biol Psychiatry 1996;39(6):400–10.
84. Goetz RR, Puig-Antich J, Dahl RE, et al. EEG sleep of young adults with major depression: a controlled study. J Affect Disord 1991;22(1–2):91–100.
85. Emslie GJ, Roffwarg HP, Rush AJ, et al. Sleep EEG findings in depressed children and adolescents. Am J Psychiatry 1987;144(5):668–70.
86. Walter TJ, Golish JA. Psychotropic and neurologic medications. In: Lee-Chiong TL, Staeia MJ, Carskadon MA, editors. Sleep medicine. Philadelphia: Hanley and Belfus; 2002. p. 587–99.
87. Sharpley AL, Cowen PJ. Effect of pharmacologic treatments on the sleep of depressed patients. Biol Psychiatry 1995;37(2):85–98.
88. Shain BN, Naylor M, Shipley JE, et al. Imipramine effects on sleep in depressed adolescents: a preliminary report. Biol Psychiatry 1990;28(5):459–62.
89. Armitage R, Emslie G, Rintelmann J. The effect of fluoxetine on sleep EEG in childhood depression: a preliminary report. Neuropsychopharmacology 1997; 17(4):241–5.
90. Buysse DJ, Schweitzer PK, Moul DE. Clinical pharmacology of other drugs used as hypnotics. In: Kryger MH, Roth T, Dement WC, editors. Principles and practice of sleep medicine. 4th edition. Philadelphia: Saunders; 2005. p. 452–67.
91. Ten Eick AP, Blumer JL, Reed MD. Safety of antihistamines in children. Drug Saf 2001;24(2):119–47.

92. Ondo WG. Restless legs syndrome. Curr Neurol Neurosci Rep 2005;5(4): 266–74.
93. Roux FJ, Kryger MH. Medication effects on sleep. Clin Chest Med 2010;31(2): 397–405.
94. Witek MW, Rojas V, Alonso C, et al. Review of benzodiazepine use in children and adolescents. Psychiatr Q 2005;76(3):283–96.
95. Vallance K, Liu W, Mandrell BN, et al. Mechanisms of dexamethasone-induced disturbed sleep and fatigue in paediatric patients receiving treatment for ALL. Eur J Cancer 2010;46(10):1848–55.
96. Moser NJ, Phillips BA, Guthrie G, et al. Effects of dexamethasone on sleep. Pharmacol Toxicol 1996;79(2):100–2.
97. Yeh CH, Chiang YC, Lin L, et al. Clinical factors associated with fatigue over time in paediatric oncology patients receiving chemotherapy. Br J Cancer 2008; 99(1):23–9.
98. Wang D, Teichtahl H. Opioids, sleep architecture and sleep-disordered breathing. Sleep Med Rev 2007;11(1):35–46.
99. Lydic R, Baghdoyan HA. Neurochemical mechanisms mediating opioid-induced REM sleep disruption. In: Lavigne GJ, Sessle BJ, Choiniere M, et al, editors. Sleep and pain. Seattle (WA): IASP Press; 2007. p. 99–122.
100. Chan J, Edman JC, Koltai PJ. Obstructive sleep apnea in children. Am Fam Physician 2004;69(5):1147–54.
101. Schechter MS. Technical report: diagnosis and management of childhood obstructive sleep apnea syndrome. Pediatrics 2002;109(4):e69.
102. Arens R, McDonough JM, Costarino AT, et al. Magnetic resonance imaging of the upper airway structure of children with obstructive sleep apnea syndrome. Am J Respir Crit Care Med 2001;164(4):698–703.
103. Marshall MJ, Bucks RS, Hogan AM, et al. Auto-adjusting positive airway pressure in children with sickle cell anemia: results of a phase I randomized controlled trial. Haematologica 2009;94(7):1006–10.
104. Regnis JA, Piper AJ, Henke KG, et al. Benefits of nocturnal nasal CPAP in patients with cystic fibrosis. Chest 1994;106(6):1717–24.
105. Gupta M, Aneja S, Kohli K. Add-on melatonin improves sleep behavior in children with epilepsy: randomized, double-blind, placebo-controlled trial. J Child Neurol 2005;20(2):112–5.
106. Phillips L, Appleton RE. Systematic review of melatonin treatment in children with neurodevelopmental disabilities and sleep impairment. Dev Med Child Neurol 2004;46(11):771–5.
107. Palm L, Blennow G, Wetterberg L. Long-term melatonin treatment in blind children and young adults with circadian sleep-wake disturbances. Dev Med Child Neurol 1997;39(5):319–25.
108. Mindell JA, Emslie G, Blumer J, et al. Pharmacologic management of insomnia in children and adolescents: consensus statement. Pediatrics 2006;117(6): e1223–32.
109. Perlis ML, Junquist C, Smith MT, et al. Cognitive behavioral treatment of insomnia. New York: Springer; 2005.
110. Degotardi PJ, Klass ES, Rosenberg BS, et al. Development and evaluation of a cognitive-behavioral intervention for juvenile fibromyalgia. J Pediatr Psychol 2006;31(7):714–23.

Sleep and Obesity in Children and Adolescents

Chantelle N. Hart, PhD[a,b,]*, Alyssa Cairns, PhD[a,b],
Elissa Jelalian, PhD[a,b]

KEYWORDS

- Sleep • Obesity • Adiposity • Eating behaviors
- Activity behaviors

Pediatric obesity is considered an epidemic, with 32% of US children and adolescents aged 2 to 19 years considered overweight or obese in 2007 to 2008.[1] The medical and psychosocial risks associated with being overweight and obese as a child or adolescent have been well documented. Multiple studies have demonstrated the increased risk for type 2 diabetes and several cardiovascular disease risks, including elevations in cholesterol, diastolic and systolic blood pressure, fasting insulin levels, and triglycerides.[2–4] Children and adolescents who are overweight and obese report lower health-related quality of life compared with their normal-weight peers, and may be at increased risk of poorer self-esteem, greater body dissatisfaction, and increased peer teasing.[5,6] The importance of addressing this epidemic is underscored by several national policy efforts and by the proposed goals for Healthy People 2020.[7]

Given the precipitous rise in pediatric obesity and its associated risks, increasing attention has been paid to efforts to enhance prevention and treatment approaches. Current prevention approaches have demonstrated variable impact on weight outcomes[8] with some efficacy shown for school-based approaches that combine diet and physical activity.[9] Several intervention approaches for children and adolescents who are overweight and obese have demonstrated efficacy, including those that combine dietary and physical activity prescriptions with the use of effective

This work was supported in part by grants 1-09-JF-22 from the American Diabetes Association, U01 CA150387 from the National Institutes of Health, and T32 HL076134 from the National Institutes of Health.
The authors have nothing to disclose.
[a] Department of Psychiatry & Human Behavior, The Warren Alpert Medical School of Brown University, Providence, RI, USA
[b] Weight Control & Diabetes Research Center, The Miriam Hospital, 196 Richmond Street, Providence, RI 02903, USA
* Corresponding author. Weight Control & Diabetes Research Center, The Miriam Hospital, 196 Richmond Street, Providence, RI 02903.
E-mail address: Chantelle_Hart@brown.edu

behavioral strategies.[10] In adolescents, both use of weight-loss medication[10] and surgical approaches[11] show some promise. However, each of these approaches has limitations and, despite their effectiveness, often do not help children and adolescents achieve nonobese status. Thus, it is imperative to identify novel targets to enhance current treatment approaches.

Several factors suggest that enhancing children's sleep may be an effective strategy for preventing and treating pediatric obesity. Over the past 20 to 30 years, as rates of pediatric obesity have climbed, children's nocturnal sleep duration has declined.[12,13] Data from the 2004 National Sleep Foundation's Sleep in America poll show that the mean sleep length for school-aged children (first to fifth grade) is 9.4 hours per night.[14] These data are in contrast to recommendations by sleep experts that children in this age group should obtain 10 to 11 hours per night.[15,16] Thus, children may not be achieving sufficient sleep length.

Experimental studies with adults have documented physiologic and behavioral changes in response to sleep deprivation, which, if chronic, may promote weight gain. The secretion of growth hormone, prolactin, cortisol, thyrotropin, and insulin, are influenced by sleep.[17] For example, studies suggest that sleep restriction leads to decreased circulating leptin[18,19] and increased ghrelin,[20] both of which are associated with increased hunger, appetite, motivation to eat, and food intake.[21–23] Further, more recent experimental studies with adults have demonstrated increases in caloric intake from both snack foods[24] and from main meals[25] when sleep is restricted, suggesting that less sleep may increase the risk of obesity via neuroendocrine changes that increase food intake. Finally, although less is known in this regard, it is hypothesized that sleep deprivation may also lead to changes in physical and sedentary activities, which could promote weight gain. Limited support for this hypothesis comes from studies with adults that have demonstrated subsequent decreases in activity level following sleep deprivation.[26,27]

To the authors' knowledge, no experimental studies involving the manipulation of sleep in children and weight-related outcomes have been reported (although there are ongoing trials). However, there are considerable epidemiologic data with children and adolescents examining the association between sleep duration (typically nocturnal sleep) and weight status. Findings from both cross-sectional and prospective studies, although limited by their inability to demonstrate causation (ie, that less sleep at night leads to increased weight status), are important for helping to shape our understanding of the potential role that sleep may play in the current obesity epidemic. Prospective studies, in particular, help to establish temporal relationships between sleep and pediatric obesity. The purpose of this review is to provide a comprehensive update of epidemiologic studies that have assessed the association between sleep and obesity risk. Although obstructive sleep apnea is also associated with obesity risk, it is beyond the scope of this review. The reader is referred to Ievers-Landis and Redline[28] as well as the article by Whitmans and Young in this special issue for a more comprehensive review. To build upon previous reviews, this review includes information on anthropometric indices (ie, waist circumference, percent body fat) other than body mass index (BMI) and findings regarding sleep timing and quality (as opposed to only focusing on sleep duration), and reviews findings regarding possible mediators of the sleep-weight relationship.

METHODS

A systematic search for publications was performed using the PubMed database that included published studies through July 2010. Combinations of key words specific to sleep (eg, sleep and sleeping), weight status (eg, BMI, overweight, obesity, adiposity, weight, fatness, food diet, and energy expenditure), and childhood and adolescence (eg, child, children, adolescent, adolescence) were used. In addition, reference lists of relevant articles and previously conducted relevant review articles/meta-analyses were reviewed to identify additional studies. Only studies that focused on children and adolescents (ie, birth to 18 years of age) and represented original empirical work (ie, reviews and editorials were excluded) were included in the present review. Questions regarding inclusion of studies were decided by consensus. This process resulted in the inclusion of 38 studies (with 2 additional duplicates) in the present review.

RESULTS
Sleep Duration and Obesity Risk

Table 1 presents findings from studies that assessed the association between sleep duration and obesity risk in children and adolescents.[29–58] It represents 30 studies from 16 countries. For ease of comparison, studies presented in **Table 1** are those in which main findings are presented as odds ratios. Two groups published subsequent studies using the same data set, but controlling for additional confounding variables. These subsequent studies were consistent with initial findings and are referenced as footnotes to **Table 1**. The majority of studies present cross-sectional findings (N = 24), with 6 studies assessing the association between sleep duration and weight status prospectively. As can be seen in the table, the majority of studies assessed the construct of sleep duration exclusively through parent or self-report (N = 28)[29–32,34–40,42–58] with 2 additional studies assessing sleep length via actigraphy.[33,41] In contrast, the majority of studies (N = 27) used measured height and weight to calculate body mass index in children with only 2 studies using parent or self-report,[38,46] and one additional study in which it was unclear whether caretaker report or measured height and weight were obtained.[56]

As can be seen in **Table 1**, for cross-sectional studies, the reference values for sleep length used to determine obesity risk varied from less than 7 hours of sleep per night to more than or equal to 12 hours per night. Despite these differences in how referents were defined, all studies demonstrated negative associations between sleep duration and obesity risk. It is important to note that most studies found significant results even after controlling for potential confounding variables (eg, parental BMI, birth weight, television viewing; see **Table 1** for specific confounders controlled for in each study). However, it is also important to note that not every category of sleep was associated with increased risk for obesity. For example, Sekine and colleagues[30] found that in comparison to children who slept 11 hours or more each night, there was no increased risk for obesity for children sleeping less than 9 hours or 10 to 11 hours per night, but that there was an increased risk for obesity for children sleeping 9 to 10 hours per night. Furthermore, when associations were examined separately in boys and girls, some studies found significant results for one gender but not the other.[37,47,49,50]

In addition to those studies presented in **Table 1**, 6 additional studies were conducted, but did not present findings in terms of odds ratios.[59–64] All 6 studies found consistent results with less sleep being associated with an increased risk for obesity. However, one study only assessed this association in adolescent girls[63] and a second study only found significant results in girls.[61]

Six prospective studies were also identified (see **Table 1**).[52–57] Findings are consistent with cross-sectional studies. For example, Snell and colleagues[53] found that for every additional hour of sleep obtained at time 1 (when children were 3–12 years of

Table 1
Findings of studies that assessed the association between sleep duration and obesity risk in children and adolescents (N = 30)

Study Country	Sample Characteristics	Sleep Measure and Reference Value	Measure of BMI Status[a]	Confounders Controlled	Main Findings
Cross-Sectional Studies					
Locard et al,[29] 1992 France	5 y old (N = 1031)	Caretaker-report Referent ≥11 h	Measured height and weight; weight-for-height and sex Zscore >2 = OB	—	OB: <11 h: OR = 1.4 (1.0–2.0)
Sekine et al,[30] 2002[b] Japan	2.5–4.3 y (N = 8941)	Caretaker-report (24-h sleep) Referent ≥11 h	Measured height and weight; OB: age/sex BMI cut-off points by Cole et al	Age, gender, parental OB, and outdoor playing time	OB: <9 h: N/S 9–10 h: ORadj = 1.34 (1.05–1.72) 10–11 h: N/S
Sekine et al,[31] 2002[b] Japan	6–7 y (N = 8274)	Caretaker-report (24-h sleep) Referent ≥10 h	Measured height and weight; OB: age/sex BMI cut-off points by Cole et al	Age, sex, parental OB, PA, TV watching, frequency of breakfast, and frequency of snack	OB: 9–10 h: ORadj = 1.49 (1.08–2.14) 8–9 h: 1.89 (1.34–2.73) <8 h: 2.87 (1.61–5.05)
Von Kries et al,[32] 2002 Germany	5.0–6.99 y (N = 6645)	Caretaker-report (WD sleep) Referent ≤10 h	Measured height and weight; OW: age/sex BMI >90th centile OB >97th centile based on local norms	Parent education, parent BMI, birth weight, first year weight gain, TV/video games, snacks while watching TV	OW: 10.5–11.0 h: ORadj = 0.77 (0.59 – 0.99) ≥11 h: 0.54 (0.40–0.73) OB: 10.5–11.0 h: ORadj = 0.53 (0.35 –0.80) ≥11 h: 0.45 (0.28–0.75)
Gupta et al,[33] 2002 USA	11–16 y old (N = 383)	Actigraphy (1 night) Referent: sleep duration as continuous	Measured height and weight; BMI >85th percentile (CDC)	—	For every additional h of sleep time, odds of OB decreased by 80%: OR = 0.20 (95th CI = 0.11)

Study	Age (N)	Sleep measure	Outcome measure	Adjustment	Results
Hui et al,[58] 2003 China	6–7 y old (N = 343)	Caretaker-reported Referent: <9 h	Measured height and weight; BMI ≥92nd centile, using Hong Kong cross-sectional growth survey as reference	Paternal and maternal obesity	OW: 9–11 h: ORadj = 0.54 (0.30–0.97) ≥11 h = 0.31 (0.11–0.87)
Padez et al,[34] 2005[d] Portugal	7.0–9.5 y (N = 4511)	Caretaker-report Referent: 8 h	Measured height and weight; age/sex BMI cut-off points by Cole et al	Sex and age	OW: 9–10 h: ORadj = 0.46 (0.40–0.51) ≥11 h: 0.44 (0.38–0.49) OB: 9–10 h: ORadj = 0.44 (0.40–0.47) ≥11 h: 0.39 (0.35–0.42)
Chen et al,[35] 2006 Taiwan	13–18 y (N = 656)	Self-report of 6–8 h of sleep (WD sleep) Referent ≥4 nights/wk	Measured height and weight; OW: BMI ≥85th percentile for age/sex (DOH)	—	OW: <4 nights/wk: OR = 1.74 (1.3–2.4)
Chaput et al,[36] 2006 Canada	5–10 y (N = 422)	Caretaker-report (WD sleep) Referent: 12–13 h	Measured height and weight; OW/OB: age/sex BMI cut-off points by Cole et al	Age, sex, parental OB, parent education, income, single parent, breakfast, media use, sport activities, and whether breastfed	10.5–11.5 h: ORadj = 1.42 (1.09 –1.98) 8–10 h: 3.45 (2.61–4.67)
Eisenmann et al,[37] 2006[c] Australia	7–15 y (N = 6324)	Self-report Referent ≥10 h	Measured height and weight; OW/OB: age/sex BMI cut-off points by Cole et al	Age	OW/OB: boys only: 9–10 h: ORadj = 1.61 (1.19–2.17) 8–9 h: 1.83 (1.30–2.58) ≤8 h: 3.06 (2.11–4.46)

(continued on next page)

Table 1
(continued)

Study Country	Sample Characteristics	Sleep Measure and Reference Value	Measure of BMI Status[a]	Confounders Controlled	Main Findings
Seicean et al,[38] 2007 USA	15.6 ± 1.23 y (N = 509)	Self-reported (WD sleep) Referent >8 h	Self-reported height and weight (30% weighed themselves using a scale on scene); OW: age/sex ZBMI >85th percentile; OB>95th percentile (CDC)	Gender, age, irregular eating, health status, and caffeine intake	OW: <5 h: ORadj = 7.65 (1.87–31.30) 5–6: N/S 6–7 h: 2.55 (1.02–6.38) 7–8: N/S
Kuriyan et al,[39] 2007 India	6 –16 y (N = 598)	Caretaker-report (younger) or self-report (older) Referent >9.5 h	Measured height and weight; OW: age/sex BMI cut-off points by Cole et al	Age, gender, living location, and SES	OW: ≦8 h: ORadj = 6.7 (1.5–30.2)
Knutson et al,[40] 2007 USA	10 –19 y (N = 1546)	A) Self-report B) Self-report using time diaries Referents: A) 9.2–19.0 h B) 10.08–16.17 h	Measured height and weight; OW: BMI ≥95th percentile for age and gender (CDC)	Race, age, gender, family income, education, TV viewing, physical activity, and media use	OW: A) 7–8 h: ORadj = 1.85: (1.01–3.38) 8.1–9.0 h: 1.93 (1.10–3.37) B) All sleep categories NS.
Nixon et al,[41] 2008 New Zealand	7.3 y (N = 519)	Actigraphy (1 night) Referent ≥9 h	Measured height and weight; OW/OB: age/sex BMI cut-off points by Cole et al	Maternal BMI, maternal age, marital status, gender, h of TV, and sedentary activity	OW/OB: <9 h: ORadj = 3.32 (1.40–7.87)
Ievers-Landis et al,[42] 2008 USA	8 –11 y (N = 819)	A) Caretaker-report of sleep duration B) Child report using 7-d sleep diary Referent: duration as continuous	Measured height and weight (PC); OB: age/sex BMI ≥95th percentile (CDC)	Age, gender, preterm status, income psychosocial functioning, and parental stress	OB: A) ORadj = 1.41 (1.12–1.76) Odd of being OB increase by 41% with every 1 h of sleep decline B) ORadj = 1.45 (1.09–1.94) Odds of being OB increase by 45% with every 1 h of sleep decline

Study	Age (N)	Sleep measure	Anthropometry	Covariates	Results
Liu et al,[43] 2008 USA	7–17 y (N = 335)	Self-reported 7-d sleep diary Referent: duration as continuous	Measured height and weight; at risk: age/sex ZBMI 85th–95th percentile; OW ZBMI ≥95th percentile (CDC)	Age, sex, SES, ethnicity, puberty, and psychiatric diagnosis	OW: Reduced sleep (1 h less of): ORadj = 2.12 (1.05–4.28)
Wells et al,[44] 2008 Brazil	10–12 y (N = 4452)	Self-report (WD sleep) Referent <9 h	Measured height & weight; IOTF guidelines used to define OW & OB	Sex, birth weight & length, maternal smoking and alcohol consumption during pregnancy, maternal pre-pregnancy BMI, SES, PA, systolic & diastolic BP, TV h	OB: ORadj = 9–10 N/S >10 h: N/S Odds of being OB decreased by 14% with every additional h of sleep
Bawazeer et al,[45] 2009 Saudi Arabia	10–19 y (N = 5877)	Caretaker-report Referent >7 h	Measured height, weight, waist circumference & hip circumference; OB defined as >95th percentile BMI for age & gender	—	OB: boys ≤7 h: OR = 1.28 (1.09–1.50) girls ≤7 h: 1.38 (1.02–1.89)
Wing et al,[46] 2009 China	5–15 y (N = 5159)	Caretaker-report Referent >10 h	Parent report of height & weight converted to ZBMI (OW ZBMI between 85th and 95th percentile; OB ZBMI >95th percentile per CDC guidelines)	Age, gender, TV viewing, time to do homework, parent education, & eating 1 h before going to bed	OW/OB: Weekdays: ≤ 8h: ORadj = 1.74 (1.23–2.45) 8.01–9 h: 1.51 (1.13–2.03) 9.01–10 h: 1.30 (0.97–1.76) Weekends: ≤8 h: ORadj = 1.80 (1.05–3.09) 8.01–9 h: 1.66 (1.30–2.13) 9.01–10 h: 1.36 (1.12–1.66)

(continued on next page)

Table 1
(continued)

Study Country	Sample Characteristics	Sleep Measure and Reference Value	Measure of BMI Status[a]	Confounders Controlled	Main Findings
Hitze et al,[47] 2009 Germany	6–19 y (N = 414)	Caretaker-report (younger) and self-report (older) (WD sleep) Referent: Long sleep (9–10 h for younger; 8–9 h for older)	Measured height & weight; German references used to define OW & OB	Parent BMI, birth weight, change in weight birth–2 y, duration of breastfeeding	OB: girls only: Short sleep: ORadj = 5.5 (1.3–23.5)
Jiang et al,[48] 2009 China	3–4 y (N = 1311)	Caretaker-report Referent ≥11 h	Measured height & weight; Country norms used to define obesity (>95th percentile)	Age, sex, appetite, birth weight, maternal age at delivery, mother & father education, household income, & geographic location	OB: <9 h: ORadj = 4.76 (1.28–17.69) 9 h: 3.42 (1.12–10.46) 9.5 h = N/S 10.0 h = N/S 10.5 h = N/S
Ozturk et al,[49] 2009 Turkey	6–17 y (N = 5358)	Caretaker-report Referent ≥10 h	Measured height & weight; IOTF guidelines used to define OW & OB	—	OW/OB: boys only: ≤8h: OR = 2.06 (1.31–3.24) 8.1–8.9 h: 1.74 (1.10–2.75) 9.0–9.9 h: 1.86 (1.17–2.97)
Sun et al,[50] 2009[b] Japan	12–13 y (N = 5753)	Self-report Referent 8–9 h	Measured height & weight; IOTF guidelines used to define OW & OB	Age, paternal overweight, maternal overweight, breakfast frequency, snacking frequency, nighttime snacking, eating speed, eating volume, physical activity, TV watching, video game playing	OW: girls only: <7h: ORadj = 1.81 (1.21–2.72) 7–8 h: 1.37 (1.00–1.88) ≥9 h = NS

Study	Age (N)	Sleep measure	BMI measure	Adjustments	Results
Anderson & Whitaker,[51] 2010 USA	~4 y (N = 8750)	Caretaker-report Referent <10.5 h	Measured height & weight; CDC guidelines used to define OB (≥95th percentile for age & gender)	Eating dinner as a family, screen viewing time, child age, gender, race/ethnic group, household income-to-poverty ratio, single-parent household, maternal education, maternal BMI, & maternal age	OB: <10.5 h: ORadj = 0.86 (0.71–1.03)
Longitudinal Studies					
Reilly et al,[52] 2005 UK	30 mo –7 y (N = 7758)	Caretaker-report (nocturnal sleep duration at 30 mo) Referent >12 h	Measured height and weight at 7 y; OB = BMI ≥95th centile using UK reference data	Maternal education, child's sex, and energy intake at 3 y	OB: <10.5 h: ORadj = 1.45 (1.10–1.89) 10.5–10.9 h 1.35 (1.02 –1.79) 11–11.9h: N/S
Snell et al,[53] 2007 USA	3 –18 y (time 1: 3–12 y; time 2: 8–18 y; N = 1441)	Caretaker-report (younger) or self-report (older)	Measured height at all time points, caretaker-reported weight at T1; OW/OB: age/sex BMI cut-off points by Cole et al	Race, age, sex, BMI at T1, parent income, and parent education	Sleeping >11 h relative to 9.0–9.9 h associated with a 17.1% reduction in OW Every additional h at T1 decreased BMI at T2 by 0.75 kg/m
Lumeng et al,[54] 2007 USA	9 y to ~12 y (N = 785)	Caretaker-report (24-h sleep) Referent: duration as a continuous variable	Measured height and weight; OW: BMI ≥95th percentile for age and gender (NCHS/CDC guidelines)	Gender, race, maternal education, ZBMI in third grade, and change in sleep duration	OW: Longitudinal: ORadj = 0.60 (0.36–0.99) For every additional h of sleep at 9 y child 40% less likely to be OW at 12 y Cross-sectional: ORadj = 0.80 (0.65–0.98) For every additional h of sleep in sixth grade, child ~20% less likely to be OW

(continued on next page)

Table 1
(continued)

Study Country	Sample Characteristics	Sleep Measure and Reference Value	Measure of BMI Status[a]	Confounders Controlled	Main Findings
Landhuis et al,[55] 2008 New Zealand	5–32 y (N = 780)	Caretaker-report (averaged over ages 5,7, 9, and 11 y) Referent: duration as a continuous variable	Measured height and weight at 32 y; BMI calculated	Sex, SES, parent BMI, TV, parental control, smoking as an adult, and adult PA	OB: ORadj = 0.65 (0.43–0.97) For every additional h of sleep in childhood, 35% less likely to be OB at 32
Touchette et al,[56] 2008 Canada	2.5–6.0 y (N = 1138)	Caretaker-report (averaged over 2.5, 3.5, 4.0, 5.0, and 6.0 y) Referent: 11-h persistent sleep duration	BMI calculated at 2.5 & 6.0 y; IOTF guidelines used to define OW and OB.	Perinatal variables (eg, birth weight, parent education), child weight & nap duration at 2.5 y; lifestyle variables (eg, child overeating, snacking, snoring, TV, PA)	OW/OB: Short persistent sleepers (<10 h/night): ORadj = 2.9 (1.0–8.5) Short increasing & 10-h persistent = NS.
Taveras et al,[57] 2008 USA	6 mo–3 y (N = 915)	Caretaker-reported (24-h sleep averaged over the 6-mo, 1-y, and 2-y assessment) Referent ≥12 h/d	Measured height and weight; OW: age/sex BMI ≥95th percentile; (NCHS/CDC guidelines)	Maternal education, income, prepregnancy BMI, marital status, prenatal smoking, breastfeeding duration, child's race/ethnicity, birth weight, 6-mo weight for length, average TV viewing, and daily active play	OW: ORadj = 2.04 (1.07–3.91)

Abbreviations: CDC, US Centers for Disease Control; DOH, US Department of Heath; IOTF, The International Obesity Task Force; NCHS, National Center for Health Statistics; OW, overweight; OB, obese; OR, odds ratio (OR, raw; ORadj, adjusted for confounders); PA, physical activity; PC, personal communication; SES, socioeconomic status; WD, weekday; ZBMI, body mass index z-score for sex and age.

[a] OR (confidence interval) reflects comparison to sleep referent for that study.

[b] Represents studies sampled from the Toyama Birth Cohort.

[c] Biggs and Dollman (2007) supported these findings on the same dataset controlling for PA and diet.

[d] Padez et al (2009) presented similar findings on the sample controlling for parent education, parent obesity, PA, and TV watching.

age), caretaker-reported BMI decreased by 0.75 kg/m^2 at time 2 (when children were 8–18 years old). Similarly, Touchette and colleagues[56] found that between 2.5 years and 6 years of age, children who consistently obtained short sleep were 2.9 times more likely to be overweight or obese than children who consistently slept 11 hours or more each night even after controlling for potential confounding factors. Consistent with these findings, but over a much longer follow-up, Landhuis and colleagues[55] found that for every additional hour of sleep obtained during childhood (averaged across 5–11 years), individuals had a 35% reduced risk of obesity at 32 years of age.

Sleep Duration and Other Anthropometric Indices

In addition to risk for overweight and obesity, more recent studies assessed the association between sleep duration and other indices of body composition. A total of 11 studies were identified, 3 of which used 2 or more measures to assess body fat.[47,49,61] Five studies used skinfold thickness,[34,49,57,62,65] 4 used waist circumference,[37,47,49,61] and 3 used bioelectrical impedance analysis (BIA).[32,41,66] Two additional studies used another measure, such as dual x-ray absorptiometry[61] and air displacement plethysmography.[47] Regardless of measure, however, an increase in sleep duration was consistently found to be associated with lower body fat.

For example, Nixon and colleagues[41] found that compared with 7-year-old children sleeping 9 hours or more per night (as measured by actigraphy), children sleeping less than 9 hours per night had an increase of 3.34% body fat (as measured by BIA). Similarly, von Kries and colleagues[32] found that when compared with children aged 5 to 6 years sleeping less than 10 hours per night, children sleeping 11.5 hours or more per night had a decreased risk for high body fat (defined as excessive fat mass > the 90th percentile for age and gender using BIA).

It should be noted that 3 studies found that significant findings varied across gender. In a sample of twins aged 10 to 20 years, Yu and colleagues[61] found that shortened sleep length (<8 hours per night) was negatively associated with total body fat and truncal fat, and positively associated with percent lean body mass as measured by DEXA in girls only. Similarly, although Hitze and colleagues[47] found that short sleep was associated with increased fat free mass in both genders (using air displacement plethysmography), they only found differences in percent body fat in girls.

Findings regarding waist circumference and nocturnal sleep length were less consistent than those previously mentioned.[37,47,49,61] For example, although Hitze and colleagues[47] found significant findings across genders in linear analyses, when comparing short versus long sleepers, only short-sleeping girls had significantly larger waist circumferences. Yu and colleagues[61] also found a significant association between sleep duration and waist circumference in girls only. In contrast, Eisenmann and colleagues[37] found that greater sleep duration was associated with decreased waist circumference in boys aged 7 to 16 years, but no consistent relationship was found in girls.

Additional Sleep Indices and Obesity Risk

In addition to the assessment of sleep duration, several studies assessed other sleep measures to determine whether additional sleep parameters may be associated with obesity risk. The primary variable of interest was the timing of sleep (ie, bedtime and rise time),[30,31,53,63,64] which was typically assessed with a single-item question (eg, "over the past week, what was your typical bedtime?"). Together, these studies suggest that later bedtimes are associated with increased risk for obesity.[31,53,63,64] However, no association between rise time and obesity risk was found in these studies.[31,53] Of note, one study with *preschool-aged* children (3 years) found that early rise time (ie, ≤7:00 AM) was associated with an increased obesity risk, but that later bedtime was not.[30]

In addition to bedtime and rise time, 3 additional studies assessed the association between irregular or problematic sleep and obesity risk. In the first study, parent report of irregular sleep habits at 2 to 4 years of age was independently associated with obesity risk in young adulthood (ie, at 21 years of age).[67] Furthermore, Wing and colleagues[46] attempted to assess how catching up on sleep on weekends and holidays may influence children's risk for obesity. The findings suggested that compared with children who slept greater than 10 hours per night, children who persistently slept 8 hours or less on weekdays and weekends or on weekdays and during holidays, were at the greatest risk for obesity (odds ratio adjusted for confounders [OR adj] = 2.59 [1.22–5.48] and 2.32 [1.00–5.53], respectively). In contrast to findings from these studies, after adjusting for potential confounding variables, no association was found between parent-reported sleep problems (using a modified version of the Children's Sleep Habits Questionnaire) in the third or sixth grades and obesity risk in the sixth grade.[54]

Finally, 2 studies assessed the association between stages of sleep and obesity risk. In the first study (which is also presented in part in see **Table 1**), Liu and colleagues[43] found that reduced rapid eye movement (REM) sleep and reduced REM density were each associated with increased obesity risk in children aged 7 to 17 years. In a second study of 52 adolescents aged 12 to 18 years who presented to a sleep clinic, greater stage 1 sleep was found for adolescents who were obese compared with those who were normal weight, and greater slow wave sleep was also found in adolescents who were categorized as overweight compared with those who were obese.[68]

Potential Mediators of the Sleep-Weight Association

Several studies have moved beyond documenting sleep-weight associations to examining variables (eg, eating) that may mediate the relationship between sleep and obesity risk. For example, Landis and colleagues[69] found that food cravings were higher in those with more daytime/less nocturnal sleep. Touchette and colleagues[56] found that parent report of child overeating (at 6 years of age) might play a small role in the association between short sleep and BMI. When removed from the statistical model to predict BMI, there was a small increase in the odds for children classified as *short persistent sleepers* to be obese (see **Table 1**). Finally, Westerlund and colleagues[70] found that shorter sleep was associated with greater consumption of energy-dense foods, such as pizza, pasta, and refined sugars. This relationship was stronger in boys and on weekdays. Additional gender differences included greater problems with waking in the morning being associated with increased intake of energy-dense foods in boys, and longer weekday sleep duration being associated with greater consumption of nutrient-dense foods (ie, fruits and vegetables) in girls.

DISCUSSION

Our understanding of the role of sleep duration in the current pediatric obesity epidemic is rapidly unfolding. Pediatric studies identified and included in the present review suggest that children who sleep less are at increased risk for being or becoming overweight/obese. This significant relationship was found in both cross-sectional and prospective studies, and persisted in most studies even after controlling for potential confounders, such as parental BMI, birth weight, and television viewing. Findings from the present review are consistent with conclusions drawn from other systematic reviews and meta-analyses,[71–76] including 2 meta-analyses that demonstrated that children with shortened sleep were at a 56% to 89% increased risk for obesity.[72,75] Findings also build upon previous reviews by demonstrating the potential influence of sleep length on other measures of adiposity, such as waist circumference and percent body fat. The consistency in findings across anthropometric measures increases confidence in findings and suggests that increased BMI associated with less sleep is likely caused by increased deposits of adipose tissue.[62]

Also building upon previous work, studies included in the present review examined the association between additional sleep indices (other than sleep duration) and weight-related outcomes. Studies with school-aged children and adolescents consistently found that later bedtimes were associated with increased obesity risk; whereas, rise times were unrelated.[31,53,63,64] It is possible that later bedtimes are simply a proxy for shorter sleep duration, which would account for their significant association with obesity risk. However, it is also possible that circadian phase-delay may play a role in establishing risk for overweight/obesity, particularly given research suggesting the importance of circadian clocks in metabolism and obesity.[77]

Beyond later bedtimes, it is unclear what other sleep indices may confer obesity risk or protection. Although findings from Wing and colleagues[46] regarding the protective benefit of catching up on sleep on weekends and holidays are interesting, it is unclear how these findings would translate into clinical practice recommendations given the importance of consistent sleep-wake habits for the promotion of healthy sleep in children. Future studies are needed to further assess the role of catching up on sleep as well as the potential influence of other irregular/problematic sleep habits, including measures of sleep quality and sleep staging, on obesity risk.

An additional focus of more recent studies is attempting to better understand the potential pathways through which sleep affects BMI. These studies have focused on eating behaviors and suggest that they may be influenced by sleep duration.[56,69,70] However, findings are largely limited by reliance on self-report measures, inconsistencies in findings both across and within studies, and lack of experimental manipulation of sleep duration. To strengthen confidence in the association between sleep and obesity risk via eating pathways, experimental or intervention research studies need to be conducted with children.

Furthermore, although change in food intake may represent one pathway through which sleep duration influences obesity risk, several additional pathways are possible. As shown in **Fig. 1**, several factors, including daytime sleepiness/fatigue and subsequent changes in activity level as well as metabolic changes, may play an important role in the sleep-weight relationship. For example, cross-sectional research demonstrate that sleep is negatively impacted by engagement in sedentary activities, such as television viewing,[78–80] and positively associated with engagement in exercise.[35] However, it remains unclear whether shortened sleep results in subsequent changes in children's activity choices. Furthermore, experimental studies with adults have demonstrated physiologic changes as a result of shortened sleep, which may promote weight gain. These changes include changes in growth hormone, prolactin, cortisol, thyrotropin, and insulin,[17] as well as leptin[18,19] and ghrelin[20] both of which are associated with increased hunger, appetite, motivation to eat, and food intake.[21–23] Studies with children in this regard are sparse, and to the authors' knowledge no experimental studies with children have been published. However, extant correlational research with children demonstrates an association between sleep and metabolic abnormalities, including lower-fasting C-peptide[81]; hyperglycemia[82]; and higher-fasting insulin,

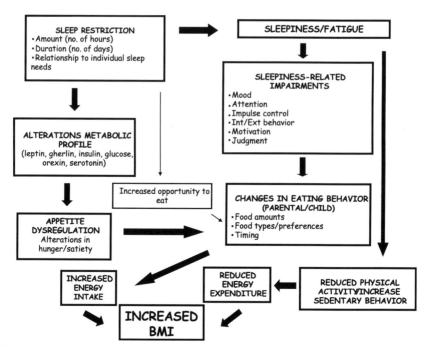

Fig. 1. Hypothesized pathways through which sleep duration may increase obesity risk. (*Courtesy of* Judith Owens, MD.)

peak insulin, and insulin resistance.[83] Taken together, study findings suggest the need to further explore the multiple pathways through which sleep duration influences obesity risk.

Despite the consistency in findings, several limitations of studies should be noted. First, the reviewed studies were predominantly cross-sectional in nature. Thus, the potential causal influence of sleep duration on obesity risk cannot be established. Although 6 prospective studies were identified and aid in our understanding of the temporal relationship between sleep length and obesity risk, they cannot demonstrate that less sleep causes increases in weight status, and hence obesity. As previously noted, future experimental research will need to be conducted before being able to determine causal links. Second, the measurement of sleep length in reviewed studies was primarily based on self-report or parent report, which calls into question reliability and validity of measures, particularly when single-item measures were used. Only 3 studies evaluated sleep length with more objective measures, such as actigraphy and polysomnography (and were often limited by having only 1 day of measurement). Third, studies often used different reference values for sleep length in analyses, which makes comparisons across studies challenging. Finally, findings across studies were not always consistent across sleep categories or across gender. Inconsistencies across sleep categories may suggest that the effect of sleep on obesity risk may be small in size. However, findings regarding inconsistencies across gender are less clear because some studies found significant results in boys rather than girls and others found contrary results. Some of these gender differences may be caused by an interaction of child gender with child age, ethnicity or race, and pubertal status. Systematic assessment of how demographic factors may interact with sleep length in conferring obesity risk could help to explain these discrepant findings.

Taken together, study findings suggest that sleep length is associated with obesity risk. Findings also point toward changes in eating pathways that may lead to increased accumulation of adipose tissue as a potential mediator of this association. However, more research is needed to establish shortened sleep duration as a true risk factor that can be targeted in pediatric weight-control interventions. Although it may not yet be prudent to prescribe changes in sleep to prevent obesity at a population level, there is ample, accumulated data that strongly argues for systematically evaluating the potential role that enhancing sleep may have in combating the current obesity epidemic. Evidence also suggests several points of intervention for providers when working with children who are overweight and obese, which are subsequently highlighted.

First, given the fact that multiple studies have shown that shortened sleep length is associated with increased BMI, assessment of sleep duration in children who are overweight and obese is important.[71] Simple questions regarding obese children's sleep habits on weekdays and weekends could identify several children who could benefit from recommendations to obtain a good night's sleep. Given the well-documented deleterious effects of sleep on children's mood and daytime functioning, such a minimal intervention could promote several benefits across multiple domains. Furthermore, given the sensitive nature of addressing weight-related concerns with families, discussion of sleep may provide a nice point of entry to begin to discuss the importance of healthy lifestyles, including eating and activity behaviors, for promoting optimal health in childhood and beyond. In addition to assessment of sleep duration, providers should also consider concurrent treatment of sleep and weight problems.[71] At the heart of treatments for both shortened sleep duration and overweight/obesity are the use of effective behavioral strategies and the importance of targeting key behaviors, such as television viewing.

It is clear from recent reviews, including the present one, that we are only beginning to understand the role of sleep in our current obesity epidemic. Consistency in study findings suggest that it is now time to begin to assess for sleep disturbances in children who are overweight and obese, to consider targeting sleep and obesity as comorbid conditions, and to begin to explore through experimental studies how changes in sleep length may influence obesity risk. Sleep duration represents an intriguing and potentially effective tool for promoting healthier weight in children and adolescents. It is time to move beyond epidemiologic studies to further our understanding regarding how effective an approach it will be.

REFERENCES

1. Ogden CL, Carroll MD, Curtin LR, et al. Prevalence of high body mass index in US children and adolescents, 2007–2008. JAMA 2010;303:242.
2. Daniels SR. The consequences of childhood overweight and obesity. Future Child 2006;16:47.
3. Freedman DS, Dietz WH, Srinivasan SR, et al. The relation of overweight to cardiovascular risk factors among children and adolescents: the Bogalusa Heart Study. Pediatrics 1999;103:1175.
4. Ludwig DS, Ebbeling CB. Type 2 diabetes mellitus in children: primary care and public health considerations. JAMA 2001;286:1427.
5. Wardle J, Cooke L. The impact of obesity on psychological well-being. Best Pract Res Clin Endocrinol Metab 2005;19:421.
6. Jelalian E, Hart CN. Pediatric obesity. In: Roberts MC, Steele RG, editors. Handbook of pediatric psychology. 4th edition. New York: Guilford Press; 2009. p. 446–63.

7. US Dept of Health and Human Services. Nutrition and Weight Status. Available at: http://www.healthypeople.gov/2020/topicsobjectives2020/overview.aspx?topicid=29. Accessed March 2, 2011.

8. Summerbell CD, Waters E, Edmunds LD, et al. Interventions for preventing obesity in children. Cochrane Database Syst Rev 2005;3:CD001871.

9. Brown T, Summerbell C. Systematic review of school-based interventions that focus on changing dietary intake and physical activity levels to prevent childhood obesity: an update to the obesity guidance produced by the National Institute for Health and Clinical Excellence. Obes Rev 2009;10:110.

10. Oude Luttikhuis H, Baur L, Jansen H, et al. Interventions for treating obesity in children. Cochrane Database Syst Rev 2009;1:CD001872.

11. Pratt JS, Lenders CM, Dionne EA, et al. Best practice updates for pediatric/adolescent weight loss surgery. Obesity 2009;17:901.

12. Iglowstein I, Jenni OG, Molinari L, et al. Sleep duration from infancy to adolescence: reference values and generational trends. Pediatrics 2003;111:302.

13. Dollman J, Ridley K, Olds T, et al. Trends in the duration of school-day sleep among 10- to 15-year-old South Australians between 1985 and 2004. Acta Paediatr 2007;96:1011.

14. National Sleep Foundation (2004). Final Report: 2004 Sleep in America Poll. Available at: http://www.sleepfoundation.org/_content//hottopics/2004SleepPollFinalReport.pdf. Accessed March 5, 2006.

15. Mindell J, Owens JA. A clinical guide to pediatric sleep. Philadelphia: Lipincott Williams & Wilkins; 2003.

16. Ferber R. Childhood sleep disorders. Neurologic Clinics 1996;14:493.

17. Copinschi G. Metabolic and endocrine effects of sleep deprivation. Essent Psychopharmacol 2005;6:341.

18. Guilleminault C, Powell NB, Martinez S, et al. Preliminary observations on the effects of sleep time in a sleep restriction paradigm. Sleep Med 2003;4:177.

19. Spiegel K, Leproult R, L'Hermite-Baleriaux M, et al. Leptin levels are dependent on sleep duration: relationships with sympathovagal balance, carbohydrate regulation, cortisol, and thyrotropin. J Clin Endocrinol Metab 2004;89:5762.

20. Taheri S, Lin L, Austin D, et al. Short sleep duration is associated with reduced leptin, elevated ghrelin, and increased body mass index. PLoS Med 2004;1:210.

21. Wren AM, Seal LJ, Cohen MA, et al. Ghrelin enhances appetite and increases food intake in humans. J Clin Endocrinol Metab 2001;86:5992.

22. Levin F, Edholm T, Schmidt PT, et al. Ghrelin stimulates gastric emptying and hunger in normal-weight humans. J Clin Endocrinol Metab 2006;91:3296.

23. Mars M, de Graaf C, de Groot CP, et al. Fasting leptin and appetite responses induced by a 4-day 65%-energy-restricted diet. Int J Obes (Lond) 2006;30:122.

24. Nedeltcheva AV, Kilkus JM, Imperial J, et al. Sleep curtailment is accompanied by increased intake of calories from snacks. Am J Clin Nutr 2009;89:126.

25. Brondel L, Romer MA, Nougues PM, et al. Acute partial sleep deprivation increases food intake in healthy men. Am J Clin Nutr 2010;91:1550.

26. Dru M, Bruge P, Benoit O, et al. Overnight duty impairs behaviour, awake activity and sleep in medical doctors. Eur J Emerg Med 2007;14:199.

27. Schmid SM, Hallschmid M, Jauch-Chara K, et al. Short-term sleep loss decreases physical activity under free-living conditions but does not increase food intake under time-deprived laboratory conditions in healthy men. Am J Clin Nutr 2009;90:1476.

28. Ievers-Landis CE, Redline S. Pediatric sleep apnea: implications of the epidemic of childhood overweight. Am J Respir Crit Care Med 2007;175:436.

29. Locard E, Mamelle N, Billette A, et al. Risk factors of obesity in a five year old population. Parental versus environmental factors. Int J Obes Relat Metab Disord 1992;16:721.
30. Sekine M, Yamagami T, Hamanishi S, et al. Parental obesity, lifestyle factors and obesity in preschool children: results of the Toyama Birth Cohort study. J Epidemiol 2002;12:33.
31. Sekine M, Yamagami T, Handa K, et al. A dose-response relationship between short sleeping hours and childhood obesity: results of the Toyama Birth Cohort Study. Child Care Health Dev 2002;28:163.
32. von Kries R, Toschke AM, Wurmser H, et al. Reduced risk for overweight and obesity in 5- and 6-y-old children by duration of sleep–a cross-sectional study. Int J Obes 2002;26:710.
33. Gupta NK, Mueller WH, Chan W, et al. Is obesity associated with poor sleep quality in adolescents? Am J Hum Biol 2002;14:762.
34. Padez C, Mourao I, Moreira P, et al. Prevalence and risk factors for overweight and obesity in Portuguese children. Acta Paediatr 2005;94:1550.
35. Chen MY, Wang EK, Jeng YJ. Adequate sleep among adolescents is positively associated with health status and health-related behaviors. BMC Public Health 2006;6:59.
36. Chaput JP, Brunet M, Tremblay A. Relationship between short sleeping hours and childhood overweight/obesity: results from the 'Quebec en Forme' Project. Int J Obes (Lond) 2006;30:1080.
37. Eisenmann JC, Ekkekakis P, Holmes M. Sleep duration and overweight among Australian children and adolescents. Acta Paediatr 2006;95:956.
38. Seicean A, Redline S, Seicean S, et al. Association between short sleeping hours and overweight in adolescents: results from a US Suburban High School survey. Sleep Breath 2007;11:285.
39. Kuriyan R, Bhat S, Thomas T, et al. Television viewing and sleep are associated with overweight among urban and semi-urban South Indian children. Nutr J 2007;6:25.
40. Knutson KL, Lauderdale DS. Sleep duration and overweight in adolescents: self-reported sleep hours versus time diaries. Pediatrics 2007;119:e1056.
41. Nixon GM, Thompson JM, Han DY, et al. Short sleep duration in middle childhood: risk factors and consequences. Sleep 2008;31:71.
42. Ievers-Landis CE, Storfer-Isser A, Rosen C, et al. Relationship of sleep parameters, child psychological functioning, and parenting stress to obesity status among preadolescent children. J Dev Behav Pediatr 2008;29:243.
43. Liu X, Forbes EE, Ryan ND, et al. Rapid eye movement sleep in relation to overweight in children and adolescents. Arch Gen Psychiatry 2008;65:924.
44. Wells JC, Hallal PC, Reichert FF, et al. Sleep patterns and television viewing in relation to obesity and blood pressure: evidence from an adolescent Brazilian birth cohort. Int J Obes (Lond) 2008;32:1042.
45. Bawazeer NM, Al-Daghri NM, Valsamakis G, et al. Sleep duration and quality associated with obesity among Arab children. Obesity (Silver Spring) 2009;17:2251.
46. Wing YK, Li SX, Li AM, et al. The effect of weekend and holiday sleep compensation on childhood overweight and obesity. Pediatrics 2009;124:e994.
47. Hitze B, Bosy-Westphal A, Bielfeldt F, et al. Determinants and impact of sleep duration in children and adolescents: data of the Kiel Obesity Prevention Study. Eur J Clin Nutr 2009;63:739.
48. Jiang F, Zhu S, Yan C, et al. Sleep and obesity in preschool children. J Pediatr 2009;154:814.

49. Ozturk A, Mazicioglu M, Poyrazoglu S, et al. The relationship between sleep duration and obesity in Turkish children and adolescents. Acta Paediatr 2009;98:699.
50. Sun Y, Sekine M, Kagamimori S. Lifestyle and overweight among Japanese adolescents: the Toyama Birth Cohort Study. J Epidemiol 2009;19:303.
51. Anderson SE, Whitaker RC. Household routines and obesity in US preschool-aged children. Pediatrics 2010;125:420.
52. Reilly JJ, Armstrong J, Dorosty AR, et al. Early life risk factors for obesity in childhood: cohort study. BMJ 2005;330:1357.
53. Snell EK, Adam EK, Duncan GJ. Sleep and the body mass index and overweight status of children and adolescents. Child Dev 2007;78:309.
54. Lumeng JC, Somashekar D, Appugliese D, et al. Shorter sleep duration is associated with increased risk for being overweight at ages 9 to 12 years. Pediatrics 2007;120:1020.
55. Landhuis CE, Poulton R, Welch D, et al. Childhood sleep time and long-term risk for obesity: a 32-year prospective birth cohort study. Pediatrics 2008;122:955.
56. Touchette E, Petit D, Tremblay RE, et al. Associations between sleep duration patterns and overweight/obesity at age 6. Sleep 2008;31:1507.
57. Taveras EM, Rifas-Shiman SL, Oken E, et al. Short sleep duration in infancy and risk of childhood overweight. Arch Pediatr Adolesc Med 2008;162:305.
58. Hui LL, Nelson EA, Yu LM, et al. Risk factors for childhood overweight in 6- to 7-y-old Hong Kong children. Int J Obes Relat Metab Disord 2003;27:1411.
59. Kagamimori S, Yamagami T, Sokejima S, et al. The relationship between lifestyle, social characteristics and obesity in 3-year-old Japanese children. Child Care Health Dev 1999;25:235.
60. Agras WS, Hammer LD, McNicholas F, et al. Risk factors for childhood overweight: a prospective study from birth to 9.5 years. J Pediatr 2004;145:20.
61. Yu Y, Lu BS, Wang B, et al. Short sleep duration and adiposity in Chinese adolescents. Sleep 2007;30:1688.
62. Bayer O, Rosario AS, Wabitsch M, et al. Sleep duration and obesity in children: is the association dependent on age and choice of the outcome parameter? Sleep 2009;32:1183.
63. Maddah M, Rashidi A, Mohammadpour B, et al. In-school snacking, breakfast consumption, and sleeping patterns of normal and overweight Iranian high school girls: a study in urban and rural areas in Guilan, Iran. J Nutr Educ Behav 2009;41:27.
64. Olds T, Blunden S, Dollman J, et al. Day type and the relationship between weight status and sleep duration in children and adolescents. Aust N Z J Public Health 2010;34:165.
65. Giugliano R, Carneiro EC. Factors associated with obesity in school children. J Pediatr (Rio J) 2004;80:17.
66. Duncan JS, Schofield G, Duncan EK, et al. Risk factors for excess body fatness in New Zealand children. Asia Pac J Clin Nutr 2008;17:138.
67. Al Mamun A, Lawlor DA, Cramb S, et al. Do childhood sleeping problems predict obesity in young adulthood? evidence from a prospective birth cohort study. Am J Epidemiol 2007;166:1368.
68. Landis AM, Parker KP. A retrospective examination of the relationship between body mass index and polysomnographic measures of sleep in adolescents. J Adolesc Health 2007;40:89 official publication of the Society for Adolescent Medicine.
69. Landis AM, Parker KP, Dunbar SB. Sleep, hunger, satiety, food cravings, and caloric intake in adolescents. J Nurs Scholarsh 2009;41:115.

70. Westerlund L, Ray C, Roos E. Associations between sleeping habits and food consumption patterns among 10-11-year-old children in Finland. Br J Nutr 2009; 102:1531.
71. Hart CN, Jelalian E. Shortened sleep duration is associated with pediatric overweight. Behav Sleep Med 2008;6:251.
72. Cappuccio FP, Taggart FM, Kandala NB, et al. Meta-analysis of short sleep duration and obesity in children and adults. Sleep 2008;31:619.
73. Marshall NS, Glozier N, Grunstein RR. Is sleep duration related to obesity? A critical review of the epidemiological evidence. Sleep Med Rev 2008;12:289.
74. Taheri S. The link between short sleep duration and obesity: we should recommend more sleep to prevent obesity. Arch Dis Child 2006;91:881.
75. Chen X, Beydoun MA, Wang Y. Is sleep duration associated with childhood obesity? a systematic review and meta-analysis. Obesity (Silver Spring) 2008; 16:265.
76. Patel SR, Hu FB. Short sleep duration and weight gain: a systematic review. Obesity (Silver Spring) 2008;16:643.
77. Bray MS, Young ME. Circadian rhythms in the development of obesity: potential role for the circadian clock within the adipocyte. Obes Rev 2007;8:169.
78. Adam EK, Snell EK, Pendry P. Sleep timing and quantity in ecological and family context: a nationally representative time-diary study. J Fam Psychol 2007;21:4.
79. Owens J, Maxim R, McGuinn M, et al. Television-viewing habits and sleep disturbance in school children. Pediatrics 1999;104:e27.
80. Thompson DA, Christakis DA. The association between television viewing and irregular sleep schedules among children less than 3 years of age. Pediatrics 2005;116:851.
81. Verhulst SL, Schrauwen N, Haentjens D, et al. Sleep duration and metabolic dysregulation in overweight children and adolescents. Arch Dis Child 2008;93:89.
82. Tian Z, Ye T, Zhang X, et al. Sleep duration and hyperglycemia among obese and nonobese children aged 3 to 6 years. Arch Pediatr Adolesc Med 2010;164:46.
83. Flint J, Kothare SV, Zihlif M, et al. Association between inadequate sleep and insulin resistance in obese children. J Pediatr 2007;150:364.

Sleep Health Education in Pediatric Community Settings: Rationale and Practical Suggestions for Incorporating Healthy Sleep Education into Pediatric Practice

Reut Gruber, PhD[a,b,]*, Jamie Cassoff, BSc[a,c], Bärbel Knäuper, PhD[c]

KEYWORDS

- Sleep education • Pediatric practice • Adolescents • Pediatrics
- Healthy sleep

A substantial body of evidence demonstrates that an appropriate level of sleep is necessary for a healthy and productive lifestyle, academic success, and emotional well-being; these are 3 key elements associated with successful development.[1] While a considerable proportion of adolescents obtain less sleep than they need, and are thus chronically sleep deprived,[2] declines in sleep time and increasingly delayed bedtimes suggest the emergence of sleep restriction in preadolescents and even younger children. Adolescents have shown a gradual decrease in weeknight sleep

The authors have nothing to disclose.

[a] Attention, Behavior and Sleep Lab, Douglas Mental Health University Institute, 6875 LaSalle Boulevard, Verdun, QC H4H 1R3, Canada
[b] Department of Psychiatry, McGill University, Douglas Mental Health University Institute, 6875 LaSalle Boulevard, Verdun, QC H4H 1R3, Canada
[c] Department of Psychology, McGill University, Stewart Biology Building, 1205 Avenue Docteur Penfield, Montreal, QC H3A 1B1, Canada
* Corresponding author. Attention, Behavior and Sleep Lab, Douglas Mental Health University Institute, 6875 LaSalle Boulevard, Verdun, QC H4H 1R3, Canada.
E-mail address: reut.gruber@douglas.mcgill.ca

Pediatr Clin N Am 58 (2011) 735–754
doi:10.1016/j.pcl.2011.03.006
0031-3955/11/$ – see front matter © 2011 Published by Elsevier Inc.

time of about 1 h, with correspondingly later weeknight bedtimes and longer sleep times on weekends.[2]

The significance of chronic sleep insufficiency is underrecognized in the context of youth health. Whereas sufficient sleep is associated with normal metabolism and appropriate physiologic functioning, sleep deprivation has been empirically linked to obesity, diabetes, hypertension, metabolic syndrome, and cardiovascular problems.[3–6] In addition, poor sleep has been shown to impair academic performance, learning, memory, and neurobehavioral functioning, especially in the context of activities essential for academic success; these include attention/response inhibition, memory, verbal creativity, problem solving, and general cognitive abilities as reflected by IQ test scores.[7] Finally, poor sleep has been linked to an increase in accidental injuries in younger children[8] and is directly related to an increased risk of motor vehicle accidents,[9,10] a topic of increasing relevance to adolescents of driving age. Collectively, therefore, the multiple negative impacts of sleep deprivation emphasize the need to provide children and their parents with education on healthy sleep and tools that assist in achieving such sleep.

The goal of this article is to offer practical ways to incorporate healthy sleep education into pediatric practice and to discuss key questions, barriers, and strategies associated with such efforts. The authors begin by presenting the rationale for incorporating healthy sleep education in pediatric practice settings. The desirable features of sleep education programs that may be implemented in pediatric practice are then identified. Next, the authors review potential barriers to implementation and offer strategies to overcome these barriers, including development of a pool of resources applicable to healthy sleep education, and practical information that may be of use to primary health care pediatricians. Key factors that increase the effectiveness of such interventional programs are highlighted. The article ends by identifying the key points relevant to successful healthy sleep education in pediatric practice.

RATIONALE FOR INCORPORATION OF HEALTHY SLEEP EDUCATION IN PEDIATRIC SETTINGS

Despite the wealth and strength of evidence demonstrating the critical importance of sleep, and the adverse impacts of sleep deprivation, such knowledge is not widely available to children and families. The existence of problems that are potentially avoidable on application of healthy sleep education, and the difficulties currently experienced in addressing such problems, represent a "translation gap." Given the critical nature of the domains that are adversely affected by sleep restriction, it has been suggested that the appropriate use and dissemination of knowledge on the importance of sleep, and of tools that allow environmental factors or habits related to sleep to be changed, may have significant positive impacts on the health, quality of life, and academic performance of youth.[1] Sleep education within the community or the consulting rooms of primary care pediatricians therefore offers a unique opportunity to close the gap associated with sleep education and, in so doing, to significantly improve youth health and well-being and reduce the preventable burden of disease caused by sleep deprivation.

THE DESIRABLE FEATURES OF SLEEP EDUCATION PROGRAMS IN PEDIATRIC PRACTICE

Healthy sleep education can be conducted at 3 complementary levels: primary, secondary, and tertiary prevention. Primary prevention encompasses interventions aimed at preventing the development of sleep deprivation by providing age-appropriate knowledge on sleep, and strategies that both ensure healthy sleep and prevent the onset of sleep disorders. To achieve this goal, the focus is typically on the provision of parental education on how sleep deprivation may affect children, information on normative developmental milestones, and how to use age-appropriate strategies to optimize sleep. Such education targets child developmental physiology and sleep needs. Secondary prevention strategies used by health care providers usually attempt to diagnose and treat existing sleep disorders at early stages, thus before significant morbidity occurs, or feature targeted interventions aimed at children at risk for sleep disorders (eg, pre-adolescents with significantly delayed bedtimes). Finally, tertiary prevention seeks to reduce the negative impact of sleep disorders using intensive individualized clinical interventions targeted to children or adolescents with serious or chronic sleep problems. This article focuses on primary prevention. The goal is to offer useful background material and to explain strategies that will help to minimize sleep deprivation, thus promoting good sleep.

THE ESSENTIAL COMPONENTS OF HEALTHY SLEEP EDUCATION PROGRAMS

Sleep education programs should provide the primary health care pediatrician with information needed to discuss with parents all aspects pertaining to healthy sleep in children. This information includes: (1) the importance of sleep and its impact on health, cognitive functions, and emotional regulation; (2) signs of child sleep deprivation; (3) the development of basic sleep processes and sleep regulation; (4) environmental factors that affect sleep and information; and (5) specific strategies to facilitate healthy sleep.

DESIRABLE ATTRIBUTES OF HEALTH CARE PROVIDERS THAT CONTRIBUTE EFFECTIVELY TO HEALTHY SLEEP EDUCATION

Primary health care pediatricians are ideally positioned to significantly contribute to sleep education efforts because they have ample opportunities to interact with families on an ongoing basis, possess a good understanding of the condition of any specific child and his or her family, and are perceived to be authorities on issues associated with health (thus parents are likely to follow their recommendations). Despite the importance of sleep to the mental and physical health of children, and the likelihood that primary health care pediatricians can effectively transfer sleep information to parents and children, a large gap in clinical practice may be discerned. This factor is problematic because until sleep information is widely disseminated, an important opportunity to significantly improve youth health will be lost.

Two key barriers to the incorporation of healthy sleep education into pediatric settings may be identified. First, pediatric providers are busy, and often lack the time and resources to actively engage in sleep health education. Primary prevention strategies are often not only time-consuming but are also less likely to be reimbursed. Second, most pediatricians have not been adequately trained regarding the importance of sleep and the impact of insufficient sleep, the recognition and evaluation of sleep disturbances, and appropriate interventions. The authors first describe these barriers in detail, and next seek to develop approaches that might lower the barriers, thereby contributing to a narrowing of the translation gap.

Barrier #1. Competing Demands for Increasingly Smaller Amounts of Time

Time pressure represents a significant barrier to the ability of the primary care pediatrician to engage in dissemination of preventative information pertaining to healthy sleep. Studies have shown that time pressure clearly affects the tolerance of providers toward added tasks or the use of new tools even when these benefit both patients and health care providers.[11–13] Hence, a busy primary care pediatrician may simply not have adequate opportunity to acquire novel relevant information, to prepare self-help tools for patients, or to deliver that information in the context of the clinical encounter.

Barrier #2. Lack of Awareness and/or Knowledge

Primary care pediatricians may lack both awareness and knowledge of the impact of sleep on several critical domains of development, and do not appreciate the need to help children and families to make healthy sleep a part of daily life. Such knowledge gaps have been reported by Papp and colleagues,[14] who found that the overall mean sleep knowledge test score of primary care physicians was 34%, and by Owens,[15] who found that primary care pediatricians correctly answered only 60% of questions testing sleep knowledge, with almost 25% of pediatricians scoring less than 50%. Such lack of knowledge may be the result of insufficient training in sleep medicine. Several studies have found that the amount and quality of sleep education included in medical student and resident training is very limited.[16–20] This lack of basic training is consistent with the minimal knowledge of sleep and sleep disorders shown by practicing physicians and pediatricians. Although the National Institutes of Health established a program to increase the sleep education component of medical training in 20 medical schools,[21] a gap between training and practice is still apparent in most schools.

Although no easy means of removing the aforementioned barriers is apparent, several strategies may increase awareness of the importance of sleep and the use of available evidence-based tools promoting healthy sleep by primary care pediatricians, enhancing integration of relevant research findings into pediatric settings with minimal impact on the workload of the pediatric primary health care provider.

Overcoming Barrier #1. Reducing the Time Demand Associated with Preparation and Dissemination of Healthy Sleep Information

First, the use of available material (brochures, pamphlets, DVDs, online resources) could save preparation time and facilitate information dissemination. For example, the information included in this article and the findings of evidence-based programs aimed at healthy sleep education have been reported in peer-reviewed journals. Most interventions have targeted the parents of infants.[22–27] A summary of results from these studies is given in **Table 1**. Second, nurses attending during regular check-ups can provide useful information, and can conduct telephone follow-up after office visits, effectively helping parents and children to develop healthy sleep education principles and to sustain good sleep behavior.[22–28] This approach minimizes time demands without compromising the quality or effectiveness of care. Third, a pediatrician or nurse could employ a group education format; both parenting programs and community maternity classes are effective in this regard.[26] Finally, screening tools such as the BEARS[29] (B = Bedtime issues, E = Excessive daytime sleepiness, A = night Awakenings, R = Regularity and duration of sleep, S = Snoring) allow for a quick assessment of sleep problems while at the same time educating parents about the importance of sleep and consequences of poor sleep habits.

Overcoming Barrier #2. Increasing Physician Awareness and/or Knowledge

Multiple information sources are available, such as pre-prepared easy-to-use material and handouts that offer families with children/adolescents useful information on the importance of sleep, and concrete strategies aimed at improving sleep behavior and preventing development of sleep problems in infants, children, and adolescents.

In this section the authors review useful information to pediatricians interested in healthy sleep education, suggest strategies that increase the effectiveness of tools or programs when applied by primary care pediatricians or practice nurses, and review online resources that provide parents and/or children with tools, information, and behavioral guidelines conducive to healthy sleep.

Content for an effective sleep education program for pediatric practice

The following information could be used by pediatricians or practice nurses to increase their level of knowledge regarding sleep and to share with interested families.

The importance of sleep and its impact on health Insufficient sleep has serious adverse consequences for those mental and physiologic processes that are vitally important during development. Moreover, it reduces effective daytime functioning of brain areas required to conduct key processes essential for academic success, and in the long term may compromise metabolic and cardiovascular function.

Evidence supporting the association between sleep and obesity Reduced sleep duration has been associated with a greater body mass index.[30] For example, a recent large-scale study in Quebec found that low sleep duration increased the developmental risk of childhood overweight status/obesity. When children reporting 12 to 13 hours of sleep per night were compared with those getting 10.5 to 11.5 hours of sleep and children sleeping for only 8 to 10 hours per night, they were 3.45-fold more likely to be obese after adjustment for age, gender, and other risk factors.[30] Studies in healthy young adults indicate that restricting sleep increases cortisol levels, induces insulin resistance,[31] and is associated with lower leptin level, elevated ghrelin concentration, and enhanced appetite.[32] In addition, sleep deprivation affects neural pathways that modulate self-control.[33] Impairments in such functions may be related to loss of willpower when faced with tempting calorie-rich food, and may increase the likelihood of impulsive food choice decisions that lead to weight gain (for additional information, Dinges and colleagues[34] and Sadeh and colleagues[35]).

Evidence supporting the association between sleep and academic performance The most common direct consequence of insufficient or disrupted sleep is increased daytime sleepiness,[36,37] which leads to reduced alertness and compromises the daytime functioning of specific brain areas that underlie key processes required for academic success. For example, sleep-deprived individuals tested on cognitive, verbal, motor, visuospatial, and creative performance measures scored poorly, thus at levels comparable to the ninth percentile of subjects who had enjoyed adequate sleep.[38] The aspects of human behavior most affected by fatigue and insufficient sleep are executive functions, learning, memory, and self-regulation, which are also the key functional domains required for academic success. Cumulative sleep restriction negatively affects cognitive performance[34,35]; consistent evidence of an inverse relationship between sleep time and school performance has been gathered. Comparison of school performance measures with reported total sleep time found that students who had grades of C, D, or F averaged 25 to 30 minutes less sleep per weeknight than did peers with better grades.[39] Most reports indicated that even when socioeconomic status, race, and other potentially important confounders were controlled, short sleep duration[40–43] and low sleep quality[41,44] were related to poorer academic performance, either when purely subjective (eg, self-reports[43,45,46]) or objective measures of sleep (eg, actigraphy[40,41,47]) and academic performance (eg, SAT scores as objective evaluations; school grades as subjective measures) were employed. In addition, not only was shorter sleep duration and low-quality sleep linked to poorer academic

Table 1
Published articles and ongoing initiatives

Author/ Organization, Country	Program Title	Age Group	Age Range	No. of Participants (Experimental/ Control)	Intervention Techniques	Mode of Delivery	Target Audience	Findings
Stremler et al,[22] 2006, Canada	n/a	Infants	6 wk	15/15	Information provision, cognitive restructuring, behavioral exercises	Informational booklet, face-to-face consultations with nurse, telephone follow-up	Parents	Fewer nighttime awakenings [7.9 vs 12.3, difference 4.4 (95% CI: 1.4–7.6), $2P = .006$], and sleep durations that were 46 min longer than the control group [217 vs 171 (95% CI: 5–88), $2P = .03$]. No effects for length of nocturnal sleep, daytime sleep
St James-Roberts et al,[23] 2001, UK	n/a	Infants	0–3 mo	202/203	Information provision, behavioral exercises	Informational booklet and face-to-face consultations with study personnel	Parents	14% reported seeking less help for problems involving infant crying or sleeping problems ($\chi^2 = 6.01, P = .049$) as compared with educational (24%) and control (21%) groups. At 12 wk, sleeping bout of >5 h was 2.61 times higher (95% CI 1.02–6.69)
Kerr et al,[24] 1996, Scotland	n/a	Infants	3 mo	86/83	Information provision	Informational booklet and face-to-face consultations with study personnel	Parents	Fewer settling difficulties ($\chi^2 = 4.88, P = .03$), less night wakings ($P = .02$), and higher overall sleep score ($P = .03$) as compared with control group

Study		Age		Sample	Intervention	Delivery	Recipient	Outcomes
Pinilla and Birch,[25] 1993, USA	n/a	Infants	Prenatal	13/13	Information provision, behavioral exercises	Face-to-face consultations with sleep specialists	Parents	Increased total sleep $F_{(1,24)} = 16.82$, $P<.01$, average duration of sleep $F_{(1,24)} = 22.45$, $P<.01$, and longest sleep episode $F_{(1,24)} = 24.29$, $P<.01$ as compared with control group. 100% slept through the night by week 8, as compared with 23% in control condition
Wolfson et al,[26] 1992, USA	n/a	Infants	0–9 wk	29/31	Information provision, cognitive restructuring, behavioral exercises	Informational booklet, question periods, group discussion, and problem-solving strategies	Parents	Increased number of sleep episodes, $F_{(1,46)} = 7.17$, $P<.01$, amount that infant sleeps for more than 300 min consecutively, $F_{(1,46)} = 9.29$, $P<.01$, and longest sleeping episode, $F_{(1,46)} = 8.56$, $P<.01$ as compared with control group. Increased parental self-efficacy
Adair et al,[27] 1992, USA	n/a	Infants	4 mo	164/172	Information provision, behavioral exercises	Informational booklet, face-to-face consultations with pediatrician, and sleep charts	Parents	At 9 mo of age, less night waking (M = 2.5) as compared with control condition (M = 3.9); $P = .02$

(continued on next page)

Table 1
(continued)

Author/ Organization, Country	Program Title	Age Group	Age Range	No. of Participants (Experimental/ Control)	Intervention Techniques	Mode of Delivery	Target Audience	Findings
Reid,[28] ongoing, Canada	Parenting Matters: Helping Parents With Young Children	Children	2–5 y	n/a	Information provision, cognitive restructuring	Informational booklet and telephone support	Parents	n/a
Gruber et al,[80] ongoing, Canada	Sleep for Success	Children	6–12 y	n/a	Information provision, cognitive restructuring, behavioral exercises	Interactive educational sessions, question periods, group discussion, and problem-solving strategies	Children, parents, educators, administrators	n/a
Blunden,[81] 2007, Australia	ACES junior sleep education package; ACES high school sleep education package	Children, adolescents	4–6, 10–12 y	n/a	Information provision	Powerpoint presentations, workbooks, teaching manuals	Educators	n/a

Study	Program	Population	Age	N	Intervention	Delivery	Providers	Outcomes
Bakotić et al,[82] 2009, Croatia	n/a	Adolescents	15–18 y	625/575	Information provision	Informational booklet	Adolescents	Increased knowledge for ages 15, $F(1,1168) = 28.46$, $P<.001$, 16, $F(1,1168) = 5.74$, $P=.017$, and 17, $F(1,1168) = 17.17$, $P<.001$, but not 18, $P=.467$. Females showed higher knowledge retention than males ($F = 95.95$, $P<.01$)
Moseley and Gradisar,[83] 2009, Australia	Improving Adolescent Well-Being: Day and Night	Adolescents	15 y	41/40	Infromation provision, cognitive restructuring, motivational interviewing, behavioral exercises	Educational sessions	Educators, adolescents	Increased total number of correct answers on sleep-related questions from preprogram ($M = 7.21$, $SD = 1.80$) to postprogram ($M = 8.52$, $SD = 1.60$), $t = 3.45$, $P = .001$. No effects on target sleep variables
De Sousa et al,[84] 2007, Brazil	n/a	Adolescents	12–18 y	58, no control	Information provision	Educational sessions	Educators, adolescents	Reduction in the index of sleep irregularity ($t = 2.18$; $P<.05$), a decrease in sleep latency ($t = 3.17$; $P<.01$) and an advanced nap schedule ($t = 1.57$; $P<.05$). No effects on sleepiness and sleep quality
Cortesi et al,[85] 2004, Italy	Crash in Bed Instead	Adolescents	17–19 y	225/200	Information provision	Powerpoint presentations and group discussion	Adolescents	Gain in correct answers $F(2.44) = 879.32$ $P<.001$ to sleep questions from baseline ($M = 4.2$) to immediately after the course ($M = 8.6$) and at follow-up periods ($M = 6.7$)

(continued on next page)

Table 1
(continued)

Author/ Organization, Country	Program Title	Age Group	Age Range	No. of Participants (Experimental/ Control)	Intervention Techniques	Mode of Delivery	Target Audience	Findings
Rossi et al,[86] 2002, USA	Young adolescent sleep-smart pacesetter program	Adolescents	12–18 y	n/a	Information provision, cognitive restructuring, behavioral exercises	n/a	Educators, adolescents	n/a
Unpublished dissemination initiatives								
Editorial review board, Sick Kids Hospital, Canada	Aboutkidshealth	Infants, children, adolescents	0–18 y	No quantitative data reported	Information provision	Web site	Parents	No quantitative data reported
American Academy of Sleep Medicine, USA	Sleepeducation	Infants, children, adolescents	0–18 y	No quantitative data reported	Information provision	Web site	Parents, adolescents	No quantitative data reported
National Sleep Foundation, USA	Pillow Talk	Infants, adolescents	0–5, 12–18 y	No quantitative data reported	Information provision	Blogging Web site	Parents, adolescents	No quantitative data reported
National Sleep Foundation, USA	Sleep for Kids	Children	5–12 y	No quantitative data reported	Information provision	Web site	Children, parents, educators	No quantitative data reported
Children's Hospital of Colorado, USA	Kids health library	Children	5–12 y	No quantitative data reported	Information provision	Interactive online Web site	Children	No quantitative data reported
The Morehouse School of Medicine, USA	Sleep and Space	Children	5–12 y	No quantitative data reported	Information provision	Television	Children	No quantitative data reported

Abbreviations: CI, confidence interval; n/a, no data available.

performance, but sleep deprivation was also associated with behavioral problems often encountered within school settings, as well as with tardiness and emotional disturbance, which may further reduce the ability of a child to perform well at school.[48]

Signs of insufficient sleep in children The required amount of sleep varies greatly among individuals, which is why provision of parental tools that help identification of insufficient sleep is important. Further, because children manifest fatigue in a manner unlike that of adults, it is important to teach parents the expected sleep durations required for optimal functioning at different ages and developmental stages, and how to identify the signs of child sleepiness. Both of these issues are discussed below. For a discussion of average child sleep duration at different ages, see Mindell and Owens.[10]

When children and adolescents are tired, rather than slowing down and asking to be allowed to sleep they may show moodiness, irritability, crankiness, and low frustration tolerance. Problems such as noncompliance, poor impulse control, and hyperactivity are apparent. In addition, the child may fall asleep in class, in the car, or in front of the TV on a regular basis. Poor weight regulation or obesity may arise; sleep-deprived children or adolescents are hungrier, tend to eat more, and may exercise less because they are tired.

A developmental perspective on basic sleep processes

Basic sleep processes Sleep is regulated by two distinct physiologic processes that interact to govern sleep timing and composition.[49–51] The homeostatic sleep process, or process S, is a regulatory mechanism whereby sleep pressure accumulates as wake time lengthens and dissipates during a sleep episode, whereas the circadian component, or process C, regulates the timing of sleep and awakening.[52–54] The circadian timing system affords the temporal organization of most neurobehavioral, physiological, and biochemical variables, including the sleep-wake cycle.[3] The timing system consists of a biological clock[4–6] that is able to distribute rhythmic messages about 24 hours in duration to the entire organism.[7] Because the rhythm of the circadian pacemaker, that is, the "biological clock," is not precisely 24 hours, it is necessary to realign it each day using the light-dark cycle.[49] This alignment process is termed entrainment.[50] Successful entrainment of sleep-wake rhythms to a 24-hour day requires the biological clock to be "reset" by an average of 1 hour each day. The most powerful synchronizer known is the light-dark cycle.[10,55] Homeostatic and circadian processes interact to determine sleep quality, quantity, and timing. Sleep timing is defined by a child's bedtime and wake-up time. Although no "correct" amount of sleep for a child has been defined, a child needs to awaken feeling well rested and alert to benefit from daily activities.

Environmental factors that affect sleep Sleep is a biological process, but sleep habits are socially learned behaviors that must be integrated with the natural rhythms of the body. By creating the children's environment parents can significantly affect their child's sleep. Several aspects of the physical environment such as light level, temperature, and the presence of objects or people that arouse the senses affect the child's ability to sleep. An appreciation and understanding of these elements are needed to provide parents with guidance on ways to optimize sleep regulation and duration. For a detailed discussion of developmental aspects of sleep, see Mindell and colleagues.[56]

Light

Our brains work on a 24-hour cycle that determines when we feel awake or sleepy; cycle timing is influenced by light. Bright light is associated with the beginning of the day (a time when it is appropriate to feel alert) and darkness signals the end of the day (a time to feel sleepy). Hence, exposure to artificial light late at night may "fool" the brain into thinking that daytime persists, and we may feel like staying up late. On the other hand, absence of exposure to bright light in the morning may make us feel drowsy on waking, in turn affecting daytime functioning and pushing back our "timing of morning." This can cause delayed bedtime and, ultimately, loss of sleep. For this reason it is important to be exposed to morning bright light, such as outdoor sun even during the winter, and to avoid nighttime bright light, such as that emitted from TV or computer screens.

Temperature

To fall asleep, our bodies cool by a few degrees. A bedroom temperature that is too warm may make it difficult to fall asleep. For this reason bedroom temperature should be less than 75°F (24°C).

Stimulation

Too much stimulation close to bedtime may inhibit the ability to fall asleep. People and objects that trigger the senses of sight, sound, touch, or smell can compromise sleep. This is the reason why interacting online with friends or playing with electronic devices in the bedroom can interfere with the ability of a child to fall asleep.

Individual Socioeconomic Status

Individual socioeconomic status (SES) is related to duration and quality of sleep. In particular, both subjective and objective measurements of sleep have indicated shorter sleep duration, and poorer sleep quality, in individuals of lower SES.[57–59] This "sleep disparity" has been attributed to a variety of psychosocial and environmental factors. For example, Van Cauter and Spiegel[60] noted that opportunities to attain adequate amounts of restorative sleep may be restricted by living conditions characterized by noise, overcrowding, and/or potential danger. Moreover, adverse economic circumstances are often associated with enhanced levels of anxiety and stress, which can also negatively affect sleep quality and duration.[61] In addition, disruptive sleep practices, such as bed-sharing, are more common among some low-SES groups, and are associated with increased incidences of childhood sleep problems including sleep anxiety, resistance, and night waking.[62,63] This is the reason why creating a quiet and comfortable sleeping environment even, and perhaps especially, in busy households, is critically important if children are to fall asleep in a timely manner and to sleep adequately during the night.

Family Processes that Affect Sleep

Parenting styles that are supportive, warm, and responsive, and family functioning characterized by effective communication and affection, promote a sense of security, whereas a coercive parenting style, or a family environment characterized by high levels of conflict and lack of trust, undermine a child's sense of security.[64–68] A threatening environment has been shown to negatively affect sleep.[69] Indeed, poor parent-child relationships,[70] insecure maternal attachment,[71] child abuse,[70–73] and conflict in the family environment,[73] are linked to sleep problems. Thus, a positive (ie, warm, responsive, and protective) parenting experience increases a child's sense of security and provides an environment conducive to prolonged sleep, whereas harsh or coercive parenting is associated with insufficient sleep.

Lifestyle Issues

Beyond the immediate environment, lifestyle factors play increasingly important roles in the life of a child as he or she grows into adolescence. Sleep deprivation often results from lifestyle-related choices made by individuals and families. For example, the idea that "more is better" causes parents to enroll children in multiple extracurricular activities and to permit attendance at late-ending social events, culminating in delayed bedtime and short sleep duration. Other lifestyle factors contributing to short sleep duration include excessive use of technology (television, Internet, instant messaging, texting, and video games) late at night, consumption of high-caffeine drinks and alcohol, and tobacco use. In addition, busy parents who work late may push dinner and family time to (say) 22:00, thus setting priorities that reduce sleep time, contribute to delayed bedtime, and result in accumulation of sleep deprivation during the week.

How to use the information effectively: making healthy sleep education work

One-on-one interventions targeting the parents of infants in person and via the phone Teaching of healthy sleep behaviors using educational materials is effective in instilling behavioral change, but guidance is required during the training process[22]; this can be done in person (see the work of Wolfson and colleagues[26]) and/or by weekly phone contact (Stremler and colleagues[22]). The goal is, first, to allow parents to express concerns and opinions regarding implementation of novel sleep practices, and second, to offer problem-solving solutions in line with family culture and values.[22] For example, various parental opinions on room sharing, cosleeping, and napping should be considered when formulating suggestions. A recent study found that, compared with a control group that received educational materials and phone contact for sleep hygiene discussion but no individualized advice, children in the experimental group displayed improvements in sleep duration and had fewer night awakenings.[22]

Telephone follow-up after routine checkups Pediatric health practitioners including pediatricians and nurses may consider implementing telephone follow-up after routine checkups; this is a valuable method by which to ensure maintenance of healthy sleep practices.[22]

Cultural sensitivity Specific educational strategies should include culturally sensitive materials appropriate for parents with a range of literacy levels, and multiple methods are available for the translation and dissemination of information; these include web-based products, handouts, and personal guidance.

Available online resources

Specialized sleep education websites and other multimedia sources[74–79] targeting parents and educators of young children and infants, or children and adolescents per se, are available and free. Sleepeducation.com[75] was developed in 2005 by the American Academy of Sleep Medicine to address the growing demand for sleep information from many members of society. The Sleep for Kids Web site[77] was later launched by the National Sleep Foundation, and is designed to directly provide information to children aged 7 to 12 years, in a comprehensible and interactive manner. Both Web sites offer detailed age-specific information relevant to sleep hygiene and sleep disorders, and describe available resources including treatment center locations and sleep study dictionaries, accessible to children of different ages (see **Table 1**). In addition, the National Sleep Foundation (NSF) offers sleep educational handouts for purchase to be distributed to parents in pediatric settings. Guide books containing information needed for prevention of sleep deprivation and promotion of healthy sleep, and printable handouts, are also available.[10]

Specific recommendations that a primary health care pediatrician might make to facilitate healthy sleep

The authors now summarize practical information that a busy primary health care pediatrician could impart during a well-baby/child visit or a check-up. Key practical points that are effective in optimizing sleep and preventing sleep deprivation are provided. The information could be reviewed with parents by a nurse before a regular check-up, and/or by a pediatrician during a visit. Information relevant to all age groups is first presented, followed by age-specific data. References to additional material on published and ongoing sleep studies[22–28,80–86] and Web sites[74–79] targeted for children and their parents are included in **Table 1**.

Bedtime routine Recommend creation of a consistent, calm, bedtime routine that includes relaxing activities over about 20 to 30 minutes in the room where the child sleeps.

Sleep schedule Recommend creation of a fixed bedtime and wake time. The body "gets used" to falling asleep at a certain time, but only if this is relatively consistent. Therefore, it is important that there should be no more than 1 hour of bedtime difference between school nights and weekends or holidays. Finally, it is important to set a bedtime that is sufficiently early to allow the child to get enough sleep.

Sleeping environment The ideal sleeping environment is quiet, dark, and cool in the evening, and well lit in the morning. If the child expresses fear of the dark, use of a nightlight is acceptable. It is important that the sleeping environment should be associated with positive experiences and emotions. Hence, parents should not use banishment to the bedroom, or early bed, as punishment.

Food before bedtime It is important that a child should not go to bed hungry. Although heavy meals within the 2 hours before bedtime should be avoided, but a small snack close to bedtime is acceptable.

Caffeine A child should avoid caffeine for at least 3 to 4 hours before bedtime. Thus, caffeinated beverages including coffee, tea, energy drinks, sodas, and hot chocolate should be avoided, as should (solid) chocolate. This restriction should be explained to adolescents who independently seek out these types of snacks or beverages.

Television, computers, and cell phones are not appropriate in the bedroom Parents should be advised to keep electronic devices out of the bedroom and limit Internet use in the evening.

Naps Napping during the day creates difficulty in nighttime sleeping. Napping should be regulated by age, with younger children having more and longer naps. For adolescents who feel sleepy during the day, a nap should be limited to 15 to 20 minutes and should be scheduled for the early afternoon.

Exercise regularly, but not directly before bedtime Regular exercise, particularly in the afternoon, can help to deepen sleep. Strenuous exercise, such as intense hockey or soccer practice, within 2 hours before bedtime can compromise the ability to fall asleep.

Light exposure Each child should spend time outside every day even during the winter.

Age-specific recommendations

Infants and toddlers As sleep processes change dramatically in infants, and as sleep is often not well regulated in infants and toddlers, it is of particular importance to help parents achieve the important milestones of sleeping throughout the night and the ability to fall asleep independently. Parents must know that infants are physiologically able to "sleep through the night" by 6 months of age, and that a drowsy but awake baby can be put down to sleep at bedtime, and during the night; this aids in acquisition of the ability to fall asleep independently.

Evidence-based interventional programs for healthy sleep education designed for parents of infants A proactive approach toward healthy sleep education has been taken by several researchers who favor the use of evidence-based interventional programs to this end.[22–27] Wolfson and colleagues[26] created a program in which parents were trained over 2 prenatal and 2 postbirth sessions; the program involved informational handouts, question-and-answer sessions, group discussion, and evolution of problem-solving strategies. Topics included the physiology of infant sleep, confident parenting, sleep routines, and sleep-wake patterns. It was found that 6 to 9 weeks after birth, the infants of informed parents were more self-reliant and had more sleep episodes, longer sleep duration, and less nighttime awakening than did infants of control parents. Pinilla and Birch[25] employed a behavioral approach; parents participated in prebirth and postbirth training sessions. The aim was to establish a breast-feeding regime to maximize differences between the day and night environments, and to extend the intervals between night feedings to teach the infant how to sleep through the night. It was sought to achieve these aims before the infant was 8 weeks of age. At this time, 100% of experimental infants were sleeping throughout the night, compared with 23% of control children. Another interventional program[22] combined the use of information booklets with follow-up discussions with pediatricians. All these programs had a significantly positive effect on infants' sleep.[22,25,26] Please refer to **Table 1** for a complete list of such research efforts, which are also sorted by the age of the child.[22–28,80–86]

School-age children and adolescents It is important to explain the importance of developing a lifestyle conducive to healthy sleep behavior,[56] thus making sleep a priority, despite the presence of competing activities. School-age children may be more receptive than are adolescents, and acquisition of appropriate habits at a younger age might help to reduce the incidence of the typical poor sleep habits seen in adolescence.

More topics specific to adolescents Given the high prevalence of sleep deprivation in adolescence and the natural tendency toward delayed rising and bedtime, it is important to advise adolescents on the importance of healthy sleep habits over the weekend. Although sleeping in on weekends is permissible, this should not be for more than 1 hour past the usual wake time, to avoid disrupting the ability to fall asleep at bedtime.

Night activities Advise adolescents to avoid stimulating activities (eg, heavy study, text messaging, engaging in prolonged conversations) around bedtime.[87]

Driving The combination of a high prevalence of sleep deprivation with the naturally increased sleep needs of adolescence renders adolescents prone to being drowsy during the day as well as tired in the evening.[88] Therefore, it is critical to inform parents and adolescents themselves to be aware of the dangers associated with drowsy driving. It is important to emphasize that accidents can happen in the middle of the afternoon as well as at night.

PRACTICE POINTS: HOW TO PROMOTE HEALTHY SLEEP EDUCATION IN PRIMARY PEDIATRIC HEALTH CARE SETTINGS

1. Help parents understand the importance of sleep for healthy and successful development
2. Help parents understand the important role they can play in optimizing child sleep and making a significant positive impact on child health and success
3. Provide parents with basic information on sleep processes and age-appropriate information on normative sleep needs and patterns
4. Help parents understand environmental factors that might affect child sleep
5. Help parents identify necessary changes in family/child routines that will maximize healthy sleep behavior
6. Help parents make necessary changes by providing concrete strategies
7. Conduct follow-up or ask your nurse to do so after parents and their child visit.

SUMMARY

In the present article, the authors emphasize the importance of incorporating healthy sleep education, transferring relevant knowledge of the impact of sleep on health and academic performance, and provision of useful tools to the busy health care provider using multiple ready-to-use information sources and strategies. This approach will result in several important benefits. First, youth sleep quality will be fundamentally improved, with positive impacts on both overall health and daytime functioning. Also, such an effort will advance partnerships among clinicians and the families they serve, resulting in significant lifestyle changes essential for healthy sleep and will promote a balanced, healthy lifestyle in families with children. Effective interventions include educational strategies offered via one-on-one interaction, either delivered face to face in the office of a clinician or health care provider by the pediatrician or the nurse, or over the phone, or via the Internet. Follow-up is recommended, and tailoring of any program to the unique needs and characteristics of a particular family will greatly enhance effectiveness. Future work should be conducted on skill-building strategies that focus on helping doctors and parents facilitate and maintain change in sleep behavior of children and adolescents.

REFERENCES

1. Gruber R, Wiebe S, Wells S, et al. Sleep and academic success: mechanisms, empirical evidence and interventional Strategies. Adolesc Med 2010;21:522–41.
2. National Sleep Foundation. Sleep in America Poll. Washington, DC: National Sleep Foundation; 2010. 2006.
3. Moore RY. The fourth C.U. Ariens Kappers lecture. The organization of the human circadian timing system. Prog Brain Res 1992;93:99–115 [discussion: 115–7].
4. Moore RY, Eichler VB. Loss of a circadian adrenal corticosterone rhythm following suprachiasmatic lesions in the rat. Brain Res 1972;42:201–6.
5. Dunlap J. Molecular bases for circadian clocks. Cell 1999;96:271–90.
6. Ralph MR, Foster RG, Davis FC, et al. Transplanted suprachiasmatic nucleus determines circadian period. Science 1990;247:975–8.
7. Van Esseveldt KE, Lehman MN, Boer GJ. The suprachiasmatic nucleus and the circadian time-keeping system revisited. Brain Res Brain Res Rev 2000;33: 34–77.
8. Koulouglioti C, Cole R, Kitzman H. Inadequate sleep and unintentional injuries in young children. Public Health Nurs 2008;25:106–14.

 9. Buysse DJ, Reynolds CF, Monk TH, et al. The Pittsburgh Sleep Quality Index: a new instrument for psychiatric practice and research. Psychiatry Res 1989; 28:193–213.
10. Mindell JA, Owens JA. Sleep problems in pediatric practice: clinical issues for the pediatric nurse practitioner. J Pediatr Health Care 2003;17:324–31.
11. Medem, Inc. Physician's use of the internet. San Francisco (CA): Medem Inc; 2000.
12. Margolis CZ, Warshawsky SS, Goldman L, et al. Computerized algorithms and pediatricians' management of common problems in a community clinic. Acad Med 1992;67:282–4.
13. Richards HM, Sullivan FM, Mitchell ED, et al. Computer use by general practitioners in Scotland. Br J Gen Pract 1998;48:1473–6.
14. Papp KK, Penrod CE, Strohl KP. Knowledge and attitudes of primary care physicians toward sleep and sleep disorders. Sleep Breath 2002;6(3): 103–9.
15. Owens JA. The practice of pediatric sleep medicine: results of a community survey. Pediatrics 2001;108:E51.
16. Rosen RC, Rosekind M, Rosevear C, et al. Physician education in sleep and sleep disorders: a national survey of U.S. medical schools. Sleep 1993;16: 249–54.
17. Rosen R, Mahowald M, Chesson A, et al. The Taskforce 2000 survey on medical education in sleep and sleep disorders. Sleep 1998;21:235–8.
18. Stores G, Crawford C. Medical student education in sleep and its disorders. J R Coll Physicians Lond 1998;32:149–53.
19. Mindell JA, Moline ML, Zendell SM, et al. Pediatricians and sleep disorders: training and practice. Pediatrics 1994;94:194–200.
20. Moline ML, Zendell SM. Sleep education in professional training programs. Sleep Research 1993;22:1.
21. Rosen R, Zozula R. Education and training in the field of sleep medicine. Curr Opin Pulm Med 2000;6:512–8.
22. Stremler R, Hodnett E, Lee K. A behavioral-educational intervention to promote maternal and infant sleep: a pilot randomized, controlled trial. Sleep 2006;29: 1609–15.
23. St James-Roberts I, Sleep J, Morris S, et al. Use of a behavioural programme in the first 3 months to prevent infant crying and sleeping problems. J Paediatr Child Health 2001;37:289–97.
24. Kerr SM, Jowett SA, Smith LN. Preventing sleep problems in infants: a randomized controlled trial. J Adv Nurs 1996;24:938–42.
25. Pinilla T, Birch L. Help me make it through the night: behavioural entrainment breast-fed infants' sleep patterns. Pediatrics 1993;91:436.
26. Wolfson A, Lacks P, Futterman A. Effects of parent training on infant sleeping patterns, parents' stress, and perceived parental competence. J Consult Clin Psychol 1992;60:41–8.
27. Adair R, Zuckerman B, Bauchner H, et al. Reducing night waking in infancy: a primary care intervention. Pediatrics 1992;89:585–8.
28. Parenting matters: helping parents with young children. Available at: http://clinicaltrials.gov/ct2/show/study/NCT00133055. Accessed March 20, 2011.
29. Owens J, Dalzell V. Use of 'BEARS' sleep screening tool in a pediatric residents continuity clinic: a pilot study. Sleep Med 2005;6:63–9.
30. Chaput JP, Brunet M, Tremblay A. Relationship between short sleeping hours and childhood overweight/obesity: results from the 'Quebec en Forme' Project. Int J Obes (Lond) 2006;30(7):1080–5.

31. Magee CA, Huang X, Iverson D, et al. Examining the pathways linking chronic sleep restriction to obesity. J Obes 2010;2010:821710.
32. Taheri S, Lin L, Austin D, et al. Short sleep duration is associated with reduced leptin, elevated ghrelin, and increased body mass index. PLoS Med 2004;1:e62.
33. Mesulam M. Large-scale neurocognitive networks and distributed processing for attention, language, and memory. Ann Neurol 1990;28:597–613.
34. Dinges DF, Pack F, Williams K, et al. Cumulative sleepiness, mood disturbance, and psychomotor vigilance performance decrements during a week of sleep restricted to 4-5 h per night. Sleep 1997;20:267–77.
35. Sadeh A, Gruber R, Raviv A. The effects of sleep restriction/extension on school-age children: what a difference an hour makes? Child Dev 2003;74:444–55.
36. Fallone G, Owens J, Deane J. Sleepiness in children and adolescents: clinical implications. Sleep Med Rev 2002;6:287–306.
37. Moore M, Meltzer LJ. The sleepy adolescent: causes and consequences of sleepiness in teens. Paediatr Respir Rev 2008;9:114–20.
38. Pilcher JJ, Huffcutt AI. Effects of sleep deprivation on performance: a meta-analysis. Sleep 1996;19:318–26.
39. Gibson ES, Powles AC, Thabane L, et al. "Sleepiness" is serious in adolescence: two surveys of 3235 Canadian students. BMC Public Health 2006;6:116.
40. Buckhalt JA, El-Sheikh M, Keller P, et al. Concurrent and longitudinal relations between children's sleep and cognitive functioning: the moderating role of parent education. Child Dev 2009;80:875–92.
41. El-Sheikh M, Buckhalk A, Cummings M, et al. Sleep disruptions and emotional insecurity are pathways of risk for children. J Child Psychol Psychiatry 2007;48:88–96.
42. Wolfson AR, Spaulding NL, Dandrowe C, et al. Middle school start times: the importance of a good night's sleep for young adolescents. Behav Sleep Med 2007;5:194–209.
43. Meijer AM. Chronic sleep reduction, functioning at school and school achievement in preadolescents. J Sleep Res 2008;17:395–405.
44. Meijer AM, Habekothe HT, Van Den Wittenboer GL. Time in bed, quality of sleep and school functioning of children. J Sleep Res 2000;9:145–53.
45. Horn JL, Dollinger SJ. Effects of test anxiety, tests, and sleep on children's performance. J Sch Psychol 1989;27:373–82.
46. BaHammam A, Al-Faris E, Shaikh S, et al. Sleep problems/habits and school performance in elementary school children. Sleep Hypn 2006;8:13–9.
47. Keller PS, El-Sheikh M, Buckhalt JA. Children's attachment to parents and their academic functioning: sleep disruptions as moderators of effects. J Dev Behav Pediatr 2008;29:441–9.
48. Pagel JF, Forister N, Kwiatkowki C. Adolescent sleep disturbance and school performance: the confounding variable of socioeconomics. J Clin Sleep Med 2007;3:19–23.
49. Moore RY. A clock for the ages. Science 1999;284:2102–3.
50. Czeisler CA, Allan JS, Strogatz S, et al. Bright light resets the human circadian pacemaker independent of the timing of the sleep-wake cycle. Science 1986;233:667–71.
51. Borbely AA. A two process model of sleep regulation. Hum Neurobiol 1982;1:195–204.
52. Ebadi M, Govitrapong P. Neural pathways and neurotransmitters affecting melatonin synthesis. J Neural Transm Suppl 1986;21:125–55.
53. Allada R, White N, Venus W, et al. A mutant *Drosophila* homolog of mammalian Clock disrupts circadian rhythms and transcription of period and timeless. Cell 1998;93:791–804.

54. Blau J, Young MW. Cycling vrille expression is required for a functional *Drosophila* clock. Cell 1999;99:661–71.
55. Czeisler CA, Duffy JF, Shanahan TL, et al. Stability, precision, and near-24-hour period of the human circadian pacemaker. Science 1999;284:2177–81.
56. Mindell J, Meltzer LJ, Carskadon MA, et al. Developmental aspects of sleep hygiene: findings from the 2004 National Sleep Foundation Sleep in America Poll. Sleep Med 2009;10:771–9.
57. Hunt SM, McEwen J, McKenna SP. Measuring health status: a new tool for clinicians and epidemiologists. J R Coll Gen Pract 1985;35(273):185–8.
58. Mezick EJ, Matthews K, Hall M, et al. Influence of race and socioeconomic status on sleep: Pittsburgh SleepSCORE project. Psychosom Med 2008;70:410–6.
59. Patel NP, Grander M, Xie D, et al. "Sleep disparity" in the population: poor sleep quality is strongly associated with poverty and ethnicity. BMC Public Health 2010;10:475.
60. Van Cauter E, Spiegel K. Sleep as a mediator of the relationship between socioeconomic status and health: a hypothesis. Ann N Y Acad Sci 1999;896:254–61.
61. Kim EJ, Dimsdale JE. The effect of psychosocial stress on sleep: a review of polysomnographic evidence. Behav Sleep Med 2007;5:256–78.
62. Liu X, Liu L, Wang R. Bed sharing, sleep habits, and sleep problems among Chinese school-aged children. Sleep 2003;26:839–44.
63. Lozoff B, Askew GL, Wolf AW. Cosleeping and early childhood sleep problems: effects of ethnicity and socioeconomic status. J Dev Behav Pediatr 1996;17:9–15.
64. Frosch CA, Mangelsdorf SC, McHale JL. Marital behavior and the security of preschooler-parent attachment relationships. J Fam Psychol 2000;14:144–61.
65. Davies PT, Cummings EM, Winter MA. Pathways between profiles of family functioning, child security in the interparental subsystem, and child psychological problems. Dev Psychopathol 2004;16:525–50.
66. Belsky J, Fearon RM. Early attachment security, subsequent maternal sensitivity, and later child development: does continuity in development depend upon continuity of caregiving? Attach Hum Dev 2002;4:361–87.
67. Belsky J, Fearon RM. Infant-mother attachment security, contextual risk, and early development: a moderational analysis. Dev Psychopathol 2002;14:293–310.
68. Nair H, Murray AD. Predictors of attachment security in preschool children from intact and divorced families. J Genet Psychol 2005;166:245–63.
69. Sadeh A. Stress, trauma and sleep in children. Child Adolesc Psychiatr Clin N Am 1996;5:685–700.
70. Liu X, Sun Z, Uchiyama M, et al. Prevalence and correlates of sleep problems in Chinese school children. Sleep 2000;23:1053–62.
71. Benoit D, Zeanah CH, Boucher C, et al. Sleep disorders in early childhood: association with insecure maternal attachment. J Am Acad Child Adolesc Psychiatry 1992;31:86–99.
72. Glod CA. Circadian dysregulation in abused individuals: a proposed theoretical model for practice and research. Arch Psychiatr Nurs 1992;6:347–55.
73. El-Sheikh M, Buckhalt J, Mize J. Marital conflict and disruption of children's sleep. Child Dev 2006;77:31–43.
74. About kids health. Available at: http://www.aboutkidshealth.ca/. Accessed November 17, 2010.
75. Sleepeducation.com. Available at: http://www.sleepeducation.com/index.aspx. Accessed November 17, 2010.
76. National Sleep Foundation Pillow Talk. Available at: http://answers.sleepfoundation.org/. Accessed November 17, 2010.

77. Sleep for kids. Available at: http://www.SleepforKids.org. Accessed November 17, 2010.
78. Kids Health Library. Available at: http://www.thechildrenshospital.org/wellness/info/results.aspx?search=sleep&id=32. Accessed November 17, 2010.
79. MacLeish M, Thomson W, Moreno N. The National Space Biomedical Research Institute's education and public outreach program: working toward a global 21st century space exploration society. Acta Astronautica 2011;68:1614–9.
80. Gruber R, Sommerville G, Brouillette D, et al. Sleep for success overview. Montreal (Quebec): McGill University; 2009.
81. Blunden S. The implementation of a sleep education program in adolescents. Sleep Biol Rhythm 2007;5:A37.
82. Bakotić M, Radošević-Vidaček B, Košćec A. Educating adolescents about healthy sleep: experimental study of effectiveness of educational leaflet. Croat Med J 2009;50:174.
83. Moseley L, Gradisar M. Evaluation of a school-based intervention for adolescent sleep problems. Sleep 2009;32:334–41.
84. De Sousa I, Araújo J, De Azevedo C. The effect of a sleep hygiene education program on the sleep–wake cycle of Brazilian adolescent students. Sleep Biol Rhythm 2007;5:251–8.
85. Cortesi F, Giannotti F, Sebastiani T, et al. Knowledge of sleep in Italian high school students: pilot-test of school-based sleep educational program. J Adolesc Health 2004;34:344–51.
86. Rossi CM, Campbell AL, Vo OT, et al. Middle school sleep-smart program: a pilot evaluation. Sleep 2002;25:A279.
87. Cain N, Gradisar M. Electronic media use and sleep in school-aged children and adolescents: a review. Sleep Med 2010;11:735–42.
88. Philip P, Ghorayeb I, Stoohs R, et al. Determinants of sleepiness in automobile drivers. J Psychosom Res 1996;41:279–88.

Cultural Issues in Children's Sleep: A Model for Clinical Practice

Oskar G. Jenni, MD*, Helene Werner, PhD

KEYWORDS

- Children • Sleep behavior and problems • Sleep regulation
- Cultural values and beliefs • Interactional • Transactional
- Goodness of fit

Sleep is a human behavior that is driven by biologic mechanisms, but also is strongly shaped and interpreted by cultural values and beliefs.[1] Over the past years, several articles have been published offering comprehensive overviews about cultural aspects of sleep in healthy children and children with medical conditions,[2–4] as well as presenting cross-cultural comparative data about sleep behaviors in different societies.[5,6] This article ties to the review by Jenni and O'Connor,[1] which was published in 2005 in *Pediatrics* as a corollary of efforts of a collaborative group of health care professionals to increase awareness of the influence of culture on sleep behavior in children.

Many "problems" with sleep behavior during childhood are based on culturally constructed definitions and expectations and not primarily founded in organic disorders (eg, sleep-disordered breathing). Children's behavioral sleep difficulties may include bedtime resistance, frequent nocturnal wakings, or the inability to sleep independently, which are typically reported by the caregivers and not by the children themselves. However, acceptability and interpretation of these sleep complaints as well as the need for treatment interventions by health care professionals are shaped by parental cultural values, norms, and beliefs. For instance, Stearns and Rowland[7] showed that sleep problems are not a matter of concern in Japan (in contrast to the United States) and are seldom the reason for a pediatric consultation. Mindell and colleagues[6] reported that only 11% of Thai parents indicated that their child had a sleep problem, whereas 76% of Chinese caregivers did so. These findings may

This work was supported by a research grant from the Swiss National Science Foundation (grant no 32473B_129956) and the Anna Mueller Grocholski-Foundation.
The authors have nothing to disclose.
Child Development Center, University Children's Hospital Zurich, Steinwiesstrasse 75, CH-8032 Zurich, Switzerland
* Corresponding author.
E-mail address: oskar.jenni@kispi.uzh.ch

reflect true cross-cultural differences, but may also point to completely different interpretations of children's sleep behavior in Japanese, Thai, and Chinese caregivers (or alternatively to a strong culturally driven reporting bias). Another example shows that Italian parents prefer to have their infants sleep in their rooms with them, irrespective of availability of separate rooms for children and parents, and consider the American norm of putting children to bed in separate rooms as not appropriate.[8] In fact, letting the child fall asleep alone in a separate room may reflect the sociocultural emphasis toward individualism with the belief in individuals' self-reliance and personal independence. These examples raise the question of whether at least some sleep problems during childhood are not primarily created by specific cultural practices, which may be incongruent with aspects of individual sleep biology or with stages of children's socioemotional development.

Culturally appropriate pediatric care is increasingly recognized as an important clinical competency, because health care professionals are confronted more and more with patients and families of widely differing cultural origins.[9] Geopolitical boundary shifts, changes in immigration patterns, and refugee relocation in response to political or economic conflicts have created large demographic changes in many countries. In addition, many ethnic groups within the countries have grown and now include large percentages of patient populations. Understanding culturally driven needs and views of patients and families may help to assess, interpret, and eventually treat children's sleep difficulties. Health care professionals should also be aware of one's own culture or at least of the culturally driven aspects of intervention procedures that they use. For instance, the developmental milestone and concept of intervention of "independent self-soothing" may not be shared by parents from all societies and cultures around the world. Health care professionals need to recognize the culture in which children and their families live, and must know how cultural beliefs and values interact with the psychosocial needs and biological characteristics of individual children, which may eventually lead to better compliance and higher success of treatment interventions.

THE DEFINITION OF CULTURE

The term "culture" is extremely difficult to define, which has led to a large proliferation of definitions.[10] Most scholars consider culture as a set of habits, values, beliefs, and practices that members of a distinct society use to interact with each other and which are learned, acquired, and transmitted through symbols, institutions, and technologies.[11] Culture may be defined at the level of an entire society (eg, referring to a group of individuals with common nationality) but also on the level of distinct groups within any society (eg, referring to a group of individuals with common religious beliefs). The term "culture" is often used erroneously in the context of race (referring to a group of individuals with the same physical characteristics, for example skin color) or when being assigned to minority populations, or is even sometimes used as a causal factor for a disorder. Despite the difficulties to define the word "culture" there seems consensus that "culture emerges in adaptive interactions between humans and environment, consists of shared elements between individuals and is transmitted across time periods and generations."[12]

Jenni and O'Connor[1] have adopted David Hufford's view that "culture is the entire non-biological inheritance of human beings."[13] In other words, everything that human beings inherit from one generation to the next that is not passed on biologically is a part of culture. To put it simply: "if you got it from other human beings and you didn't get it through biology, then you got it through culture."[1] We are all included in this broad definition of culture: culture is not something that comes through the door with patients. It means that not only values, languages, religions, arts, cuisines, modes of dress, family structures, authority relationships, gender roles, social behavioral norms, and modes of communication are elements of culture, but also economic and political structures, sciences, modern information technologies, bodies of knowledge and texts, reference works, and health care resources. All are products of culture, and all reflect cultural shaping.

There are many cultural differences that may be described in multiple dimensions.[14] As a typical example, cultures may be distinguished on the basis of their individualism/collectivism or independency/interdependency dimension (although this classification is rather simplistic because not all members of a culture may share the same tendencies and behave in different manner[15]). Individualism refers to when individuals view themselves as separate and autonomous from each other, whereas collectivism refers to when individuals view themselves as interconnected and defined by their relations and social context.[16] Asian countries predominantly rely on collectivism, whereas Euroamerican (Caucasian) countries rely on individualism. Cultural differences or cultural standards may also be described in the dimension of uncertainty avoidance (to which extent rules are used to live together) or power distance (how it is expected that power is equally or unequally distributed).[16] Cultural standards always indicate how members of a specific culture should behave and how objects and actions should be valued and coped with.[17] It is important to bear in mind, however, that all cultures are partial, in the sense that they select for certain human preferences and omit (or never even imagine) others. In addition, while cultures provide some guidelines for regulating human behavior, in reality there are considerable individual differences in the behavior within a culture.

CROSS-CULTURAL COMPARATIVE ASPECTS

Cross-cultural comparative research among societies of different political, economic, and ideological backgrounds is a straightforward approach for the study of the roles of culture on sleep behavior and its interpretation. Previous studies have primarily focused on key aspects of sleep behavior: sleep duration and sleep need; bedtime routines; napping; children's use of sleep aids; sleeping arrangements, particularly cosleeping of children and parents; sleep problems including bedtime resistance, nighttime awakenings, and sleep terrors. For detailed information the reader is referred to previous work.[1–6]

However, do the variations in sleep behavior across cultures reflect the true cultural differences or rather differences based on the methodology used? The scientific pediatric sleep literature cited in previous articles illustrates some of the inherent difficulties in comparative and cross-cultural research. For example, studies within and across countries and cultures have used different recruitment strategies (eg, population randomly selected from national surveys or from clinical, urban, or rural populations), and have examined different numbers of subjects and descriptions of age ranges. In addition, the variation of reported sleep behavior across decades limits comparability between studies performed at different times. Problems in cross-cultural research particularly arise in the attempt to compare studies of cultural groups conducted with instruments (eg, questionnaires sent by mail or filled out in the pediatrician's office, or face-to-face or telephone interviews) that have not been cross-culturally standardized, appropriately translated, or validated for the populations under study (see also Sagheri and colleagues[18]).

Another problem lies in the numerous definitions of key terms. For example, "sleep amount," "sleep need," "sleep duration," and "time in bed" are terms that often are used interchangeably in the literature. Apart from the obvious problem that "time in bed" may be different from actual sleep time and thus is not a reliable proxy for "sleep amount or duration," these common research terms may have different conceptual meanings across the cultures in which the studies were conducted. In a substantial number of studies, sleep behavior and practices have not been assessed with appropriate validated instruments or qualitative inquiry.[18] Rather, general cultural influences have been assumed or inferred according to the investigators' own (often tacit) guiding assumptions.

True cross-cultural comparative studies of children's sleep behavior are extremely rare. There is currently only one large-scale survey available that describes parent-reported sleep patterns and behaviors, sleep problems, and sleeping arrangements of children using the same method in 17 Caucasian and Asian countries.[6] If we bear in mind that countries should not be equated with culture (because of the large cultural heterogeneity that exists within any country), this Internet-based study by Mindell and colleagues[6] shows that infants and toddlers in Asian countries may obtain less overall sleep, have later bedtimes, are more likely to room-share, and are perceived to have more sleep problems than children of the same age in Caucasian countries. However, the investigators may not answer the question as to whether these variations reflect true differences in children's sleep behavior or rather indicate culturally driven reporting biases. Individuals living in diverse cultural value systems may demonstrate different types of response biases when completing behavioral surveys. Thus, objective methods for assessing sleep behavior should be included in future cross-cultural studies.[16] By the comparison of agreement rates between objective measures and subjective reports of different cultures, the reporting biases may be operationalized and described.[19] It is interesting that the study by Mindell and colleagues[5] also indicates that not all aspects of sleep are influenced by cultural beliefs and practices to the same extent: daytime sleep seems to be less likely influenced than nocturnal sleep, which may point to a strong biological drive for sleeping during the day.

SLEEP BIOLOGY AND SLEEP CULTURE
Sleep Biology

Over the past decades much has been learned about the structure of sleep, its regulation, and its purpose. Among the explanations for the biological function of sleep, 2 hypotheses have dominated the field: sleep is restorative for brain metabolism and sleep serves memory consolidation, learning and brain plasticity. Considering such vital functions for the organism, sleep must be regulated by biological processes.[20] In fact, deprivation from or restriction of sleep lead to a higher degree of sleepiness and a compensatory response with increased need for sleep. Specific biological processes (ie, circadian and homeostatic) and the interaction between these two processes play an important role in determining the duration and timing of individuals' sleep.[21,22] The endogenous nature of sleep and its regulation have been well described based on the basis of general mechanisms, but human beings obviously demonstrate considerable interindividual differences in their sleep patterns as well as in their ability to compensate for insufficient sleep. The large variability between individuals is also reflected in their habitual sleep duration (long sleepers vs short sleepers) and their preferred bedtime.[23,24] "Larks" or "morning people" show a preference for waking at an early hour and find it difficult to remain awake beyond their usual bedtime, as compared with "owls" or "night people," who show a preference for sleeping at later hours and often find it difficult to get up in the morning. Theoretically, interindividual differences may be related to differences in both or only one of the two biological processes as well as to differences in the interaction between the two processes.

However, one study indicated that the between-subject variability of habitual sleep duration has a biological basis through the individually programmed circadian clock.[23] The circadian pacemaker programs the daily cyclic change in the body's internal milieu (eg, neuroendocrine function, body temperature) and is synchronized by periodic stimuli acting on the clock (eg, light). Circadian rhythms arise from autoregulatory transcriptional and translational feedback cycles of clock genes in cells of the suprachiasmatic nucleus.[25] So it is conceivable that polymorphisms in one or several of these genes result in differences in the duration of the circadian rhythm's nocturnal interval and thus in the duration of sleep.

Even though most research on sleep biology has been performed either in adults or animals, an increase of interest is also apparent in how sleep is regulated in children and adolescents and in what function(s) sleep serves during development.[26] It is most likely that children, like adults, exhibit large interindividual differences in their ability to regulate sleep and in their particular "natural" sleep rhythms. Differences in sleep patterns as a function of development (sleep duration across childhood declines and the timing of sleep undergoes a gradual shift to later bedtimes[24]) and the fact that children's sleep is much more embedded in the context of the family compared with adolescents and adults add to the complexity of understanding sleep behavior in children.

Sleep Culture

Interindividual differences in sleep behavior are not only based on genetic variations or age-related and health-related issues (eg, medication), but may also be associated with differences in environmental circumstances. For example, work or school schedules, acting as strong social "zeitgebers" on individual's sleep, vary substantially across societies. Social institutional demands, such as the requirement that school is standardized to begin at specific times, that children who attend them be on time, and that there are special days (vacations, days of rest, or days of special religious or social obligation) in which the typical pattern is permitted or required to be broken, substantially influence the regulation of sleep.

Children's sleep, however, is also embedded in the context of the family with its characteristics of size, composition, family lifestyle, parental personality, and parenting styles (a well-articulated overview of the involved components in children's sleep behavior gives the transactional model of Sadeh and Anders[27]). The family may be seen as the "development niche" in which children's behavior is conditioned and regulated.[28] Children learn what is expected of them, how they are expected to engage in activities, the ways other individuals will deal with them, and the ways in which they are expected to deal with others.[11] Or in brief, children become skilled in the cultural practices and learn the values, concepts, and ways of behaving that are valued in the culture in which children are living.[11] In the context of sleep behavior, this means for example that some parents have strict and rigid views about their children's bedtime, whereas others are less strict. In some families, there is a routine around the time of bed with a fixed order of events, culminating in a bedtime story while the child drops off to sleep. In other families, parents are much more likely just to wait for the child to become tired and fall off to sleep wherever the child is or allow the children to watch a DVD tape in order to settle down and fall asleep (see the vignettes in Tudge,[11 pp247–56]). The examples cited in the study by Tudge[11] indicate that there are large differences in parenting practices across different cultures (eg, control of children, degree of parental authority, expression and involvement of affection, and values of achievement).

The previously mentioned study of Mindell and colleagues[5] also explored the differences in sleep-related parenting behaviors (eg, parental involvement at bedtime by holding, rocking, feeding) in Caucasian and Asian infants and toddlers. These investigators reported that parents of Asian cultures engage more at bedtime, whereas children of Caucasians fall asleep more frequently independently in their own crib or bed. But what do these findings means for the individual child and his or her sleep quality and overall well-being? Do children of parents who engage more at bedtime sleep better than those who engage less? Self-soothing and falling asleep independently are seen as key components in the development of consolidated sleep. In line with this view, the study of Mindell and colleagues[5] indicates that children of parents who engage more have more fragmented sleep than children of parents who engage less, although we still do not know whether children with longer and less fragmented sleep are really better sleepers and perform better during the day or not.

Sleeping too little, too late, too much, too fragmented, at wrong times, or in wrong places may be indicators of "abnormality." However, the boundaries between "normal" and "problematic" are often defined by cultural norms and values. The authors believe that indicators of abnormality are typically based on the extent to which individuals conform to sleep schedule and sleep behavior expectations.

INTERACTION BETWEEN BIOLOGY AND CULTURE IN SLEEP BEHAVIOR

Actual sleep behavior and problems are the result of the complex interplay of biological, psychological, developmental, environmental, and social influences. However, the relative contributions of each of these individual aspects are often difficult to separate.[4] Over the past century, several developmental theorists have conceptualized the bidirectional interplay of culture and biology in human behavior by interactional (or transactional) models.[29] These models stress that all aspects of complex systems are mutually interinfluential, covariant, and constantly dynamic. As spelled out by Chess and Thomas,[29] application of this approach to human behavior requires that "behavioral attributes must always be considered in their reciprocal relationship with other characteristics of the organism and in their interaction with environmental demands, opportunities and stresses."

Chess and Thomas[29] have provided an integrative analysis of the nature and dynamics of interactional processes in their concept of "goodness of fit," which means specifically that culturally defined expectations of how the child is taught and permitted to sleep match well with the individual child's sleep biology or individual characteristics (eg, emotional needs). Culturally guided parental strategies around bedtime that best satisfy adult interests and needs, for example, may not be in accord with those that best serve the child's needs ("poor fit" for the child). For example, the situation in which the parents biologically prefer to go to bed late and it is an expected cultural custom to eat dinner late at night, as observed in many regions around the world, is considered a "good fit." If their child's biological preference for waking up in the morning is early, it may not be in harmony with the parent's demands and cultural expectations. Or as another example, Euroamerican parents generally seek to provide confidence and emotional security and to accommodate individual needs of the child during the day[30]; but on the other hand they expect their child to go to bed at a specified time, irrespective of evidence of sleepiness, and to sleep alone and isolated in a dark room, as culturally anticipated. The Euroamerican child whose individual emotional needs might be for close proximity to parents or other family members while sleeping or for a bedtime congruent with his or her internal biological clock might find a "better fit" for sleeping in the normative practices of Italy or in Japan than in his or her own culture.[8,31]

We know that cultural values and beliefs may shape biology to some extent, and that neurobiological processes may also facilitate the emergence and transmission of cultural traits.[16] Children grow up in a family that is embedded in a culture and learn the specific sleep routines (eg, cosleeping, bedtime rituals, sleeping environment) as the normal and appropriate ones. Whereas some parents shape their parenting strategies and sleep routines in response to their children's behaviors, others may follow the accepted cultural standards (eg, letting the child to fall asleep alone). Most children can adapt and cope with a certain approach well, but a significant number of children struggle. In fact, a "poor fit" between culturally normative bedtime or sleep practices and individual sleep biology or individual emotional needs may eventually lead to behavioral sleep problems such as sleep-onset difficulties. Current clinical recommendations in pediatric sleep medicine are often based on changing the individual child (extinction of the undesired behavior) or altering parental behavior (eg, reducing parental involvement around bedtime) toward accepted cultural standards, rather than trying to find a balance between both the child's and parent's individual needs, and thus to transfer a "poor fit" into a "good fit" (or at least a "better fit").

SUMMARY AND PRACTICAL CONCLUSIONS

Health care professionals dealing with children's sleep problems need to recognize the cultural environment in which children live and how cultural habits, values, beliefs, and practices interact with the psychosocial needs of the individual child and with the biological characteristics of his or her sleep patterns. It is not necessary to know everything about cultural diversity or to be an "expert" on culture, but it is important to know that key aspects of children's sleep behavior are influenced by culture. Knowing that children "typically" exhibit a particular behavior at a specific developmental stage (eg, separation anxiety) or that children of a certain age must sleep for a specific time period is not enough; to best meet the needs of patients and families, it is imperative to acknowledge individual psychosocial and biological/physiological needs in the context of the cultural background and social circumstances. The authors believe that notions like sleeping to little, too late, too fragmented, at wrong places, and so forth are related to cultural expectations and norms, which should be primarily assessed on the basis of the individual sleep patterns and sleep difficulties of the child.

The description of cross-cultural differences in children's sleep patterns and practices (in the view of the aforementioned methodological problems) may provide an important basis for the awareness of difference and the reconsideration of our own culture. Culturally appropriate pediatric care includes the systematic reflection of one's own culture's values and preferences, and to the ways in which these conditions influence responses and expectations, both in the clinic and in all aspects of research design and interpretation.

The large diversity of children's sleep behaviors among societies and cultures may in fact indicate that one "optimal cultural standard" does not exist. The "goodness of fit" between individual children's biologic and socioemotional needs and their cultural environments may provide a conceptual model for clinical practice.

REFERENCES

1. Jenni OG, O'Connor BB. Children's sleep: an interplay between culture and biology. Pediatrics 2005;115(Suppl 1):204–16.
2. Boergers J, Koinis-Mitchell D. Sleep and culture in children with medical conditions. J Pediatr Psychol 2010;35(9):915–26.

3. Giannotti F, Cortesi F. Family and cultural influences on sleep development. Child Adolesc Psychiatr Clin N Am 2009;18(4):849–61.

4. Owens J. Sleep in children: cross-cultural perspectives. Sleep Biol Rhythm 2004; 2:165–73.

5. Mindell JA, Sadeh A, Kohyama J, et al. Parental behaviors and sleep outcomes in infants and toddlers: a cross-cultural comparison. Sleep Med 2010;11(4):393–9.

6. Mindell JA, Sadeh A, Wiegand B, et al. Cross-cultural differences in infant and toddler sleep. Sleep Med 2010;11(3):274–80.

7. Stearns PN, Rowland P. Children's sleep: sketching historical change. J Soc Hist 1996;30(2):345–67.

8. Wolf AW, Lozoff B, Latz S, et al. Parental theories in the management of young children's sleep in Japan, Italy, and the United States. In: Harkness S, Super CM, editors. Parents' cultural belief systems: their origins, expressions, and consequences. New York: Guilford Press; 1996. p. 364–84.

9. Lynch WE, Hanson MJ. Developing cross-cultural competence. Baltimore (MD): Paul H. Brookes Publishing Co; 2004.

10. Matsumoto D. Culture and cultural worldviews: do verbal descriptions about culture reflect anything other than verbal descriptions of culture? Cult Psychol 2006;12(1):33–62.

11. Tudge J. The everyday lives of young children: culture, class, and child rearing in diverse societies. New York: Cambridge University Press; 2008.

12. Triandis HC. Culture and psychology: a history of the study of their relationships. In: Kitayama S, Cohen D, editors. Handbook of cultural psychology. New York: Guilford Press; 2007. p. 59–76.

13. Hufford DJ. Culturally sensitive delivery of health care and human services. In: Staub S, editor. Proceedings of the governor's conference on ethnicity. Harrisburg (PA): Pennsylvania Heritage Affairs Commission; 1990. p. 35–7.

14. Hofstede G. Culture's consequences: comparing values, behaviors, institutions and organisations across nations. Thousand Oaks (CA): Sage Publications; 2001.

15. Strauss C. The culture concept and the individualism-collectivism debate: dominant and alternative attributions for class in the United States. In: Saxe GB, Turiel E, editors. Culture, thought, and development. Mahwah (NJ): Erlbaum; 2000. p. 85–114.

16. Chiao JY. Cultural neuroscience: a once and future discipline. Prog Brain Res 2009;178:287–304.

17. Thomas A. Kulturvergleichende Psychologie. Eine Einführung. Göttingen: Hogrefe; 1993.

18. Sagheri D, Wiater A, Steffen P, et al. Applying principles of good practice for translation and cross-cultural adaptation of sleep-screening instruments in children. Behav Sleep Med 2010;8:151–6.

19. Werner H, Molinari L, Guyer C, et al. Agreement rates between actigraphy, diary, and questionnaire for children's sleep patterns. Arch Pediatr Adolesc Med 2008; 162(4):350–8.

20. Achermann P, Borbély AA. Sleep homeostasis and models of sleep regulation. In: Kryger M, Roth T, Dement W, editors. Principles and practices of sleep medicine. 5th edition. St Louis (MO): Elsevier Saunders; 2010. p. 431–44.

21. Borbély AA. A two process model of sleep regulation. Hum Neurobiol 1982;1(3): 195–204.

22. Daan S, Beersma DG, Borbély AA. Timing of human sleep: recovery process gated by a circadian pacemaker. Am J Physiol 1984;246(2 Pt 2):R161–83.

23. Aeschbach D, Sher L, Postolache TT, et al. A longer biological night in long sleepers than in short sleepers. J Clin Endocrinol Metab 2003;88(1):26–30.
24. Iglowstein I, Jenni OG, Molinari L, et al. Sleep duration from infancy to adolescence: reference values and generational trends. Pediatrics 2003;111:302–7.
25. Brown SA, Kunz D, Dumas A, et al. Molecular insights into human daily behavior. Proc Natl Acad Sci U S A 2008;105(5):1602–7.
26. Jenni OG, LeBourgeois M. Understanding sleep-wake behavior and sleep disorders in children: the value of a model. Curr Opin Psychiatry 2006;19(3):982–7.
27. Sadeh A, Anders TF. Infant sleep problems: origins, assessment, interventions. Infant Ment Health J 1993;14(1):17–34.
28. Super CM, Harkness S. The developmental niche: a conceptualization at the interface of child and culture. Int J Behav Dev 1986;9:545–69.
29. Chess S, Thomas A. Origins and evolution of behavior disorders. New York: Brunner/Mazel; 1984.
30. Brazelton TB, Greenspan SI. The irreducible needs of children: what every child must have to grow, learn, and flourish. Boulder (CO): Perseus Publishing; 2000.
31. Steger B. Negotiating sleep patterns in Japan. In: Steger B, Brunt L, editors. Night-time and sleep in Asia and the west: exploring the dark side of life. London: Routledge Curzon; 2003. p. 65–86.

Sleep in the Family

Lisa J. Meltzer, PhD[a],*, Hawley E. Montgomery-Downs, PhD[b]

KEYWORDS
• Sleep • Family • Children • Parents

Family systems are dynamic, with reciprocal interactions among family members, including interactions at night and during the day. When children have sleep problems, they often awaken a parent, affecting parent sleep and subsequent parent daytime functioning. Parent behaviors, which are shaped by parental cognitions and beliefs about sleep, as well as external stressors (eg, work or marital problems), can also disrupt child sleep patterns. Thus sleep among children cannot be understood in isolation, but rather it is important to view sleep from a family context.[1] This article reviews the relationship between sleep among children and their parents from infancy through adolescence. It also reviews the added complexity for sleep in the family when a child has a chronic illness or development disorder. For the sake of brevity, we summarize all primary care roles as parents.

PREGNANCY, NEONATES, AND INFANTS

Hormonal changes contribute to alterations in maternal sleep as early as the first trimester,[2] resulting in less total sleep, lower sleep efficiency, more frequent night wakings, and less deep sleep than before pregnancy.[3,4] However, sleep is most disrupted in the immediate postpartum period. Compared with pregnancy, the postpartum period is characterized by a self-report of 3 times the number of nighttime awakenings, a decrease in sleep efficiency, and twice the level of daytime sleepiness.[5] Most postpartum mothers' sleep disturbances are caused by the newborns' sleep and feeding schedules.[6,7]

Newborn sleep is distributed almost equally across the day and night.[8] To match their newborns' polyphasic sleep pattern, mothers report having to adjust their own sleep schedule, often attempting to sleep when the baby sleeps. However, this can be challenging, often because of household chores, caring for other children, or simply the inability to fall asleep on demand for short periods of time. New mothers report being surprised by their level of sleep disturbance and daytime exhaustion.[9]

This work was supported by grant no. MH077662 from the National Institutes of Health.
The authors have nothing to disclose.
[a] Department of Pediatrics, National Jewish Health, 1400 Jackson Street, G311, Denver, CO 80206, USA
[b] Department of Psychology, West Virginia University, 53 Campus Drive, Morgantown, WV 26506-6040, USA
* Corresponding author.
E-mail address: meltzerl@njhealth.org

Despite the common belief that new mothers are significantly sleep deprived, recent evidence shows that mothers experience significant sleep fragmentation and low sleep efficiency rather than sleep loss per se. Their average total sleep time of 7.2 hours per night throughout the first 4 months after giving birth is within the recommended range.[10]

Sleep fragmentation can have a significant impact on women, most notably on mood. During the first week following childbirth, most women report baby blues, a risk factor for the onset of postpartum depression.[11,12] One of the major contributors to the baby blues is the fatigue caused by disrupted sleep. For example, one study found that the negative mood effects during the first postpartum week were mediated by the amount of time mothers spent awake during the night.[13] Another study found a strong association between fatigue caused by chronic sleep disruptions and the onset of depressive symptoms.[14]

Although sleep disruption is linked to the onset of postpartum depression and depressive symptoms, there is a bidirectional and interactive relation between sleep disruption and negative affect. Although infant sleep disruptions contribute to maternal sleep disruption and subsequent depressive symptoms, prenatal depressive symptoms or negative cognitions may also contribute to infant sleep problems. Maternal cognitions related to infant distress at night have been associated with poorer infant sleep quality.[15] One complicating factor is that sleep disruption during pregnancy may contribute to an accumulated sleep debt that then facilitates the onset of symptoms not directly attributable to childbirth or childcare.[16]

Fathers can also experience significant sleep disruptions in the postnatal period, including less total sleep time[2] and increased fatigue.[2,17,18] Research has shown that paternal cognitions about infant sleep were associated with infant sleep patterns,[19] but when fathers were involved with overall infant care, infants had fewer night awakenings.[20] Because they play an important role in infant sleep and development, it is important for future research studies and interventions to include fathers.

The dynamic relation between infant sleep and parent mood continues for infants 6 to 12 months of age. Although multiple studies have found an association between infant sleep problems and maternal depression,[14,21–23] longitudinal studies have shown that infant sleep problems contribute to maternal depressive symptoms.[24,25] In addition, maternal sleep quality has been shown to mediate the relation between infant sleep disturbances and maternal mood,[23,26] whereas resolution of infant sleep problems from the first to the second year after birth is more likely among mothers with lower depression and anxiety.[27]

For most infants, sleep begins to consolidate by 6 months of age, with infants establishing a circadian rhythm and no longer needing to feed during the night. However, for 17% to 46% of families, bedtime problems and night wakings persist.[23,28,29] If left untreated, infant sleep problems can continue into childhood.[25,30]

Most interventions to address sleep problems have focused on infants more than 6 months old, but preventative behavioral-educational interventions have also been found to promote maternal and infant sleep.[31–34] For infants 6 months and older, several behavioral treatment approaches have been recommended and shown to be efficacious, producing reliable and durable changes.[29] Behavioral intervention for infant sleep problems have also been shown to improve maternal mood,[35–38] decrease caregiver fatigue,[35,36] and reduce distress in both mothers and fathers,[39] with benefits for maternal depression maintained for up to 2 years.[37]

TODDLERS, PRESCHOOLERS, AND SCHOOL-AGED CHILDREN

A national survey of sleep in American children reported more than 50% of parents losing an average of 30 minutes of sleep per night because of their child's night awakenings.[40] The negative association between child sleep disruptions and parent sleep and health has also been reported in population studies of Australian preschoolers and Swedish school children. Sleep problems in Australian children were associated with psychological distress among mothers and poor general health among both mothers and fathers[28]; frequent night wakings in Swedish children were associated with maternal sleep problems, whereas difficulties falling asleep or sleep disordered breathing were associated with paternal sleep problems.[41]

Parental sleep schedules may also be influenced by children's sleep. One study of young children found that maternal chronotype was influenced by children's sleep patterns.[42] However, a study of school-aged children found no relation between parent and child sleep schedules.[43] Differences in the results from these studies are likely caused by child age, with parents becoming less involved with sleep routines as children get older. Furthermore, older children require less supervision when they awaken in the morning, reducing the impact of their sleep schedules on parent sleep schedules.

Beyond sleep schedules, 2 studies examined the impact of children's sleep disorders and sleep disturbances on parent sleep and parent functioning. One found daytime sleepiness in both mothers and fathers to be associated with child sleep problems, child sleep duration, and child daytime sleepiness.[44] Another study reported that maternal sleep quality, mood, parenting stress, fatigue, and daytime sleepiness were all worse when children had significant sleep disruptions.[45] Children's sleep disruptions were reported to have an indirect association with maternal daytime functioning, with children's sleep disruptions predicting maternal sleep quality, whereas maternal sleep quality predicted maternal negative daytime functioning (eg, depression, parenting stress).

Behavioral interventions for younger children (toddlers and preschooler) have been shown to be effective for improving both child sleep and family functioning, including parental depression, marital satisfaction, and parenting stress.[29,35,46,47] A recent study also found that the simple implementation of a consistent bedtime routine for infants and toddlers was associated with decreased maternal tension, anger, and fatigue.[48] A brief behavioral sleep intervention among 8 to 10 month olds was associated with not only fewer child sleep problems 2 years after treatment but also fewer symptoms of maternal depression.[37] Together these studies show the effectiveness and durability of changes to the child's sleep, parent's sleep, and family functioning. However, few studies have examined treatments for sleep problems in typically developing school-aged children, with a recent call for more research in this area.[49]

This article has primarily focused on the premise that children's sleep problems disrupt parent sleep and family functioning. However, several recent studies have also examined aspects of families that may influence a child's sleep. One group has found marital conflict to be associated with disruptions to sleep quantity and quality among third graders.[50,51] In a 2-year follow-up of these youth, initial emotional security predicted later sleep duration and quality, with emotional security about marital relationships negatively associated with child sleepiness, sleep-wake problems, and increased sleep onset latency.[52] In a cross-sectional nationally representative study, parental warmth was related to increased total sleep time among school-aged children.[53] Although more research is needed in this area, it is clear that family functioning plays an important role in children's sleep.

ADOLESCENTS

In general, adolescents in the United States are sleep deprived, averaging only 7.6 hours, considerably less than the required 9.2 hours.[54,55] This sleep deprivation is primarily caused by academic and social demands that result in late bedtimes and early wake times, as well as a circadian shift in the underlying biologic clock. This shortened sleep opportunity may also influence parent sleep, although few studies have examined this issue. For example, parents may have difficulties initiating and maintaining sleep if they are waiting for their teen to come home late at night, or parent sleep may be delayed if an adolescent needs to be picked up after a late night extracurricular activity or social event.

Only a handful of studies have examined the relationship between adolescent sleep and either parent sleep or family functioning. Parents are typically not involved with adolescent sleep routines. However, one study reported that adolescent total sleep time increased with parental rules (including an earlier bedtime).[53] Another study found that psychological distress mediated the relationship between parental involvement and sleep efficiency in adolescents with a history of substance abuse.[56] When parents were more involved with monitoring, adolescents experienced less psychological distress and greater sleep efficiency. In addition, a study of undergraduate students found that family stressors predicted insomnia, even after controlling for depression.[57]

Three other studies have examined the association between adolescent and parent sleep.[58–60] Each of these studies reported that adolescent sleep quantity, sleep quality, and/or sleep problems were associated with family factors, including parenting style, family problems, and the atmosphere in the home. Together, these studies suggest a dynamic relationship between adolescent and parent sleep, with adolescent sleep affected by poor parenting or family functioning. In turn, poor parenting may result from poor parent sleep, which may be a result of poor or insufficient adolescent sleep. However, each of these studies was limited by relying solely on the adolescent's report of both their own and their parents' sleep. More research is needed that examines the association between adolescent sleep, parent sleep, and family functioning.

CHRONIC ILLNESS

A chronic illness affects family functioning in many ways, including sleep disruptions for both children and caregivers. Sleep problems among children can be caused by disease symptoms (eg, pain, itching, wheezing) or medical management of the disease (eg, nocturnal blood glucose monitoring).[61–67] Parent sleep may be disrupted because of heightened vigilance (eg, monitoring for a seizure), worries about the child's health, or changes to sleeping arrangements (eg, increased cosleeping).[61,68–70]

Together, these factors result in significant sleep deprivation in parental caregivers, with studies reporting an average of less than 6 hours of sleep for many parents.[68,69,71] With research showing significant declines in alertness and memory after 18 cumulative hours of wakefulness,[72] the significant sleep loss experienced by caregivers may interfere with the parents' ability to provide the best medical care in the home or make critical medical decisions.[73,74]

Sleep disruptions in parents of children with chronic illnesses have also been associated with increased symptoms of depression and anxiety, less marital satisfaction, poorer parent health, and more days of missed work.[62,68,75,76] Two studies have shown that sleep quality in parental caregivers mediates the relationship between child health and negative caregiver outcomes (ie, depression, anxiety, fatigue).[67,69]

Although disease management should be the primary intervention to alleviate child night wakings caused by illness factors, additional interventions are needed to improve both child and parent sleep. Behavioral interventions that work for healthy children should also be used for children with chronic illnesses. However, many parents struggle with consistency and limit setting when a child is ill. Interventions such as respite care should also be examined for parents. One recent study of parents of ventilator-assisted children found that regular night nursing was associated with increased parent total sleep time (>1 hour), as well as fewer symptoms of parent depression and sleepiness.[77]

As suggested in a recent review article focusing on sleep in parental caregivers, future studies need to include objective assessments of sleep (ie, actigraphy), longitudinal study designs to assess changes in sleep associated with disease factors (eg, flares, remission), and appropriate control groups (eg, children with other illnesses, children with developmental delays, healthy children).[78] Interventions are needed to alleviate caregiver burden and reduce sleep disruptions. Siblings' sleep can also be affected when there is a child in the home with a chronic illness, so sibling sleep should also be examined in future studies.

DEVELOPMENTAL DISORDERS

For children with developmental disorders (including intellectual disabilities, autism spectrum disorder [ASD], and attention-deficit/hyperactivity disorder [ADHD]), sleep problems are common and can include difficulties initiating sleep, frequent and/or prolonged night waking, as well as early morning sleep termination.[79–84] Because many of these children cannot go unsupervised, if the child is not sleeping, parents are typically also not sleeping.

Multiple studies have found associations between sleep problems in children with developmental disorders and parent sleep disruptions.[82,85,86] One study using actigraphy found that parents of children with ASDs slept 1 hour less than parents of typically developing children.[87] Along with sleep disruptions, parent daytime functioning has also been associated with sleep problems among children with developmental disorders, including increased parenting stress,[88,89] as well as increased symptoms of depression and anxiety.[90,91] Parent work attendance and family functioning have also been associated with sleep problems among children with ADHD.[90]

Although only a handful of studies have examined the benefits for parents of treatments that address sleep problems among children with developmental disorders, improvements were reported in parent satisfaction with their own sleep, as well as their ability to manage their child's sleep.[92,93] Together, these studies highlight the need to include parent sleep and functioning as an important outcome for interventions that primarily target sleep problems in children with developmental disorders.

SUMMARY

Because the family system is a central part of a child's life, child sleep problems can have a significant impact on family functioning, in particular parent sleep and daytime functioning (eg, mood, stress, and marital satisfaction). Likewise, family functioning (eg, parent stress, marital conflict) may affect child sleep. Behavioral treatments that improve sleep in children are also likely to result in improvements to parental sleep and subsequent daytime functioning, although more research is needed in this area. Clinicians and researchers who work with children of all ages, both healthy and those with a chronic illness or developmental disorder, need to be aware not only of the causes and consequences of sleep problems among children but also how these sleep problems affect the entire family system.

REFERENCES

1. Dahl RE, El-Sheikh M. Considering sleep in a family context: introduction to the special issue. J Fam Psychol 2007;21(1):1–3.
2. Gay CL, Lee KA, Lee SY. Sleep patterns and fatigue in new mothers and fathers. Biol Res Nurs 2004;5(4):311–8.
3. Kang MJ, Matsumoto K, Shinkoda H, et al. Longitudinal study for sleep-wake behaviours of mothers from pre-partum to post-partum using actigraph and sleep logs. Psychiatry Clin Neurosci 2002;56(3):251–2.
4. Lee KA, Zaffke ME, McEnany G. Parity and sleep patterns during and after pregnancy. Obstet Gynecol 2000;95(1):14–8.
5. Nishihara K, Horiuchi S. Changes in sleep patterns of young women from late pregnancy to postpartum: relationships to their infants' movements. Percept Mot Skills 1998;87(3 Pt 1):1043–56.
6. Nishihara K, Horiuchi S, Eto H, et al. Mothers' wakefulness at night in the postpartum period is related to their infants' circadian sleep-wake rhythm. Psychiatry Clin Neurosci 2000;54(3):305–6.
7. Hunter LP, Rychnovsky JD, Yount SM. A selective review of maternal sleep characteristics in the postpartum period. J Obstet Gynecol Neonatal Nurs 2009;38(1):60–8.
8. Kleitman N. Sleep and wakefulness. Chicago: University of Chicago Press; 1963.
9. Kennedy HP, Gardiner A, Gay C, et al. Negotiating sleep: a qualitative study of new mothers. J Perinat Neonatal Nurs 2007;21(2):114–22.
10. Montgomery-Downs HE, Insana SP, Clegg-Kraynok MM, et al. Normative longitudinal maternal sleep: the first 4 postpartum months. Am J Obstet Gynecol 2010; 203(5):465.e1–7.
11. Kendell RE, McGuire RJ, Connor Y, et al. Mood changes in the first three weeks after childbirth. J Affect Disord 1981;3(4):317–26.
12. Cox JL, Holden JM, Sagovsky R. Detection of postnatal depression. Development of the 10-item Edinburgh Postnatal Depression Scale. Br J Psychiatry 1987;150:782–6.
13. Swain AM, O'Hara MW, Starr KR, et al. A prospective study of sleep, mood, and cognitive function in postpartum and nonpostpartum women. Obstet Gynecol 1997;90(3):381–6.
14. Dennis CL, Ross L. Relationships among infant sleep patterns, maternal fatigue, and development of depressive symptomatology. Birth 2005;32(3):187–93.
15. Tikotzky L, Sadeh A. Maternal sleep-related cognitions and infant sleep: a longitudinal study from pregnancy through the 1st year. Child Dev 2009;80(3):860–74.
16. Hedman C, Pohjasvaara T, Tolonen U, et al. Effects of pregnancy on mothers' sleep. Sleep Med 2002;3(1):37–42.
17. Damato EG, Burant C. Sleep patterns and fatigue in parents of twins. J Obstet Gynecol Neonatal Nurs 2008;37(6):738–49.
18. Elek SM, Hudson DB, Fleck MO. Couples' experiences with fatigue during the transition to parenthood. J Fam Nurs 2002;8(3):221–40.
19. Sadeh A, Flint-Ofir E, Tirosh T, et al. Infant sleep and parental sleep-related cognitions. J Fam Psychol 2007;21(1):74–87.
20. Tikotzky L, Sadeh A, Glickman-Gavrieli T. Infant sleep and paternal involvement in infant caregiving during the first 6 months of life. J Pediatr Psychol 2011;36(1):36–46.
21. Armstrong KL, O'Donnell H, McCallum R, et al. Childhood sleep problems: association with prenatal factors and maternal distress/depression. J Paediatr Child Health 1998;34(3):263–6.

22. Goodlin-Jones B, Eiben LA, Anders TF. Maternal well-being and sleep-wake behaviors in infants: an intervention using maternal odor. Infant Ment Health J 1997;18(4):378–93.
23. Hiscock H, Wake M. Infant sleep problems and postnatal depression: a community-based study. Pediatrics 2001;107(6):1317–22.
24. Karraker KH, Young M. Night waking in 6-month-old infants and maternal depressive symptoms. J Appl Dev Psychol 2007;28(5–6):493–8.
25. Lam P, Hiscock H, Wake M. Outcomes of infant sleep problems: a longitudinal study of sleep, behavior, and maternal well-being. J Pediatr 2003;111(3):203–7.
26. Bayer JK, Hiscock H, Hampton A, et al. Sleep problems in young infants and maternal mental and physical health. J Paediatr Child Health 2007;43(1–2): 66–73.
27. Morrell J, Steele H. The role of attachment security, temperament, maternal perception, and care-giving behavior in persistent infant sleeping problems. Infant Ment Health J 2003;5(447):468.
28. Martin J, Hiscock H, Hardy P, et al. Adverse associations of infant and child sleep problems and parent health: an Australian population study. Pediatrics 2007; 119(5):947–55.
29. Mindell JA, Kuhn BR, Lewin DS, et al. Behavioral treatment of bedtime problems and night wakings in infants and young children. Sleep 2006;29(10): 1263–76.
30. Gaylor EE, Burnham MM, Goodlin-Jones BL, et al. A longitudinal follow-up study of young children's sleep patterns using a developmental classification system. Behav Sleep Med 2005;3(1):44–61.
31. Stremler R, Hodnett E, Lee K, et al. A behavioral-educational intervention to promote maternal and infant sleep: a pilot randomized, controlled trial. Sleep 2006;29(12):1609–15.
32. Wolfson A, Lacks P, Futterman A. Effects of parent training on infant sleeping patterns, parents' stress, and perceived parental competence. J Consult Clin Psychol 1992;60(1):41–8.
33. Kerr S, Jowett SA, Smith LN. Preventing sleep problems in infants: a randomized controlled trial. J Adv Nurs 1996;24:938–42.
34. St James-Roberts I, Sleep J, Morris S, et al. Use of a behavioural programme in the first 3 months to prevent infant crying and sleeping problems. J Paediatr Child Health 2001;37:289–97.
35. Eckerberg B. Treatment of sleep problems in families with young children: effects of treatment on family well-being. Acta Paediatr 2004;93(1):126–34.
36. Hall WA, Clauson M, Carty EM, et al. Effects on parents of an intervention to resolve infant behavioral sleep problems. Pediatr Nurs 2006;32(3):243–50.
37. Hiscock H, Bayer JK, Hampton A, et al. Long-term mother and child mental health effects of a population-based infant sleep intervention: cluster-randomized, controlled trial. Pediatrics 2008;122(3):e621–7.
38. Hiscock H, Wake M. Randomised controlled trial of behavioural infant sleep intervention to improve infant sleep and maternal mood. Br Med J 2002;324(7345): 1062–5.
39. Thome M, Skuladottir A. Evaluating a family-centred intervention for infant sleep problems. J Adv Nurs 2005;50(1):5–11.
40. Sleep in America poll. National Sleep Foundation; 2004. Available at: http://www.sleepfoundation.org/. Accessed May 11, 2007.
41. Smedje H, Broman JE, Hetta J. Sleep disturbances in Swedish pre-school children and their parents. Nord J Psychiatry 1998;52(1):59–67.

42. Leonhard C, Randler C. In sync with the family: children and partners influence the sleep-wake circadian rhythm and social habits of women. Chronobiol Int 2009;26(3):510–25.

43. Gau SS, Merikangas KR. Similarities and differences in sleep-wake patterns among adults and their children. Sleep 2004;27(2):299–304.

44. Boergers J, Hart C, Owens JA, et al. Child sleep disorders: associations with parental sleep duration and daytime sleepiness. J Fam Psychol 2007;21(1):88–94.

45. Meltzer LJ, Mindell JA. Relationship between child sleep disturbances and maternal sleep, mood, and parenting stress: a pilot study. J Fam Psychol 2007; 21(1):67–73.

46. Adams LA, Rickert VI. Reducing bedtime tantrums: comparison between positive routines and graduated extinction. Pediatrics 1989;84(5):756–61.

47. Mindell JA, Durand VM. Treatment of childhood sleep disorders: generalization across disorders and effects on family members. J Pediatr Psychol 1993;18(6): 731–50.

48. Mindell JA, Telofski L, Wiegand B, et al. A nightly bedtime routine: impact on sleep in young children and maternal mood. Sleep 2009;32(5):599–606.

49. Tikotzky L, Sadeh A. The role of cognitive-behavioral therapy in behavioral childhood insomnia. Sleep Med 2010;11(7):686–91.

50. El-Sheikh M, Buckhalt JA, Mize J, et al. Marital conflict and disruption of children's sleep. Child Dev 2006;77(1):31–43.

51. Keller P, Buckhalt JA, El-Sheikh M. Links between family functioning and children's sleep. In: Ivanenko A, editor. Sleep and psychiatric disorders in children and adolescents. New York: Informa Healthcare; 2008. p. 49–60.

52. Keller P, El-Sheikh M. Children's emotional security and sleep: longitudinal relations and directions of effects. J Child Psychol Psychiatry 2011;52(1):64–71.

53. Adam EK, Snell EK, Pendry P. Sleep timing and quantity in ecological and family context: a nationally representative time-diary study. J Fam Psychol 2007;21(1): 4–19.

54. Sleep in America poll. National Sleep Foundation; 2006. Available at: http://www.sleepfoundation.org/. Accessed March 31, 2006.

55. Carskadon MA. When worlds collide: adolescent need for sleep versus societal demands. Phi Delta Kappan 1999;80(5):348–53.

56. Cousins JC, Bootzin RR, Stevens SJ, et al. Parental involvement, psychological distress, and sleep: a preliminary examination in sleep-disturbed adolescents with a history of substance abuse. J Fam Psychol 2007;21(1):104–13.

57. Bernert RA, Merrill KA, Braithwaite SR, et al. Family life stress and insomnia symptoms in a prospective evaluation of young adults. J Fam Psychol 2007; 21(1):58–66.

58. Brand S, Gerber M, Hatzinger M, et al. Evidence for similarities between adolescents and parents in sleep patterns. Sleep Med 2009;10(10):1124–31.

59. Tynjala J, Kannas L, Levalahti E, et al. Perceived sleep quality and its precursors in adolescents. Health Promot Int 1999;14(2):155–66.

60. Vignau J, Bailly D, Duhamel A, et al. Epidemiologic study of sleep quality and troubles in French secondary school adolescents. J Adolesc Health 1997; 21(5):343–50.

61. Chamlin SL, Mattson CL, Frieden IJ, et al. The price of pruritus: sleep disturbance and cosleeping in atopic dermatitis. Arch Pediatr Adolesc Med 2005;159(8):745–50.

62. Diette GB, Markson L, Skinner EA, et al. Nocturnal asthma in children affects school attendance, school performance, and parents' work attendance. Arch Pediatr Adolesc Med 2000;154(9):923–8.

63. Fiese BH, Winter MA, Sliwinski M, et al. Nighttime waking in children with asthma: an exploratory study of daily fluctuations in family climate. J Fam Psychol 2007; 21(1):95–103.

64. Gedaly-Duff V, Lee KA, Nail LM, et al. Pain, sleep disturbance, and fatigue in children with leukemia and their parents: a pilot study. Oncol Nurs Forum 2006;33(3):641–6.

65. Hinds PS, Hockenberry M, Rai SN, et al. Nocturnal awakenings, sleep environment interruptions, and fatigue in hospitalized children with cancer. Oncol Nurs Forum 2007;34(2):393–402.

66. Monaghan MC, Hilliard ME, Cogen FR, et al. Nighttime caregiving behaviors among parents of young children with type 1 diabetes: associations with illness characteristics and parent functioning. Fam Syst Health 2009;27(1):28–38.

67. Moore K, David TJ, Murray CS, et al. Effect of childhood eczema and asthma on parental sleep and well-being: a prospective comparative study. Br J Dermatol 2006;154(3):514–8.

68. Cottrell L, Khan A. Impact of childhood epilepsy on maternal sleep and socioemotional functioning. Clin Pediatr (Phila) 2005;44(7):613–6.

69. Meltzer LJ, Mindell JA. Impact of a child's chronic illness on maternal sleep and daytime functioning. Arch Intern Med 2006;166:1749–55.

70. Williams J, Lange B, Sharp G, et al. Altered sleeping arrangements in pediatric patients with epilepsy. Clin Pediatr (Phila) 2000;39(11):635–42.

71. McCann D. Sleep deprivation is an additional stress for parents staying in hospital. J Spec Pediatr Nurs 2008;13(2):111–22.

72. Van Dongen HP, Maislin G, Mullington JM, et al. The cumulative cost of additional wakefulness: dose-response effects on neurobehavioral functions and sleep physiology from chronic sleep restriction and total sleep deprivation. Sleep 2003;26(2):117–26.

73. Balas MC, Scott LD, Rogers AE. Frequency and type of errors and near errors reported by critical care nurses. Can J Nurs Res 2006;38(2):24–41.

74. Scott LD, Hwang WT, Rogers AE. The impact of multiple care giving roles on fatigue, stress, and work performance among hospital staff nurses. J Nurs Adm 2006;36(2):86–95.

75. Yilmaz O, Sogut A, Gulle S, et al. Sleep quality and depression-anxiety in mothers of children with two chronic respiratory diseases: asthma and cystic fibrosis. J Cyst Fibros 2008;7(6):495–500.

76. Hatzmann J, Heymans HS, Carbonell A, et al. Hidden consequences of success in pediatrics: parental health-related quality of life–results from the care project. Pediatrics 2008;122(5):e1030–8.

77. Meltzer LJ, Boroughs DS, Downes JJ. The relationship between home nursing coverage, sleep, and daytime functioning in parents of ventilator-assisted children. J Pediatr Nurs 2010;25(4):250–7.

78. Meltzer LJ, Moore M. Sleep disruptions in parents of children and adolescents with chronic illnesses: prevalence, causes, and consequences. J Pediatr Psychol 2008;33(3):279–91.

79. Didden R, Korzilius H, van Aperlo B, et al. Sleep problems and daytime problem behaviours in children with intellectual disability. J Intellect Disabil Res 2002; 46(7):537–47.

80. Owens JA. The ADHD and sleep conundrum: a review. J Dev Behav Pediatr 2005;26(4):312–22.

81. Patzold LM, Richdale AL, Tonge BJ. An investigation into sleep characteristics of children with autism and Asperger's disorder. J Paediatr Child Health 1998;34(6): 528–33.

82. Robinson AM, Richdale AL. Sleep problems in children with an intellectual disability: parental perceptions of sleep problems, and views of treatment effectiveness. Child Care Health Dev 2004;30(2):139–50.

83. Wiggs L, Montgomery P, Stores G. Actigraphic and parent reports of sleep patterns and sleep disorders in children with subtypes of attention-deficit hyperactivity disorder. Sleep 2005;28(11):1437–45.

84. Wiggs L, Stores G. Severe sleep disturbance and daytime challenging behaviour in children with severe learning disabilities. J Intellect Disabil Res 1996;40(Pt 6): 518–28.

85. Chu J, Richdale AL. Sleep quality and psychological wellbeing in mothers of children with developmental disabilities. Res Dev Disabil 2009;30(6):1512–22.

86. Lopez-Wagner MC, Hoffman CD, Sweeney DP, et al. Sleep problems of parents of typically developing children and parents of children with autism. J Genet Psychol 2008;169(3):245–59.

87. Meltzer LJ. Brief report: sleep in parents of children with autism spectrum disorders. J Pediatr Psychol 2008;33(4):380–6.

88. Doo S, Wing YK. Sleep problems of children with pervasive developmental disorders: correlation with parental stress. Dev Med Child Neurol 2006;48(8):650–5.

89. Richdale A, Francis A, Gavidia-Payne S, et al. Stress, behaviour, and sleep problems in children with an intellectual disability. J Intellect Dev Dis 2000;25(2): 147–61.

90. Sung V, Hiscock H, Sciberras E, et al. Sleep problems in children with attention-deficit/hyperactivity disorder: prevalence and the effect on the child and family. Arch Pediatr Adolesc Med 2008;162(4):336–42.

91. Meltzer LJ. Factors associated with depressive symptoms in parents of children with autism spectrum disorders. Research in Autism Spectrum Disorders 2011; 5(1):361–7.

92. Wiggs L, Stores G. Behavioural treatment for sleep problems in children with severe learning disabilities and challenging daytime behaviour: effect on sleep patterns of mother and child. J Sleep Res 1998;7(2):119–26.

93. Wiggs L, Stores G. Behavioural treatment for sleep problems in children with severe intellectual disabilities and daytime challenging behaviour: effect on mothers and fathers. Br J Health Psychol 2001;6(Pt 3):257–69.

Index

Note: Page numbers of article titles are in **boldface** type

Pediatr Clin N Am 58 (2011) 775–785
doi:10.1016/S0031-3955(11)00054-X
0031-3955/11/$ – see front matter © 2011 Elsevier Inc. All rights reserved.

pediatric.theclinics.com

Printed and bound by CPI Group (UK) Ltd, Croydon, CR0 4YY

13/10/2024

01773585-0001